Patient Unit Safety and Care Quality: Promotion of Self-Healing Systems during Hospital Stays

Patient Unit Safety and Care Quality: Promotion of Self-Healing Systems during Hospital Stays

Huey-Ming Tzeng, PhD, RN
School of Nursing, The University of Michigan
Ann Arbor, Michigan

AND

Chang-Yi Yin, MS
Department of History
Chinese Culture University, Taipei, Taiwan

Nova Biomedical Books
New York

Library of Congress Cataloging-in-Publication Data

Tzeng, Huey-Ming, 1968-
 Patient unit safety and care quality : promotion of self-healing systems during hospital stays / Huey-Ming Tzeng and Chang-Yi Yin (authors).
 p. ; cm.
 Includes bibliographical references and index.
 ISBN 978-1-60456-670-3 (hardcover : alk. paper)
 1. Hospitals--Safety measures. 2. Hospital patients--Wounds and injuries--Prevention. 3. Medical errors--Prevention. I. Yin, Chang-Yi, 1944- II. Title.
 [DNLM: 1. Hospitals. 2. Safety Management--methods. 3. Accidental Falls--prevention & control. 4. Medical Errors--prevention & control. WX 185 T998p 2008]
 RA969.9.T947   2008
 362.11028'9--dc22   2008019252

Published by Nova Science Publishers, Inc. ✦ New York

We dedicate this book to Professor Beatrice J. Kalisch, PhD, RN

Contents

List of Tables   ix

List of Figures   xv

About the Author   xvii

Preface   xix

Handy Reminders to be Used during Hospital Stays   1

Section I: Setting the Scene   5

Chapter 1.1.   Demanding a Safe Hospital Stay   7

Chapter 1.2.   The Caring Philosophy in Acute Hospital Settings   19

Chapter 1.3.   No Safety, No Quality: Initiatives for Promoting
                Patient Safety in Hospitals   29

Chapter 1.4.   Problematic Patient Safety Areas in Hospitals   47

Section II: Preventing Harms and Errors   67

Chapter 2.1.   Inpatient Falls   69

Chapter 2.2.   Health Care-associated Pressure Ulcers   99

Chapter 2.3.   Serious Injury or Death in Physical Restraints or Seclusion   117

Chapter 2.4.   Inpatient Suicide   135

Chapter 2.5.   Medication Errors   147

Chapter 2.6.   Transfusion Errors   177

Chapter 2.7.   Wrong-Site Surgery   191

Chapter 2.8.   Treatment Delays   205

Chapter 2.9.   Operative and Postoperative Errors and Complications   **215**

Chapter 2.10.   Health Care-associated Infections   **229**

Chapter 2.11.   The Impact of Hospital Human Resource
                    Management on Patient Outcomes   **253**

Chapter 2.12.   Unsafe Design of Patient Rooms   **259**

Section III: **Knowing Why**   **269**

Chapter 3.1.   Say NO to Poor Care Safety I: Poor Communication
                    among Health Care Providers   **271**

Chapter 3.2.   Say NO to Poor Care Safety II: Incorrect Patient
                    Identification in the Process of Providing Care   **275**

Chapter 3.3.   Learning the Facts from Research I: The Family
                    Involvement Culture in the US Hospital Environment   **279**

Chapter 3.4.   Learning the Facts from Research II: Historical Human
                    Resource Issues Related to Hospital Nursing   **287**

Chapter 3.5.   Learning the Fact from Research III: The Linkage
                    between Nurse Staffing and Inpatient Fall Rates   **295**

Epilogue   **303**

Glossary of Terms Commonly Used in Hospital Care   **307**

Index   **313**

List of Tables

Preface

Table 1.   The number of sentinel events reported to the Joint
Commission by year, from all types of health care institutions   **xx**

Table 2.   Type of sentinel events reported to the Joint Commission
from all types of health care institutions   **xx**

Table 3.   Root causes of the sentinel events reported to the Joint Commission
from all types of health care institutions, on all types of events   **xxi**

Chapter 1.1.

Table 1.   Learning to speak up for our health care needs during hospital stays   **11-14**

Table 2.   Knowing our rights before, during, and after our hospital stays   **15-16**

Chapter 1.2.

Table 1.   A comparison among the commonly adopted terms, newly
invented terms, and the modified terms as related to nursing   **20**

Table 2.   The nine provisions and the outline of the accompanying
interpretive statement for each provision as indicated
in the *Code of Ethics for Nurses with Interpretive Statements*   **22**

Table 3.   The Agency for Healthcare Research and
Quality inpatient quality indicators   **24**

Table 4.   The Agency for Healthcare Research and
Quality pediatric quality indicators   **25**

Table 5.   The Agency for Healthcare Research and
Quality patient safety indicators   **25**

Chapter 1.3.

Table 1.　　The four categories and the suggested high leverage changes as indicated in the initiative of "Transforming Care at the Bedside"　　**30**

Table 2.　　The 2008 National Patient Goals for hospital programs　　**32**

Table 3.　　The International Patient Safety Goals as developed by the Joint Commission International　　**35**

Table 4.　　The Joint Commission International's nine patient safety solutions　　**36**

Table 5.　　Number of articles by year: 1996 to March 31, 2007　　**38**

Table 6.　　Descriptive information on each identified safety dimension and category: From 1996 to March 31, 2007[*]　　**38**

Table 7.　　Frequency table on each identified safety category (indicated in code number) by year ($n = 6569$)　　**40**

Table 8.　　A comparison between the interventions set for the "100,000 Lives Campaign" in 2004 and the "5 Million Lives Campaign" in 2006 as initiated by Institute for Healthcare Improvement　　**42**

Chapter 1.4.

Table 1.　　Domains of ergonomics approaches to address patient safety issues　　**48**

Table 2.　　Additional types of sentinel events　　**50**

Table 3.　　The most frequently cited root causes, potential problems, and possible solutions for nurses working in acute inpatient care units　　**51-24**

Table 4.　　A comparison table across the patient safety dimensions in hospitals as identified in Tzeng and Yin's study (2007), types of sentinel events, and the 2008 National Patient Safety Goals for hospital programs　　**57-58**

Table 5.　　The 14 priority areas in the Joint Commission's accreditation process for hospitals　　**60-62**

Table 6.　　Patient safety actions as recommended by the World Health Professions Alliance　　**65**

Chapter 2.1.

Table 1.　　The commonly seen intrinsic and extrinsic risk factors for inpatient falls　　**73-74**

Table 2.　　The locus-stability classification scheme in the attributional theory of success and failure　　**75**

Table 3.　　The extrinsic risk factors for inpatient fall abstracted from a total of 104 fall incident reports　　**76**

Table 4. The extrinsic risk factors for inpatient falls elicited from the interview transcriptions of nine nurses and four nursing attendants **78-80**

Table 5. The major root causes of the reported sentinel events related to patient falls and the corresponding prevention strategies for nurses **81-84**

Table 6. A comparison between the intervention strategies toward preventing patient falls as identified by the Joint Commission and the ones abstracted from the nurse interview transcriptions **85-90**

Table 7. Preventing falls: Critical tips for hospital and nursing leaders, and nurses, who work in acute inpatient care units **94**

Table 8. Preventing falls: Critical tips for patients and families **95-96**

Chapter 2.2.

Table 1. The commonly seen intrinsic and extrinsic risk factors for health care-associated pressure ulcers **103**

Table 2. The suggested tips from the Joint Commission to help prevent pressure ulcers **104**

Table 3. The six essential steps of pressure ulcer prevention as suggested by the Institute for Healthcare Improvement **105-106**

Table 4. The educational program for health care professionals and the one for patients and their families as suggested by the National Pressure Ulcer Advisory Panel **108**

Table 5. Preventing the development of pressure ulcers: Critical tips for hospital and nursing leaders and nurses who work in acute inpatient care units **109-110**

Table 6. Preventing the development of pressure ulcers during hospital stays: Critical tips for patients and their families **111-112**

Chapter 2.3.

Table 1. The standards for restraint use and elements of performance for acute medical and surgical inpatient care settings **120-122**

Table 2. The standards for restraint and seclusion use and elements of performance for behavioral health care settings or psychiatric hospitals **122-124**

Table 3. The major root causes of the reported sentinel events related to restraint or seclusion use and the corresponding prevention strategies for nurses **127-128**

Table 4. Preventing physical restraint- and seclusion-related serious injuries or deaths: Critical tips for nurses who work in acute, medical, and surgical inpatient care units **130**

Table 5.   Preventing physical restraint- and seclusion-related serious
injuries or deaths: Critical tips for accompanying families   **131-132**

Chapter 2.4.

Table 1.   The commonly mentioned suicide risk factors   **138**

Table 2.   The major root causes of the reported sentinel events
related to inpatient suicides and the corresponding
prevention strategies for nurses   **139-140**

Table 3.   Preventing inpatient suicides: Critical tips for nurses
who work in acute inpatient care units   **142**

Table 4.   Preventing inpatient suicides: Critical tips for patients and families   **144**

Chapter 2.5.

Table 1.   The six processes in a commonly seen medication
use system for inpatient care services   **150**

Table 2.   The major root causes of the reported sentinel
events related to medication errors and the corresponding
prevention strategies for nurses   **151-154**

Table 3.   Symbols and Braille for instructing patients about medication use   **168**

Table 4.   Preventing medication errors: Critical tips for nurses
who work in acute inpatient care units   **170**

Table 5.   Critical information to know to help avoid mistakes with
medications: For hospitalized patients and their families   **173-174**

Chapter 2.6.

Table 1.   The major root causes of the reported sentinel events on transfusion
errors and the corresponding prevention strategies for nurses   **182-184**

Table 2.   Preventing transfusion errors: Critical tips for nurses
who work in acute inpatient care units   **186**

Table 3.   Critical information to know to help avoid transfusion errors:
Tips for patients and families   **188**

Chapter 2.7.

Table 1.   The major root causes of the reported sentinel
events related to wrong-site surgery   **197-198**

Table 2.   Preventing wrong-site surgery: Critical tips for nurses
who work in acute inpatient care units   **200**

Table 3.   Ensuring a safe surgery: Essential information
for patients and families to know   **201-202**

Chapter 2.8.

Table 1.   The major root causes of the reported sentinel events
                  related to treatment delays and the corresponding
                  prevention strategies for nurses   **207-208**

Table 2.   Preventing treatment delays: Critical tips for nurses
                  who work in acute inpatient care units   **210**

Table 3.   Preventing treatment delays: Tips for patients and families   **212**

Chapter 2.9.

Table 1.   The major root causes of the reported sentinel events related
                  to operative and postoperative errors and complications
                  and the corresponding prevention strategies for nurses   **221-222**

Table 2.   Preventing operative and postoperative errors and complications:
                  Critical tips for nurses who work in acute inpatient care units   **224**

Table 3.   Preventing operative and postoperative errors and
                  complications: Tips for patients and families   **226**

Chapter 2.10.

Table 1.   The major root causes of the reported sentinel events
                  related to health care-associated infections and the
                  corresponding prevention strategies for nurses   **240-244**

Table 2.   Preventing health care-associated infections:
                  Critical tips for nurses who work in acute inpatient care units   **247-248**

Table 3.   Preventing health care-associated infections:
                  Tips for patients and families   **248**

Chapter 3.3.

Table 1.   Descriptive information on family involvement-related variables   **282**

Chapter 3.4.

Table 1.   Descriptive information on the eight human
                  resource themes and corresponding issues   **290**

Table 2.   Descriptive information on the eight
                  identified human resource themes by year   **291**

List of Figures

Figure 1.	The prone position was used to get out of the bed.	**91**
Figure 2.	The traditional sitting-standing position was used to get out of the bed.	**91**
Figure 1.	Repositioning on a hospital patient bed.	**113**
Figure 2.	Repositioning on a hospital patient bed.	**113**
Figure 1.	A patient with only the wrist restraint being used.	**119**
Figure 2.	A patient in both the wrist and vest restrains.	**119**
Figure 1.	A patient rests on the patient bed after taking her medications.	**172**
Figure 2.	A patient sits on the edge of the bed with her two IV infusion pumps.	**172**
Figure 1.	The high-low horizontal grab bars/hand rails.	**264**
Figure 2.	The U-shaped support stand to be used to enhance patient safety when performing the toileting movements.	**265**
Figure 1	The dynamic balance model of family ecology.	**280**

About the Author

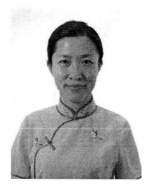

Huey-Ming Tzeng, PhD, RN, graduated from The University of Michigan, School of Nursing, Ann Arbor, Michigan, in 1997. Currently, she is an Associate Professor, The University of Michigan, School of Nursing, Division of Nursing Business and Health Systems, Ann Arbor, Michigan. Dr. Tzeng became interested in patient safety issues and ethics when Taiwan was seriously attached by Severe Acute Respiratory Syndrome (SARS) in 2003. H5N1 avian flu can be the next one. Since then, she has been concerned about the safety of patients and clinical staff in the process of delivering health care across the care continuum. She took both macro- and micro-approach to address health care quality issues. Her research areas involve patient safety in hospitals, health care management and delivery systems, religions, cultures and care quality, newly emerging infectious diseases and global health, and research methodology. Promoting safe hospital stays with a focus on inpatient fall prevention is her current research theme. Dr. Tzeng has published 65 articles on peer-reviewed journals, and several book chapters.

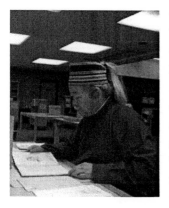

Chang-Yi Yin, MA, graduated from the National Taiwan University, Department of History, Taipei, Taiwan, in 1971. Currently, he is a Professor at Chinese Culture University, Department of History, Taipei, Taiwan. He has been interested and researched in the subjects of history of China, area and culture studies, theology, medicine, and psychology. As a social activist, he has led and been the leader of several social actions in Taiwan. At the beginning of the SARS outbreak in Taiwan in 2003, his inner voice urged him to study human responses to help human beings survive from SARS and any future newly emerging infectious diseases, like H5N1 avian flu. Since then, promoting global health has been the theme of his research. He has published more than 300 journal articles in English or Mandarin, and 30 professional books, including 11 in area studies.

Preface

Hospitalized patients (also called inpatients) in acute care settings are generally weaker than outpatients who live in the community. At some point during patients' hospital stays, they are at their most vulnerable. This may occur when they first come in for treatment with acute, life-threatening medical conditions or immediately after treatments, procedures, or surgeries (Reiling, 2006). In addition, during acute hospital stays, deconditioning, a complex process of physiologic change, may follow after a period of inactivity, bed rest, or sedentary lifestyle. Deconditioning often has an impact on the musculoskeletal system (e.g., diminished muscle mass and decreases of muscle strength by 2-5% per day). The decline in muscle mass and strength has been linked to inpatient falls, functional decline, increased frailty, and immobility. Good nursing care should include strategies to prevent deconditioning and restore patients to their maximum level of functioning so that they may return to their prehospital state (Gillis & MacDonald, 2005).

Inpatients have most contacts with nurses, who are legally responsible for the safety of patient. Patients expect a safe care environment to heal during their hospital stays. Let's face the fact that a hospital can be a dangerous and erratic place for patients because of the unfamiliar physical environment and changes in their medical conditions. In addition, most hospitals are not explicitly designed to enhance patient safety (e.g., Reiling, 2006; Runy, 2006).

The Joint Commission is a national private, nonprofit organization whose purpose is to foster the attainment of uniformly high standards of institutional medical care. The Joint Commission accredits the care quality of the health care institutions across the care continuum and acts as the "guardian angel" for patients. The accredited health care institutions must report the sentinel events (also called serious adverse events or serious errors occurring within health care organizations) to the Joint Commission (Joint Commission, 2007a). In the sentinel event report announced by the Joint Commission (2007b) on June 30, 2007, a total of 4473 sentinel events were reviewed by the Joint Commission for the period from January 1995 to June 30, 2007. In the most recent 3 years, an average of 556 sentinel events was reported per year (Table 1).

Table 1. The number of sentinel events reported to the Joint Commission by year, | from all types of health care institutions

Year	No. of events
1995	23
1996	34
1997	139
1998	180
1999	333
2000	357
2001	437
2002	415
2003	487
2004	561
2005	582
2006	526
2007 (January 1 to June 30)	399 (798 events for the entire year of 2007, estimated)
Total	4473

Source: Joint Commission (2007b). Sentinel event statistics: As of June 30, 2007. Available at: http://www.jointcommission.org/NR/rdonlyres/D7836542-A372-4F93-8BD7-DDD11D43E484/0/se_stats_063007.pdf (accessed November 7, 2007).

Table 2. Type of sentinel events reported to the Joint Commission from all types of health care institutions

Types of sentinel event	No. of events	Percentage
Wrong-site surgery	592	13.2%
Suicide	555	12.4%
Operation or postoperative complication	534	11.9%
Medication error	416	9.3%
Delay in treatment	336	7.5%
Fall	257	5.7%
Assault, rape, or homicide	164	3.7%
Death or injury in restraints	164	3.7%
Perinatal death or loss of function (unanticipated death of full-term infant)	138	3.1%
Transfusion error	108	2.4%
Unintended retention of foreign body	107	2.4%
Infection-related event	93	2.1%
Anesthesia-related event	79	1.8%
Elopement death	74	1.7%
Medical equipment-related	72	1.6%
Fire	68	1.5%
Maternal death	66	1.5%
Ventilator death or injury	50	1.1%
Abduction	25	0.6%
Utility systems-related event	20	0.4%
Infant discharge to wrong family	7	0.2%
Other less frequent types	548	12.3%

Source: Joint Commission (2007b). Sentinel event statistics: As of June 30, 2007. Available at: http://www.jointcommission.org/NR/rdonlyres/D7836542-A372-4F93-8BD7-DDD11D43E484/0/se_stats_063007.pdf (accessed November 7, 2007).

Patients and their family want to heal. When we are hospitalized, we trust and sincerely hope that physicians, nurses, and pharmacists will work diligently and provide safe care, services, treatments, or procedures. Still, we must aware and watch for problematic safety areas and learn to report our complaints or concerns related to potential harms or risk, if our safety is endangered during our hospital stays. We must say No to harms and YES to heal.

Table 3. Root causes of the sentinel events reported to the Joint Commission from all types of health care institutions, on all types of events

Root cause	Ranking of the root causes based on events that occurred in 2006
Communication among health care providers	1 (the most often indicated cause)
Patient assessment	2
Leadership	3
Procedural compliance	4
Environmental safety or security	5
Competency or credentialing of the health care providers	6
Staff orientation or training related	7
Availability of information	8
Care planning	9
Organizational culture	9
Staffing	11
Continuum of care	12 (the least often indicated cause)

Source: Joint Commission (2007c). Root causes of sentinel events. Available at: http://www. jointcommission.org/NR/rdonlyres/FA465646-5F5F-4543-AC8F-E8AF6571E372/0/root_cause_ se.jpg (accessed November 7, 2007).

Why Should we All Read the Book?

This book is designed for inpatients, their families, and anyone who wants to advocate promoting safer hospital stays. The hospital and nurse leaders, clinical nurses, physicians, and pharmacists are also the intended audience for this book because they are legally responsible for harms and errors that befall inpatients, but each to a different extent depending on the types of harms and errors.

In the process of receiving medical care, physicians play the most critical role in curing the diseases or lessening the medical symptoms. However, nurses have the most contact with hospitalized patients and are most responsible for keeping patients safe during their entire hospital stays. Among the health care providers employed in hospitals, nurses know best the kind of safety features that would work well in patient rooms. Patient unit safety is the area that is closest to nurses and needs to be addressed first.

From the time a patient is admitted to an inpatient care unit, nurses who work in this unit are, indeed, the gatekeeper for the safety of this patient's entire hospital stay. For this reason, this book focuses on the duties and responsibilities of nurses who work in acute inpatient care units. However, this approach should not be interpreted as ignorance of the responsibilities of other staff members in the health care team. The other health care providers (e.g., physicians, pharmacists, nursing attendants, physical therapists, occupational therapists, respiratory therapists, and medical technicians) are also responsible for ensuring the safety of patients and their care, treatments, or procedures.

No safety, no quality! We all may be hospitalized at some time during our life. Health care providers may also become inpatients or the family visitors of their hospitalized loved ones. Consequently, we wrote this book to show current and potential patients and their families the safety issues to pay attention to and care about. The ultimate aim is to help patients and their families be their own consultants to minimize preventable harms and errors during hospital stays and promote the process of healing from within.

Description of Contents

This book includes three sections: Setting the scene (Section I), Preventing harms and errors (Section II), and Knowing why (Section III). In Section I, we first illustrate patients' desperate need for a safer hospital stay and the caring philosophy in inpatient, acute care settings. Then, we use the findings from our previous study to show the initiatives being promoted to improve patient safety in hospitals and areas needing more attention from researchers and medical communities.

In Section II, we discuss in depth a total of 12 safety issues with a focus on preventing patient harms and errors occurring during hospital stays. Included safety issues are inpatient falls, health care-associated pressure ulcers, serious injury or death in physical restraints and seclusion, inpatient suicide, medication errors, transfusion errors, wrong-site surgery, treatment delays, operative and postoperative errors and complications, health care-associated infections, the impact of hospital human resource management on patient outcomes, and unsafe design of patient rooms. For each chapter, patient stories or medical malpractice legal cases on related errors or harms are used to illustrate possible situations that can put patients at risk.

In Section III, the first two chapters address two critical causes of patient harms and errors: poor communication among health care providers (Say NO to poor care safety I) and incorrect patient identification in the process of providing care (Say NO to poor care safety II). For the other three chapters, we use our recent research findings to illustrate the family involvement culture in the US hospital environment (Learning the facts from research I), critical issues related to human resource allocation (Learning the facts from research II), and the linkage between human resource allocation and inpatient fall rates as one of the patient outcomes (Learning the facts from research III).

References

Gillis, A., & MacDonald, B. (2005). Deconditioning in the hospitalized elderly. *Canadian Nurse, 101*(6), 16-20.

Joint Commission (2007a). Sentinel event statistics. Available at: http://www.jointcommission.org/SentinelEvents/Statistics/ (accessed November 1, 2007).

Joint Commission (2007b). Sentinel event statistics: As of June 30, 2007. Available at: http://www.jointcommission.org/NR/rdonlyres/D7836542-A372-4F93-8BD7-DDD11D43E484/0/se_stats_063007.pdf (accessed November 7, 2007).

Joint Commission (2007c). Root causes of sentinel events. Available at: http://www.jointcommission.org/NR/rdonlyres/FA465646-5F5F-4543-AC8F-E8AF6571E372/0/root_cause_se.jpg (accessed November 7, 2007).

Reiling, J. (2006). Safe design of healthcare facilities. *Quality & Safety in Health Care, 15*(Suppl. 1), i34-i40.

Runy, L. A. (2006). Patient rooms come of age. *Hospitals & Health Networks, 80(4)*, 34.

Handy Reminders to be Used during Hospital Stays

During hospitalization, most of us are afraid to question our health care providers about, for instance, potentially wrong medications or reminding them to wash their hands before approaching us. We often worry that if we do so, they may become offended and angry. Then, our care quality may suffer as a consequence. We know such a feeling is ridiculous! We are being hospitalized for professional care to get better, regain our health, and heal. An inpatient care environment should be error-free and safe and should promote our health. As patient advocates for inpatient unit safety and care quality, we must say no to harms and errors.

Alternative Ways to Communicate our Concerns

We created several reminders that are meant for inpatients and their families to show their concerns to their health care providers during hospitalization. We may show any of these reminders to our physician, nurses, or other health care providers (abbreviated as clinicians) to speak for our safety needs or concerns. These reminders are:

1. Watch out for fall! No fall-related injury.
2. Lower my bed! No fall-related injury.
3. Demand a safe patient room! Keep it clean and tidy.
4. Wash your hands! No infections.
5. Keep me clean and dry! No pressure ulcers.
6. Check my wristband and ask for my name! No wrong-patient error.
7. Mark my surgical site! No wrong-site surgery.
8. Explain my medications to me! Written medication information is needed.
9. Explain my treatments and procedures! Written information is needed.

We may turn to the page with the words we want to tell our clinician and place it on our bedside table where our clinician can see it. By using any of the included reminders, we should be able to get the actions we demand from our clinicians without verbally relaying our safety concerns. Speaking up about our concerns (though politely) is still needed and important to effectively resolve our immediate safety worries.

Creating Additional Reminders

We understand that each individual patient may have different or specific concerns during the entire hospital stay. Several reminder templates are also included after the ready-to-use reminders. To effectively communicate our concerns with clinicians, we must indicate our expected actions (What?) and specific concerns (Why?). If needed, our family or a friend can help us develop the reminders to be used to communicate with our doctor, nurse, or the other health care providers.

Reminder 1: Watch out for fall! No fall-related injury

Watch Out for FALL!

No Fall-Related Injury.

Reminder 2: Lower my bed! No fall-related injury

Lower My Bed!

No Fall-Related Injury.

Reminder 3: Demand a safe patient room! Keep it clean and tidy

Demand a SAFE Patient Room!

Keep it Clean and Tidy.

Reminder 4: Wash your hands! No infections

Wash Your Hands!

No Infections.

Reminder 5: Keep me clean and dry! No pressure ulcers

Keep Me Clean and Dry!

No Pressure Ulcers.

Reminder 6: Check my wristband and ask for my name! No wrong-patient error

Check My Wristband
and
Ask for My Name!

No Wrong-Patient Error.

Reminder 7: Mark my surgical site! No wrong-site surgery

Mark My Surgical Site!

No Wrong-Site Surgery.

Reminder 8: Explain my medications to me! Written medication information is needed

Explain My Medications to Me!

Written Medication Information is Needed.

Reminder 9: Explain my treatments and procedures! Written information is needed

Explain My Treatments
and Procedures!

Written Information is Needed.

Reminder Template 1: Write down the expected actions under "What?" and the reasons or concerns under "Why?"

What?

Why?

Reminder Template 2: Write down the expected actions under "What?" and the reasons or concerns under "Why?"

What?

Why?

Reminder Template 3: Write down the expected actions under "What?" and the reasons or concerns under "Why?"

What?

Why?

Section I:
Setting the Scene

Demanding a Safe Hospital Stay

Modern Medicine is Not the Answer to Most of our Health Problems

Regardless of the advancement in technology and pharmacology, Western medicine still cannot resolve or partially resolve our physical and psychological problems. To date, 70% of the diseases cannot be cured by medicines (Bäumler, 1992). For example, AIDS, HIV positivity, most of the cancers, and Alzheimer's disease still cannot be cured by medications or procedures. Some diseases, such as diabetic mellitus, may be controlled by medications.

Western medicine is still searching for cures for these commonly seen devastating diseases. Regardless, medical diagnostic technology has advanced dramatically in the past 20 years.

Boosting our Self-healing System to Live

Patients may regain health only if they stay in a safe environment that promotes their self-healing system. Surgeries, medical procedures, and medications may remove pathogens, but often cannot cure the diseases. Our immune and internal systems of repair are keys to healing our physical malfunctions, as long as the malfunctions are not permanent. These repair systems have existed within our bodies since our birth as our self-healing system. Malfunctions may include fighting a cold, healing from minor cuts or bruises, and recovering from major surgery or a heart attack. Permanent malfunctions refer to, for instance, limb amputation or being deaf or blind.

Every recovering process takes time and demands an environment that promotes our self-healing functions. This process may start as soon as the onset of a malfunction, accelerate during hospital stays after receiving appropriate medical or surgical treatments, and continue after being discharged from the hospital. Lacking a self-healing system may result in the inability to sustain the existing physical condition or to retain the preexisting physical condition. Any external or added threats (e.g., medication errors, health care-associated infections) may interrupt our self-healing process and result in delayed recovery.

Being Hospitalized to Live, Not to Be Harmed

Hospitals are supposed to provide a safe care environment for the purpose of promoting patients' self-healing systems during their hospital stays. Despite the consequences, patients and their families have to trust their physicians and nurses for regaining health or living longer. After being admitted to a hospital, patients are practically at the mercy of the health care providers. For hospital leaders, providing a safe and quality inpatient care environment is crucial to patients' healing and involves creating a safety-focused practice culture within hospitals along with the processes to sustain continued improvement in patient safety (Joint Commission Resources, 2007).

Indeed, if 70% of the diseases cannot be cured by modern medicine (Bäumler, 1992), we would expect no preventable harms or errors to occur during our hospital stays. However, it was estimated that medical errors would injure as many as 1 of every 25 hospitalized patients and that 48,000 to 98,000 patients would die from medical errors each year (Agency for Healthcare Research and Quality, 2000; Brennan et al., 1991; Institute of Medicine, 2000). Another report estimated that 1.5 million patients would be injured each year due to medication errors. These errors would cost hospitals nearly $3.5 billion annually. In fact, medication errors have been so widespread that patients could suffer one error every day during their hospital stays (Institute of Medicine Report, 2007). McCaughey (2005) also estimated that health care-associated infections would cost about $30 billion each year in the United States.

Medicine is a caring science. Human beings, similar to the other species, primarily depend on their self-healing systems to recover and to sustain their health. Caring is important during the self-healing process. If we are hospitalized, a safe hospital care environment is key to allowing our self-healing system to function. Nursing is a caring profession. Promoting safe hospital stays should a nurse's first priority. Safety is always the first priority!

Patient Satisfaction versus Care Quality

Safe hospital stays are critical to promote our self-healing system in recovering and repairing our physical malfunctions. Safety should always come first, followed by quality (do better) and patient and family satisfaction (do more). We should speak up if we have any doubts or concerns related to the safety and quality of the care we receive.

We all may have wondered: If we go to a medical facility located in the center of a metropolitan city, which is more expensive, has more advanced technology, and demands more copayment for health care services, would we necessarily receive better care? Would we have better outcomes? Would our safety during a hospital stay be guarded more effectively? We often believe that if we pay more, we will receive better services. When we are sick, we often are willing to pay extra for more services and better care.

Thus far, no evidence shows that longer hospital stays, more staff, and more intensive treatment would better prolong patients' lives (Wennberg et al., 2005). Ironically, the patients who were most satisfied with the care they received may not actually be getting better health care compared with those who were least satisfied. It is arguable that patient satisfaction may not be the best indication of hospital care quality (Roohan et al., 2003).

As we have observed, patient satisfaction and quality measures may decline as the level or amount of care increases (e.g., receiving unnecessary care as suggested by our doctors and longer length of stay). Quality measures refer to improvements in patients' health conditions, the occurrences or rates of health care-associated infections, serious injuries and harms, or surgical complications. It is understandable that we often wish for more care to recover more fully and more quickly.

Patients' Perceptions Do Matter!

Patient satisfaction, defined as an individual patient's or the family's subjective perspective toward received medical services, has long been adopted as one of the references of care quality. During hospital stays, we have more interactions with nursing staff than with our doctors and other health care providers (e.g., pharmacists, nutritionists, and medical technicians). Our perceptions toward the care we received mostly reflect our perceptions toward the nursing care provided and our interactions with our nurses.

In most cases, each patient's level of satisfaction with nursing care primarily depended on the perception on how well the nurses were able to meet the individual's needs in both humanistic (e.g., a nurse's ability to anticipate the patient's needs, smiles, humor, reassurance, kindness, compassion, and gentle touch) and relatively concrete behaviors (e.g., correct and prompt attention to physical needs, timely administration of medication, and pain assessment) (Dozier et al., 2001; Fagerstrom, Eriksson, & Engberg, 1999; Meade, Bursell, & Ketelsen, 2006; Nguyen Thi et al., 2002). Our satisfaction levels do reflect our subjective evaluations on the care we received, which are usually based on our knowledge about health care and associated with our previous hospitalization experiences and expectations (e.g., clinical outcomes).

The safety and quality measures of patient care are more objective than the levels of patient satisfaction. The extent to which a hospital is providing safe and quality care primarily depends on whether this hospital and its health care providers comply with professional practice standards and guidelines. Someone must have the health care professional knowledge to make judgments about the levels of care safety and quality (Tzeng & Yin, 2008). If there is no safety for inpatient care, there would be no quality at all.

Unsafe care, which may lead to harms and errors, often results in patients' dissatisfaction. If patients suffered from preventable hospital harms and errors, an apology and explanation from their health care providers are needed. In fact, long illness and frequent hospitalizations will not make anyone a physician although we may become quite knowledgeable about our own illness, treatments, and medications. Regardless of self-learning, without professional medical or nursing training, we will not acquire the capability and professional knowledge to examine whether professional practice standards have been followed.

Care safety and quality go beyond the humanistic behaviors of the health care providers. We often can easily tell the differences in the physical environment, facilities, and equipment across hospitals. However, we often do not have choices on the layout and equipment included in hospital patient rooms because the design and equipment are given. We can only use and adapt to what we get.

Patients in an Unfamiliar Hospital Environment

Inpatients in acute care settings are weaker than outpatients who live in the community. At some point during a hospitalization, we, as patients, are at our most vulnerable. This may occur when we first come in for treatment with acute, life-threatening medical conditions or immediately after treatments, procedures, or surgeries (Reiling, 2006). During acute hospital stays, deconditioning, a complex process of physiologic change, may follow after a period of inactivity, bed rest, or sedentary lifestyle. Deconditioning often has an impact on the musculoskeletal system, including diminished muscle mass and decreases of muscle strength by 2% to 5% per day. The decline in muscle mass and strength has been linked to inpatient falls, functional decline, increased frailty, and immobility (Gillis & MacDonald, 2005).

Good nursing care should include strategies to prevent deconditioning and restore patients to their maximum level of functioning, such that they may return to their prehospital physical condition (Gillis & MacDonald, 2005). Nurses should also ensure that patients will not be harmed by falls, medication or medical procedure errors, or acquiring infectious disease during the process of health care delivery.

Avoiding Preventable Hospital Harms and Errors

If we pay attention to the health education related to our treatment, procedure, or medications as given by our doctor, nurse, clinical pharmacist, or the other health care providers, we may be able to assist in promoting a safe hospital stay for ourselves. As we have observed, patients who are more involved with their care tend to have better outcomes. For this reason, we should not hesitate to talk to our doctor or nurse if we have any safety concerns. Sometimes, we have to ask two or three times before our questions are answered or concerns resolved. We should always speak up when we have concerns related to the safety of the care we are receiving or have received.

In March 2002, the Joint Commission and the Centers for Medicare & Medicaid Services together launched a national campaign to urge patients to take a role in preventing medical errors by becoming actively involved in their health care during hospital stays. This campaign included a program, Speak Up™, that features a variety of patient safety topics (Joint Commission, 2007a). The Speak Up program was meant to help us become more involved in and informed about our health care during our hospital stays and help prevent errors in our care. The meaning of Speak Up and the rationale for each suggested action are summarized in Table 1. Speak Up (Joint Commission, 2007a) includes eight initiatives:

1. Four things we can do to prevent infection
2. Helping avoid mistakes in our surgery
3. Helping avoid mistakes with our medications
4. Helping prevent medical test mistakes
5. Information for living organ donors
6. Knowing our rights
7. Planning our follow-up care
8. What we should know about research studies

Table 1. Learning to speak up for our health care needs during hospital stays

Speak Up	Statement	Rationale and Interpretations
S	Speak up if we have questions or concerns. If we still don't understand or our concerns are not resolved, ask again. It's our body and we have a right to know.	1. Our health is important. We should not worry about being embarrassed if we don't understand something that our doctors, nurses, or other health care professionals tell us. 2. We should not be afraid to ask about our care safety. If we are having surgery or an invasive procedure, we should ask our doctor to mark the area that is to be operated on. 3. We should not be afraid to tell our nurse or the doctor if we think we are about to get the wrong medicine. 4. We should not be afraid to tell health care professionals if we think they have confused us with another patient.
P	Pay attention to the care we are receiving. Always make sure we are getting the right treatments and medications by the right health care professionals. Don't assume anything.	1. We should tell our nurse or doctor if something doesn't seem right. 2. We would expect our health care providers to introduce themselves to us (e.g., job title and how we can address them). We should look for their identification badges. For example, a new mother should know the person she hands her baby to. 3. We should pay attention to whether our health care providers have washed their hands. Hand washing is the most important way to prevent health care-associated infections. We should not be afraid to remind our doctors or nurses to wash their hands. 4. We should know what time of day we normally get our medications or treatments. If we do not get them, we must tell our nurse or doctor. 5. We should make sure that our nurses or doctors check our identification on our wristband and ask our name before they give us our medications or treatments.

Table 1. Continued

Speak Up	Statement	Rationale and Interpretations
E	Educate ourselves about our illness and diagnosis. We should try our best to learn about the medical tests that we are undergoing as well as our treatment and care plans.	1. We should ask our doctors about the special training and experience that qualifies them to treat our illness. 2. We may look for information about our medical problem or condition. Good places to get that information are from our doctor, nearby library, respected Web sites, and support groups. 3. We must write down important facts our doctors tell us. We should also ask our doctors if they have any written information we can keep. 4. We or our family should read all medical forms and make sure that we understand the information on these forms before we sign anything. If we don't understand, we should ask our doctors or nurses to explain them. 5. We must make sure that we know how to respond to any equipment that is being used in our care. At least, we need to know the signs or alarms that indicate malfunctioning and what to do if the alarm sounds. We should write down the instructions as given by our health care providers in the way we understand.
A	Ask a trusted family member or friend to be our advocate.	1. Our advocate can ask questions that we may not think about when we are stressed. 2. We may ask our advocate to stay with us, even overnight, when we are hospitalized. If we are not staying in a private room, we may need to ask our nurse for the hospital policies regarding having our advocate stay overnight. 3. Our advocate can help make sure we get the right medicines and treatments. 4. Our advocate can also help remember answers to questions we have asked our doctors or nurses. When it is needed, our advocate can speak up for us when we cannot speak up for ourselves. 5. We must make sure that our advocate understands the kind of care we want. We have to make sure that our advocate knows what we want done about life support and other lifesaving efforts, if we are unconscious and not likely to get better. 6. We may have our advocate go over the consents for treatments, procedures, or surgeries with us before we sign any consent form. We must make sure that we and our advocate understand exactly what we are about to agree to. 7. We and our advocate should understand the type of care we will need when we get home. Once we are discharged, our advocate should know what to look for if our condition worsens. Our advocate must also know who to call for help.

Speak Up	Statement	Rationale and Interpretations
K	Know what medications we take, and why we take them, because medication errors are the most common health care mistakes.	1. We should ask about the reason we should take any of the medications prescribed by our doctor and ask for written information about each one of them, including brand and generic names and any side effects for each of our medications. We should ask for written information whenever there are any changes on our medications or treatments. 2. If we do not recognize a medication given by our nurse, we should double check and ask our nurse whether it is for us. We should routinely ask about the medications that we are about to take by mouth before we swallow them. 3. If we are given IV fluids, we or our advocate should ask about and read the contents of the bags of IV fluids. We should also ask our nurse how long it should take for the liquid to run out. We must tell our nurse if our IV fluid seems not to be dripping correctly, that is, too fast or too slow. 4. Whenever we get a new medication, we should tell our doctor and nurse about allergies we have or the side effects and negative reactions we have had to other medicines. 5. If we are taking several medications, we should ask our doctor, nurse, or pharmacist whether it is safe to take all medications together at the same time. We should do the same thing if we are taking vitamins, herbs, and over-the-counter drugs during our hospital stays. 6. If we have to fill a prescription at a pharmacy, we have to make sure that we can read the handwriting on the prescription written by our doctor. We may ask our doctor or someone at the doctor's office to print the prescription, if necessary. We want to make sure that the pharmacist will be able to read it.
U	Use a hospital that has undergone a rigorous on-site evaluation against established state-of-art quality and safety standards.	1. The Joint Commission visits hospitals to see if they are meeting the Joint Commission's quality standards. We may go to Quality Check at www.qualitycheck.org to find out whether our hospital is 'accredited' by the Joint Commission. 'Accredited' means that the hospital works by rules that make sure that patient safety and quality standards are followed. 2. Before being admitted into a hospital, we may ask our doctor about this hospital's and our doctor's experience in taking care of patients with our type of illness. How often do this hospital and our doctor perform the procedure we need? What special care do this hospital and our doctor provide to help patients get well? 3. If we have more than one hospital to choose from, we should ask our doctor which one has the best care for our condition. We should ask about follow-up care and make sure that we understand all of the instructions.

Table 1. Continued

Speak Up	Statement	Rationale and Interpretations
P	Participate in all decisions about our treatments because we are the center of the health care team.	1. We and our doctor should agree on exactly what will be done during each step of our care. 2. We should know who will be taking care of us, how long the treatment will last, and how we should feel. 3. We have to understand that more tests or medicines may not always be better for us. We may ask our doctor how a new test or medication will help our condition. 4. We should keep copies of our medical records from previous hospital stays and share them with our doctors and nurses. This will give them better information about our health history. 5. We should not be afraid to ask for a second opinion. If we are unsure about the best treatment for our illness, we should talk with one or two additional doctors. The more information we have about all the kinds of treatment available to us, the better we will feel about the decision made. We may bring our advocate with us when we are seeking a second opinion. 6. We may ask to speak with someone who has the same treatment or operation we may need. This person may be able to tell us what to expect, what worked best, and help us prepare for the days and weeks ahead.

Sources: Joint Commission (2007a). Speak up: Facts about Speak Up Initiatives. Available at: http://www.jointcommission.org/GeneralPublic/Speak+Up/about_speakup.htm (accessed November 11, 2007). Joint Commission (2007b). Speak Up: Help Prevent Errors In Your Care. Available at: http://www.jointcommission.org/NR/rdonlyres/484AD48F-C464-4B5B-8D70-AA79179B3970/0/Speakup.pdf (accessed November 11, 2007).

Our Rights to Demand a Safe Hospital Stay

The health care environment throughout the world currently is under enormous pressure to improve the safety and quality of health care, while at the same time restraining the increasing costs in medical care. In a cost-containment practice environment, there will always be an ethical dilemma for hospital executives to justify resource allocation priorities between those resources that affect the safety and quality of care and those that influence patient satisfaction (Tzeng & Yin, 2008).

From a patient's viewpoint, satisfaction is about a desire and more is usually better. However, patients always wish to pay less money to obtain more satisfaction and higher quality. This situation results in a gap between the quality of care and the level of patient satisfaction. Most hospitals can only provide services at a reasonable price. However, safe patient care is the minimum requirement. Our "bottom line" should be to ensure that we are housed in a safe care environment without compromising our healing and recovery.

Therefore, we must know our rights in the process of receiving health care during hospitalization. The Speak Up program also urges all patients to know their rights (Table 1). Consequently, the Joint Commission developed a set of questions to help us know our rights before, during, and after our hospitalization (Joint Commission, 2007c; Table 2). Knowing our rights during a hospitalization can be the first and most important step to be involved in our care and promote our own self-healing system to heal ourselves from within.

Table 2. Knowing our rights before, during, and after our hospital stays

Main question	Rationale and interpretations
What are our rights?	1. We have the right to be informed about the care we will receive. 2. We have the right to get information about our care in our language. 3. We have the right to make decisions about our care, including refusing the care suggested by our doctor. 4. We have the right to know the names of the health care providers who treat us. 5. We have the right to receive safe care. 6. We have the right to have our pain treated. 7. We have the right to know when something goes wrong with our care. 8. We have the right to get an up-to-date list of all of our current medications. 9. We have the right to be listened to. 10. We have the right to be treated with courtesy and respect. 11. We have the right to ask for written information about all of our rights as patients.
What is our role as patients in our health care?	1. We should be active in our health care. 2. We should ask the questions that concern our condition and care. 3. We should pay attention to the instructions given to us by our doctor or nurse. 4. We should share as much information as possible about our health with our doctor and nurse, including an up-to-date list of our medications and our allergies.
Questions to ask our doctor before we enter the hospital	Can we have an advocate? Do we need to sign a document so our advocate can get important information about our care? What will be done to make sure we don't get a health care-associated infection during our hospitalization? Is there a form we need to sign about lifesaving actions, such as resuscitation, before being admitted to the hospital? Is there a form we need to sign about life support? Does the hospital allow the members of our religion to visit and pray with us? What kind of security does the hospital have, such as a 24-hour guard or alarm system? Whom should we speak to if a problem or safety concern arises? How does the hospital handle complaints? Are there any procedures that can't be done at our chosen hospital, for example, for religious reasons? Can we get a copy of our medical record and test results during hospitalization and after being discharged?
Questions to ask our doctor during hospital stays	How often will our doctor see us during our hospital stay? Who is responsible for our care when our designated doctor is not available? How about during weekends and at night? If my test or procedure shows that I need another procedure right away, can I get it done here in this hospital? Or will I need to go to a different hospital?

Table 2. Continued

Main question	Rationale and interpretations
Questions related to our advocate	
Can our family or friends help with our care?	We should ask our doctor or nurse if there is a form we need to fill out to name our advocate (also called a personal representative).
How can our advocate help with our care?	Our advocate can get information, ask questions for us when we can't, and find out whom to go to if we are not getting the care we need. Our advocate can remind us about instructions and help us make decisions.
Can our advocate make decisions for us?	Our advocate cannot make decisions for us unless our advocate is our legal guardian or we have given them that responsibility by signing a legal document, such as a health care power of attorney.
Can other people find out about our condition or disease?	Our health care providers should keep information about our health private. We may need to sign a form if we want our doctor or nurse to share information with our advocate or others.
What is "informed consent?"	A signed informed consent means that our doctor, surgeon, or nurse has talked to us about our treatment and its risks. Our doctor also has talked to us about options for treatment and what can happen if we aren't treated.
If something goes wrong with my care	
What will happen if something goes wrong with my care or during treatment?	If something goes wrong, we have the right to an honest explanation and an apology from our health care providers. The explanation and apology should be made within a reasonable amount of time.
How do we file a complaint?	If we have been discharged from the hospital, we can call the appropriate hospital personnel so that they can correct the problem. If we still have concerns, our complaints can be sent to the licensing authority or the Joint Commission. The Web site of the Joint Commission provides a complaint form at http://www.jointcommission.org/GeneralPublic/Complaint/.

Source: Joint Commission (2007c). Speak Up: Know your rights. Available at: http://www.joint commission.org/NR/rdonlyres/58A5230D-3E58-48D8-8114-C95AF53ECA27/0/Speakup_Rights. pdf (accessed November 12, 2007).

References

Agency for Healthcare Research and Quality (2000). Reducing errors in health care: Translating research into practice. Available at: http://www.ahrq.gov/research/errors.htm (accessed October 31, 2007).

Bäumler, E. (1992). *Die großen Medikamente*. Forscher und ihre Entdeckungen schenken uns Leben. Munich: Grunwald [in German].

Brennan, T. A., Leape, L. L., Laird, N. M., Hebert, L., Localio, A. R., Lawthers, A. G., Newhouse, J. P., Weiler, P. C., & Hiatt, H. H. (1991). Incidence of adverse events and negligence in hospitalized patients. Results of the Harvard Medical Practice Study I. *New England Journal of Medicine, 324*(6), 370-376.

Dozier, A. M., Kitzman, H. J., Ingersoll, G. L., Holmberg, S., & Schultz, A. W. (2001). Development of an instrument to measure patient perception of the quality of nursing care. *Research in Nursing & Health, 24*(6), 506-517.

Fagerstrom, L., Eriksson, K., & Engberg, I. B. (1999). The patient's perceived caring needs: Measuring the unmeasurable. *International Journal of Nursing Practice, 5*(4), 199-208.

Gillis, A., & MacDonald, B. (2005). Deconditioning in the hospitalized elderly. *Canadian Nurse, 101*(6), 16-20.

Institute of Medicine Report (2000). Executive summary. In L. T. Kohn, J. M. Corrigan, & M. S. Donaldson (Eds.), *To err is human: Building a safer health systems.* Available at: http://www.nap.edu/catalog.php?record_id=11623 (accessed October 31, 2007).

Institute of Medicine Report (2007). Executive summary. In P. Aspden, J. Wolcott, J. L. Bootman, & L. R. Cronenwett (Eds.), *Preventing medication errors: Quality chasm series.* Available at: http://www.nap.edu/catalog.php?record_id=11623 (accessed October 31, 2007).

Joint Commission (2007a). Speak up: Facts about Speak Up initiatives. Available at: http://www.jointcommission.org/GeneralPublic/Speak+Up/about_speakup.htm (accessed November 11, 2007).

Joint Commission (2007b). Speak Up: Help prevent errors in your care. Available at: http://www.jointcommission.org/NR/rdonlyres/484AD48F-C464-4B5B-8D70-AA79179B3970/0/Speakup.pdf (accessed November 11, 2007).

Joint Commission (2007c). Speak Up: Know your rights. Available at: http://www.jointcommission.org/NR/rdonlyres/58A5230D-3E58-48D8-8114-C95AF53ECA27/0/Speakup_Rights.pdf (accessed November 12, 2007).

Joint Commission Resources (2007). New consulting services from JCR. Available at: http://www.jcrinc.com/ (accessed on September 30, 2007).

McCaughey, B. (2005). *Unnecessary deaths: The human and financial costs of hospital infections* (2nd ed.). Published by National Center for Policy Analysis, Committee to Reduce Infection Death. Available at: http://www.pall.com/pdf/Unnecessary_Deaths_booklet.pdf (accessed on October 31, 2007).

Meade, C. M., Bursell, A. L., & Ketelsen, L. (2006). Effects of nursing rounds on patients' call light use, satisfaction and safety. *American Journal of Nursing, 106*(9), 58-70.

Nguyen Thi, P. L., Briancon, S., Empereur, F., & Guillemin, F. (2002). Factors determining inpatient satisfaction with care. *Social Science & Medicine, 54*(4), 493-504.

Reiling, J. (2006). Safe design of healthcare facilities. *Quality & Safety in Health Care, 15*(Suppl. 1), i34-i40.

Roohan, P. J., Franko, S. J., Anarella, J. P., Dellehunt, L. K., & Gesten, F. C. (2003). Do commercial managed care members rate their health plans differently than Medicaid managed care members? *Health Services Research, 38*(4), 1121-1134.

Tzeng, H. M., & Yin, C. Y. (2008). Patient satisfaction versus quality. *Nursing Ethics, 15*(1), 112-115.

Wennberg, J. E., Fisher, E. S., Baker, L., Sharp, S. M., & Bronner, K. (2005). Evaluating the
    efficiency of California providers in caring for patients with chronic illness. *Health
    Affairs (Millwood),* July-December, W5-526-43.

The Caring Philosophy
in Acute Hospital Settings

Medical Resources and Care Quality

Expenditures by the Medicare program in the United States have demonstrated a trend of being flat-of-the-curve medicine, where incremental spending above a certain point produces no incremental health benefits (Fuchs, 2004). Since 1996, acute myocardial infarction survival gains have stagnated although Medicare costs have continued to increase (Skinner, Staiger, & Fisher, 2006). Medicare enrollees in higher-spending regions of the United States received more care than those residing in lower-spending regions, but these enrollees did not have greater improvements in survival and functional status or in satisfaction with care (Fisher et al., 2003). A recent study of hospitals in California also reported that some hospitals spent up to four times more than others in that state to treat patients with similar conditions. Yet, these additional costs did not result in any gains in quality, patient satisfaction, or health outcomes (Benko, 2005).

In reality, whenever physicians and nurses treat their patients by following procedures based on their most current knowledge and best judgment, patients would not die or be harmed from the consequences of negligence (e.g., medication or procedure errors). Advanced medical technology may, for example, assist physicians and nurses to identify problems, maintain a patient's vital signs, extend a patient's life, and allow more time for the patient to heal. Any gains in quality are always built on comprehensively following professional practice standards, not on technology alone (Tzeng & Yin, 2008).

Occupational Identity of Nurses

Landon and associates (2006) examined the quality of care for the treatment of acute medical conditions in US hospitals (e.g., acute myocardial infarction, congestive heart failure, and pneumonia). Based on the study findings, they concluded that patients were more likely to receive high-quality care in not-for-profit hospitals, in teaching hospitals, and in hospitals with high registered nurse staffing ratios and more investment in technology. As we have observed, during hospitalization, nurses often play an important role in providing a communication bridge between physicians and inpatients. High levels of registered nurse staffing allow for more counseling and other activities to be performed (Tzeng & Yin, 2008).

Nursing is well recognized as a professional, specialized field of study. As indicated in the Old Testament of the Holy Bible, nurses and physicians were considered as two independent occupations with different responsibilities. In the time of the Old Testament (from the 17th century B.C. to the 1st century B.C.), nurses practiced independently as wet nurses, dry nurses, midwives, or the ones who cared for the sick. They looked after, fostered, or advised healthy or sick people (Tzeng & Yin, 2007). Being midwives and caring for women's health problems were nurses' unique functions. Physicians, who were primarily men, could not get close to women and care for female patients. At that time, nurses did not practice under physicians' supervision and did not need to follow physicians' orders for delivering care (Tzeng & Yin, 2007).

Table 1. A comparison among the commonly adopted terms, newly invented terms, and the modified terms as related to nursing

Popularly adopted terms	Newly invented terms	Modified terms
"Nursing" as a *noun* indicates the profession of a nurse (e.g., School of Nursing) or the duties of a nurse.	"Nurstry" as a *noun* indicates the profession of a nurse (e.g., School of Nurstry) and the science and caring art dealing with the maintenance of health and the prevention and alleviation of diseases.	
"Nurse" as a *noun* refers to: (1) a person who looks after, fosters, or advises someone or (2) a person who is skilled or trained in caring for the sick under the supervision of a physician.	"Nurstrist" as a *noun* refers to a scholar or scientist who is involved in the academic research of "nurstry" as his or her primary responsibility.	"Nurse" as a *noun* refers to a person who is skilled or trained in: (1) caring for the sick or people in rehabilitation, (2) promoting the community health of the population, or (3) preventing disease by providing health counseling or education.
"Nurse" as a *verb* means to care for and wait on a sick person or to attempt to cure a sick person by care and treatment.		"Nurse" as a *verb* means: (1) to care for and wait on a sick person or (2) to promote the health of the population. "Nursing" as an *adjective* means relating to "nurstry."

Sources: Tzeng, H. M., & Yin, C. Y. (2007). Seeing the nursing profession from a different perspective: Nurstry? Why not! *Nursing Forum, 42*(4), 185-188. Merriam-Webster Online (2007). Merriam-Webster online dictionary. Springfield, MA: Merriam-Webster, Inc. Available at: http://www.m-w.com/cgi-bin/dictionary (accessed November 10, 2007).

Nurses should be treated as equals with physicians and as professionals who are capable of independent practice. The term "nursing" has been popularly used to refer to the profession, but it is not enough to demonstrate the nature of an independent discipline in practice and academia (Tzeng & Yin, 2007). As a result, we proposed the term *Nurstry* to be used to refer to the science and caring art of nursing (Table 1). *Nurstry* includes nursing knowledge developed by *nurstrists* and nurses in the global nursing village.

Caring Philosophy: Code of Ethics for Nurses

Patients come to hospitals because they want to live and expect their health care providers to save their lives. They rely heavily on nurses' professional training, knowledge, and lifesaving practices (Tzeng & Yin, 2008).

In July 2001, the Congress of Nursing Practice and Economics approved the *Code of Ethics for Nurses with Interpretive Statements* (American Nurses Association, 2007a). This code has been disseminated by the American Nurses Association, which represents the nation's 2.9 million registered nurses through its 54 constituent member associations (American Nurses Association, 2007b). Table 2 summarizes the nine provisions indicated in the *Code of Ethics for Nurses with Interpretive Statements* (American Nurses Association, 2001).

This *Code of Ethics for Nurses* was developed to provide a succinct statement of the ethical obligations and duties of every individual who enters the nursing profession. It serves as the nursing profession's nonnegotiable ethical standard and as the expression of the nursing profession's own understanding of its commitment to society. The *Code of Ethics for Nurses* is a dynamic document. Because nursing and its social context may change over time, revisions to the *Code of Ethics for Nurses* may be required. For each provision, interpretive statements provide greater specificity for practice and are responsive to the contemporary context of nursing (American Nurses Association, 2001).

Nursing, as a profession, has its philosophy, and the code of ethics is their caring philosophy. Professional nurses working in different regions and types of hospitals are expected to practice the same standardized procedures competently, such as universal precautions, disinfection measures, and turning patients to prevent pressure ulcers. In other words, a commonly recognized caring philosophy, like the *Code of Ethics for Nurses*, leads to the development of practice principles and ethics that are used to judge whether any activities are ethical or being practiced in a competent manner (Tzeng & Yin, 2008). Nurses may use different levels of medical technology and equipment for patient care, but their skills and clinical judgment should not differ.

**Table 2. The nine provisions and the outline of the accompanying interpretive statement
for each provision as indicated in the
*Code of Ethics for Nurses with Interpretive Statements***

Domain	Provision*	Outline of the accompanying interpretive statement
Fundamental values and commitments	Provision 1 The nurse, in all professional relationships, practices with compassion and respect for the inherent dignity, worth, and uniqueness of every individual, unrestricted by considerations of social or economic status, personal attributes, or the nature of health problems.	1. Relationships to patients 2. Relationships with colleagues and others 3. Respect for human dignity 4. The nature of health problems 5. The right to self-determination
	Provision 2 The nurse's primary commitment is to the patient, whether an individual, family, group, or community.	1. Collaboration 2. Conflict of interest for nurses 3. Primacy of the patient's interests 4. Professional boundaries
	Provision 3 The nurse promotes, advocates for, and strives to protect the health, safety, and rights of the patient.	1. Acting on questionable practice 2. Addressing impaired practice 3. Confidentiality 4. Privacy 5. Protection of participants in research 6. Standards and review mechanisms
Boundaries of duty and loyalty	Provision 4 The nurse is responsible and accountable for individual nursing practice and determines the appropriate delegation of tasks consistent with the nurse's obligation to provide optimum patient care.	1. Acceptance of accountability and responsibility 2. Accountability for nursing judgment and actions 3. Delegation of nursing activities 4. Responsibility for nursing judgment and actions
	Provision 5 The nurse owes the same duties to self as to others, including the responsibility to preserve integrity and safety, to maintain competence, and to continue personal and professional growth.	1. Moral self-respect 2. Preservation of integrity 3. Professional growth and maintenance of competence 4. Wholeness of character
	Provision 6 The nurse participates in establishing, maintaining, and improving health care environments and conditions of employment conducive to the provision of quality health care and consistent with the values of the profession through individual and collective action.	1. Influence of the environment on ethical obligations 2. Influence of the environment on moral virtues and values 3. Responsibility for the health care environment

Domain	Provision*	Outline of the accompanying interpretive statement
Aspects of duties beyond individual patient encounters	Provision 7 The nurse participates in the advancement of the profession through contributions to practice, education, administration, and knowledge development.	1. Advancing the profession by developing, maintaining, and implementing professional standards in clinical, administrative, and educational practice 2. Advancing the profession through active involvement in nursing and in health care policy 3. Advancing the profession through knowledge development, dissemination, and application to practice
	Provision 8 The nurse collaborates with other health professionals and the public in promoting community, national, and international efforts to meet health needs.	1. Health needs and concerns 2. Responsibilities to the public
	Provision 9 The profession of nursing, as represented by associations and their members, is responsible for articulating nursing values, for maintaining the integrity of the profession and its practice, and for shaping social policy.	1. Assertion of values 2. Intra-professional integrity 3. Social reform 4. The profession carries out its collective responsibility through professional associations

* Reprinted with permission from American Nurses Association, Code of Ethics for Nurses with Interpretive Statements (c)2001, Nursesbooks.org, Silver Spring, MD.

Source: American Nurses Association (2001). Codes of ethics for nurses with interpretative statements. Available at: http://nursingworld.org/ethics/code/protected_nwcoe831.htm (accessed November 11, 2007).

Do any Government Agencies Oversee the Safety and Quality of Hospital care?

Yes, the Agency for Healthcare Research and Quality (AHRQ) is the primary gatekeeper for the safety of our hospital care. In February 2006, the AHRQ developed a set of inpatient quality indicators to be used with the hospital inpatient discharge data to provide a perspective on quality. These inpatient quality indicators (a total of 32 measures) can be used to help hospitals identify potential problem areas in the quality of care that may need further investigation (Agency for Healthcare Research and Quality, 2006a, 2006b; Table 3).

Table 3. The Agency for Healthcare Research and Quality inpatient quality indicators

Dimension	Indicator
Mortality rates for inpatient medical conditions (7 indicators): These measures include the conditions for which mortality has been shown to vary substantially across hospitals. For these indicators, there is evidence that high mortality may be associated with deficiencies in the quality of care.	1. Acute myocardial infarction mortality rate, all cases 2. Acute myocardial infarction mortality rate, without transfer cases 3. Congestive heart failure mortality rate 4. Gastrointestinal hemorrhage mortality rate 5. Hip fracture mortality rate 6. Pneumonia mortality rate 7. Stroke mortality rate
Mortality rates for inpatient surgical procedures (8 indicators): These measures include the procedures for which mortality has been shown to vary across hospitals. For these indicators, there is evidence that high mortality may be associated with poorer quality of care.	1. Abdominal aortic aneurysm repair mortality rate 2. Carotid endarterectomy mortality rate 3. Coronary artery bypass graft mortality rate 4. Craniotomy mortality rate 5. Esophageal resection mortality rate 6. Hip replacement mortality rate 7. Pancreatic resection mortality rate 8. Percutaneous transluminal coronary angioplasty mortality rate
Hospital-level procedure utilization rates (7 indicators): These measures examine procedures whose use varies significantly across hospitals. Questions related to the volume have been raised about overuse, underuse, or misuse of these procedures.	1. Bilateral cardiac catheterization rate 2. Cesarean section delivery rate 3. Incidental appendectomy in the elderly rate 4. Laparoscopic cholecystectomy rate 5. Primary cesarean delivery rate 6. Vaginal birth after cesarean rate, all cases 7. Vaginal birth after cesarean rate, uncomplicated
Area-level utilization rates (4 indicators): These measures provide the rate of hospitalization in the area for specific procedures. They represent procedures whose use varies widely across relatively similar geographic areas with substantial inappropriate use.	1. Coronary artery bypass graft rate 2. Hysterectomy area rate 3. Laminectomy or spinal fusion area rate 4. Percutaneous transluminal coronary angioplasty area rate
Provider-level volume of procedures (6 indicators): These indicators are indirect measures of quality, and simply represent counts of admissions in which these procedures were performed. These measures are based on evidence suggesting that hospitals performing more of certain highly complex, high-technology, or intensive procedures may have better outcomes for those procedures.	1. Abdominal aortic aneurysm repair volume 2. Carotid endarterectomy volume 3. Coronary artery bypass graft volume 4. Esophageal resection volume 5. Pancreatic resection volume 6. Percutaneous transluminal coronary angioplasty volume

Sources: Agency for Healthcare Research and Quality (2006a). Inpatient quality indicators overview: AHRQ quality indicators (updated February 2006). Available at: http://www. qualityindicators.ahrq.gov/iqi_overview.htm (accessed November 12, 2007). Agency for Healthcare Research and Quality (2006b). Inpatient quality indicators (updated February 2006). Available at: http://www.qualityindicators.ahrq.gov/downloads/iqi/2006-Feb-InpatientQuality Indicators .pdf (accessed November 12, 2007).

Table 4. The Agency for Healthcare Research and Quality pediatric quality indicators

Dimension	Indicator
Provider-level pediatric quality indicators (13 indicators): These measures examine potentially preventable complications for patients who received their initial care and the complications of care within the same hospitalization. These indicators include only those cases where a secondary diagnosis code flags a potentially preventable complication.	1. Accidental puncture or laceration 2. Decubitus ulcer 3. Foreign body left during procedure 4. Iatrogenic pneumothorax in neonates at risk 5. Iatrogenic pneumothorax in non-neonates 6. Pediatric heart surgery mortality 7. Pediatric heart surgery volume 8. Postoperative hemorrhage or hematoma 9. Postoperative respiratory failure 10. Postoperative sepsis 11. Postoperative wound dehiscence 12. Selected infections due to medical care 13. Transfusion reaction
Area-level pediatric quality indicators (5 indicators): These measures are specified to include principal and secondary diagnoses for the complications of care. These indicators also add the cases where a patient's risk of the complication occurred in a separate hospitalization.	1. Asthma admission rate 2. Diabetes short-term complication rate 3. Gastroenteritis admission rate 4. Perforated appendix admission rate 5. Urinary track infection admission rate

Sources: Agency for Healthcare Research and Quality (2006c). Inpatient quality indicators overview: AHRQ quality indicators (updated February 2006). Available at: http://www.qualityindicators. ahrq.gov/pdi_overview.htm (accessed November 13, 2007). Agency for Healthcare Research and Quality (2006d). Pediatric quality indicators (updated February 2006). Available at: http://www.qualityindicators.ahrq.gov/downloads/pdi/2006-Feb-PediatricQualityIndicators.pdf (accessed November 13, 2007).

Table 5. The Agency for Healthcare Research and Quality patient safety indicators

Dimension	Indicator
Provider-level indicators (20 indicators): These measures examine the potentially preventable complications for patients who received their initial care and the complications of care within the same hospitalization. These indicators include only those cases where a secondary diagnosis code flags a potentially preventable complication.	1. Accidental puncture and laceration 2. Birth trauma, injury to neonate 3. Complications of anesthesia 4. Death in low-mortality diagnoses, based on diagnostic-related groups (DRGs) 5. Decubitus ulcer 6. Failure to rescue 7. Foreign body left in during procedure 8. Iatrogenic pneumothorax 9. Obstetric trauma, cesarean delivery 10. Obstetric trauma, vaginal delivery with instrument 11. Obstetric trauma, vaginal delivery without instrument 12. Postoperative hemorrhage or hematoma 13. Postoperative hip fracture 14. Postoperative physiologic and metabolic derangements 15. Postoperative pulmonary embolism or deep vein thrombosis 16. Postoperative respiratory failure 17. Postoperative sepsis 18. Postoperative wound dehiscence in abdominopelvic surgical patients 19. Selected infections due to medical care 20. Transfusion reaction

Table 5. (Continued)

Dimension	Indicator
Area-level indicators (7 indicators): These measures capture all cases of the potentially preventable complications that occur in a given area (e.g., a county or a metropolitan area), and these cases can happen either during hospitalization or result in subsequent hospitalization. These indicators include both principal diagnosis and secondary diagnoses for the complications of care. These measures also add the cases where a patient' risk of the complication occurred in a different hospitalization.	1. Accidental puncture and laceration 2. Foreign body left in during procedure 3. Iatrogenic pneumothorax 4. Postoperative hemorrhage or hematoma 5. Postoperative wound dehiscence in abdominopelvic surgical patients 6. Selected infections due to medical care 7. Transfusion reaction

Sources: Agency for Healthcare Research and Quality (2006e). Patient safety indicators: AHRQ quality indicators (updated February 2006). Available at: http://www.qualityindicators.ahrq.gov/psi_ overview.htm (accessed November 12, 2007). Agency for Healthcare Research and Quality (2006f). Patient safety indicators (updated February 2006). Available at: http://www.quality indicators.ahrq.gov/downloads/psi/2006-Feb-PatientSafetyIndicators.pdf (accessed November 12, 2007).

Pediatric quality indicators were also developed with a focus on children's health care quality using routinely collected hospital discharge data as the basis for indicator specifications. These pediatric inpatient measures (a total of 18 measures) examine potentially preventable complications, iatrogenic events for pediatric patients treated in hospitals, and preventable hospitalizations. The population for the pediatric quality indicators includes youngsters under the age of 18 years, not yet considered part of an adult diagnostic-related group (DRG), and not in the major diagnostic category 14 (pregnancy, childbirth, and the puerperium; Agency for Healthcare Research and Quality, 2006c, 2006d; Table 4).

In addition, the AHRQ created a set of patient safety indicators as a tool to help identify potentially preventable complications or adverse events occurring in hospitalized patients. These patient safety indicators (a total of 27 indicators) provide the opportunity to assess the incidence of adverse events and complications using the hospital inpatient discharge data (Agency for Healthcare Research and Quality, 2006e, 2006f; Table 5).

These three sets of inpatient quality, pediatric quality, and patient safety indicators are meant to monitor the safety and quality of hospital care as a whole. Hospital care involves *all* members of the health care team. Physicians, nurses, and pharmacists have the main roles in delivering inpatient care services. Currently, there is a widespread consensus in the US medical community that hospitals can reduce patient injuries by improving the care environment for safety. Possible interventions include implementing electronic medical record systems and improving staff awareness of patient safety risks (Agency for Healthcare Research and Quality, 2006f).

Are the Safety and Quality of Nursing Care being Monitored?

Yes, the American Nurses Association (ANA) monitors the safety and quality of nursing care provided in acute inpatient settings (e.g., hospitals). As a matter of fact, nursing is the only health care discipline that cares for hospitalized patients 24 hours a day, 7 days a week. Because of this, it is reasonable to assume that the quality of nursing care would have an impact on patient safety in inpatient care.

Consequently, the ANA instituted the *Nursing Care Report Card for Acute Care* in which 10 specific nursing quality indicators were developed and defined to guide and improve care (Duffy & Korniewicz, 2000; Table 6). These 10 quality indicators were categorized into three domains: (1) safety measures, (2) patient satisfaction measures, and (3) human resource management measures. Health care-associated infection rates, patient falls, and maintenance of skin integrity were identified as safety quality indicators for the nursing care delivered in the inpatient care settings.

References

Agency for Healthcare Research and Quality (2006a). Inpatient quality indicators overview: AHRQ quality indicators (updated February 2006). Available at: http://www. qualityindicators.ahrq.gov/iqi_overview.htm (accessed November 12, 2007).

Agency for Healthcare Research and Quality (2006b). Inpatient quality indicators (updated February 2006). Available at: http://www.qualityindicators.ahrq.gov/downloads/ iqi/2006-Feb-InpatientQualityIndicators.pdf (accessed November 12, 2007).

Agency for Healthcare Research and Quality (2006c). Inpatient quality indicators overview: AHRQ quality indicators (updated February 2006). Available at: http://www. qualityindicators.ahrq.gov/pdi_overview.htm (accessed November 13, 2007).

Agency for Healthcare Research and Quality (2006d). Pediatric quality indicators (updated February 2006). Available at: http://www.qualityindicators.ahrq.gov/downloads/pdi/ 2006-Feb-PediatricQualityIndicators.pdf (accessed November 13, 2007).

Agency for Healthcare Research and Quality (2006e). Patient safety indicators: AHRQ quality indicators (updated February 2006). Available at: http://www.qualityindicators. ahrq.gov/psi_overview.htm (accessed November 12, 2007).

Agency for Healthcare Research and Quality (2006f). Patient safety indicators (updated February 2006). Available at: http://www.qualityindicators.ahrq.gov/downloads/ psi/2006-Feb-PatientSafetyIndicators.pdf (accessed November 12, 2007).

American Nurses Association (2001). Codes of ethics for nurses with interpretative statements. Available at: http://nursingworld.org/ethics/code/protected_nwcoe831.htm (accessed November 11, 2007).

American Nurses Association (2007a). About the code. Available at: http://nursingworld. org/MainMenuCategories/ThePracticeofProfessionalNursing/EthicsStandards/CodeofEth ics/AboutTheCode.aspx (accessed November 11, 2007).

American Nurses Association (2007b). About ANA. Available at: http://nursingworld.org/ FunctionalMenuCategories/AboutANA.aspx (accessed November 11, 2007).

Benko, L. B. (2005). Big spending. *Modern Healthcare, 35*(48), 14.

Duffy, J. R., & Korniewicz, D. M. (2000). Quality indicators: Outcomes measurement using the ANA safety and quality indicators. Available at: http://nursingworld.org/mods/ archive/mod72/ceomfull.htm (accessed November 11, 2007).

Fisher, E. S., Wennberg, D. E., Stukel, T. A., Gottlieb, D. J., Lucas, F. L., & Pinder, E. L. (2003). The implications of regional variation in Medicare spending. Part 1: The content, quality, and accessibility of care. *Annals of Internal Medicine, 138*(4), 288-298.

Fuchs, V. R. (2004). Perspective: More variation in use of care, more flat-of-the-curve medicine. Health Affairs Web Exclusive (October 7, 2004). Available at: http://content. healthaffairs.org/cgi/reprint/hlthaff.var.104v1.pdf (accessed on December 21, 2006).

Landon, B. E., Normand, S. L. T., Lessler, A., O'Malley, A. J., Schmaltz, S., Leob, J. M., & McNeil, B. (2006). Quality of care for the treatment of acute medical conditions in US hospitals. *Archives of Internal Medicine, 166*(22), 2511-2517.

Merriam-Webster Online (2007). Merriam-Webster online dictionary. Springfield, MA: Merriam-Webster, Inc. Available at: http://www.m-w.com/cgi-bin/dictionary (accessed November 10, 2007).

Skinner, J. S., Staiger, D. O., & Fisher, E. S. (2006). Is technological change in medicine always worth it? The case of acute myocardial infarction. *Health Affairs (Millwood), 25*(2), w34-47.

Tzeng, H. M., & Yin, C.Y. (2007). Seeing the nursing profession from a different perspective: Nurstry? Why not! *Nursing Forum, 42*(4), 185-188.

Tzeng, H. M., & Yin, C. Y. (2008). What's our philosophy? *Journal of Professional Nursing, 24*(1), 5-6.

No Safety, No Quality: Initiatives for Promoting Patient Safety in Hospitals

Care Safety versus Care Quality

Patient safety always comes first, followed by the quality of care. Quality has been commonly defined as the degree to which health services for individuals and populations increase the likelihood of desired health or medical outcomes and are consistent with current professional knowledge (Institute of Medicine, 2007a). Hospital quality improvement initiatives often were approached through building or maintaining a facility and policies that promote provision of care under safe conditions (National Academy of Sciences, 2004a). Safety is, indeed, the basis of a quality hospital environment and the minimum requirement to satisfy patients and their families.

We Expect a Safe Hospital Stay
Patient Safety Initiatives

The Initiative of Transforming Care at the Bedside

In 2003, the Robert Wood Johnson Foundation and Institute for Healthcare Improvement started an initiative called *Transforming Care at the Bedside* and created a framework for changes on medical and surgical inpatient care units. The Robert Wood Johnson Foundation, as the nation's largest philanthropy organization, is devoted exclusively to improving the health and health care of all Americans. The Institute for Healthcare Improvement is a not-for-profit organization that was created in 1991 to help lead the improvement efforts of health care systems for the purpose of increasing their quality and value (Institute for Healthcare Improvement, 2007a).

The Institute for Healthcare Improvement built the framework of *Transforming Care at the Bedside* around improvement in four main categories. This initiative has involved a total of 10 participating hospitals in testing, refining, and implementing change ideas within each category. Table 1 lists these four categories and the suggested high-level changes (Institute for Healthcare Improvement, 2007a, 2007b, 2007c).

Table 1. The four categories and the suggested high leverage changes as indicated in the initiative of "Transforming Care at the Bedside"

Category	Change
Safe and reliable care: Improving the safety and quality of patient care on medical and surgical patient care units	*Best practices existed on 25 medical or surgical patient care units* 1. Creating early detection and response systems 2. Developing hospice and palliative care programs 3. Preventing adverse drug events through medication reconciliation 4. Preventing deep vein thrombosis for surgical patients 5. Preventing high hazard drug errors 6. Preventing pressure ulcers *Best practices existed on 5 medical or surgical patient care units* 1. Preventing harm from falls 2. Preventing health care-associated infections
Patient-centered care: Engaging and improving patients' and their families' experience of care	*Best practices existed on 25 medical or surgical patient care units* 1. Creating patient-centered healing environments *Best practices existed on 5 medical or surgical patient care units* 1. Involving patients and their families in all quality improvement teams 2. Optimizing transitions to home or other facility
Vitality and teamwork: Increasing the vitality and retention of nurses	*Best practices existed on 25 medical or surgical patient care units* 1. Building capability of front-line staff in innovation and process improvement *Best practices existed on 5 medical or surgical patient care units* 1. Identifying competencies and developing mid-level managers and clinical leaders to lead transformation 2. Optimizing communications among health care providers
Value-added care processes: Improving the effectiveness of the entire health care team.	*Best practices existed on 25 medical or surgical patient care units* 1. Creating acuity adaptable beds 2. Eliminating waste and improving work flow in admission process, medication administration, hand-off, and discharge process 3. Improving work environment through physical space design. *Best practices existed on 5 medical or surgical patient care units* 1. Moving value-added activities to the bedside

Sources: Institute for Healthcare Improvement (2007a). Transforming care at the bedside: Overview. Available at: http://www.ihi.org/IHI/Programs/StrategicInitiatives/TransformingCareAtThe Bedside.htm (accessed November 13, 2007). Institute for Healthcare Improvement (2007b). Transforming care at the bedside: The framework for change on medical/surgical units. Available at: http://www.ihi.org/NR/rdonlyres/F81270CD-B8BC-47D5-B2A6-BDA550096AA9/5802/Visio TCABframework0907.pdf (accessed November 13, 2007). Institute for Healthcare Improvement (2007c). Transforming care at the bedside: TCAB overview. Available at: http://www.ihi. org/NR/rdonlyres/BD24233D-6328-4F1E-9197-151628F1EA35/0/TCABvideotape907.pdf (accessed November 13, 2007).

Other promising changes cannot be strictly classified into any one of the four main categories (Institute for Healthcare Improvement, 2007a) and include:

1. Using rapid response teams to rescue patients before a crisis occurs
2. Liberalizing diet plans and meal schedules for patients
3. Adopting specific communication models that support consistent and clear communication among health care providers
4. Offering professional support programs (e.g., preceptorships and educational opportunities)
5. Redesigning the workspace to enhance efficiency and reduce waste

As described in the initiative of *Transforming Care at the Bedside*, we should expect safe, reliable, effective, and equitable care without preventable harms and complications of care during hospitalization. Truly patient-centered care on medical and surgical patient care units should honor the whole person and the family, respect individual values and choices, and ensure continuity of care. We should also expect that nurses are available to meet our needs. Nurses who work in an acute inpatient care unit are expected to spend 70% of their total working hours per shift in direct patient care and these direct patient care hours must be reasonably distributed among patients (Institute for Healthcare Improvement, 2007a).

From a patient safety advocate's perspective, after a patient is discharged home, this patient would really hope to be able to tell family and friends that "my doctor and nurse gave me exactly the help I wanted and needed exactly when I wanted and needed it." However, such a wish seldom comes true. The Institute for Healthcare Improvement (2007a) urged the health care industry to recognize that such a wish from patients is a reasonable expectation from hospital care.

The Institute of Medicine's Initiatives

The Institute of Medicine (IOM) is a private, non-for-profit institution that provides objective, timely, authoritative information and advice relating to health science policy to the government, corporate sector, professions, and public as a component of the National Academy of Sciences under a congressional charter. In 1996, the IOM launched an initiative on assessing and improving the nation's quality of care. To date, three phases have been implemented and the initiative is currently in its third phase (Institute of Medicine, 2007a). These three phases are:

1. Phase 1 (1996-1998). The first phase focused on understanding the scope of issues as one of overuse, misuse, and underuse of health care services.
2. Phase 2 (1999-2001). This phase targeted the demands on the health care system and called for transformations to close the gap between what was known to be good quality care and what actually existed in practice.

3. Phase 3 (2002-present). The current phase focuses on reforming three different overlapping levels of the system: (1) the environmental level, (2) the level of the health care organization, and (3) the interface between clinicians and patients.

Since 1995, the IOM has published 116 reports addressing health care and quality (Institute of Medicine, 2007b). These health care and quality-related reports can be further categorized into the following five care quality issues (Tzeng & Yin, 2007):

1. Promoting health
2. Accessing health care
3. Treating disease
4. Developing quality standards
5. Enhancing health care or hospital administration systems

Setting up the National Patient Safety Goals

The Joint Commission in the United States is an accreditation agency that constantly monitors hospitals and the other types of health care institutions (e.g., home care programs). Each year, a broadly representative sentinel event advisory group works with the Joint Commission staff on a continuing basis to prioritize and develop national patient safety goals (Joint Commission, 2007a, 2007b). The Joint Commission's national patient safety goals aim to promote specific improvements in patient safety. The 2008 National Patient Safety Goals for hospital programs are summarized in Table 2 (Joint Commission, 2007d).

Table 2. The 2008 National Patient Goals for hospital programs

Goal	Implementation expectation
Improve the accuracy of patient identification (Goal 1)*	1. Using at least two patient identifiers, when providing care, treatment or services
Improve the effectiveness of communication among caregivers (Goal 2)	1. For verbal or telephone orders, verifying the complete order by having the person receiving the information record and "read-back" the complete order
	2. For telephonic reporting of critical test results, verifying the test result by having the person receiving the information record and "read-back" the test result
	3. Standardizing a list of abbreviations, acronyms, symbols, and dose designations that are not to be used throughout the hospital
	4. Measuring, assessing, and if appropriate, taking action to improve the timeliness of reporting and receipt of critical test results and values, by the responsible licensed caregiver
	5. Implementing a standardized approach to "hand off" communications, including an opportunity to ask and respond to questions

Goal	Implementation expectation
Improve the safety of using medications (Goal 3)	1. Identifying and, at a minimum, annually reviewing a list of look-alike or sound-alike medications prescribed by doctors within a hospital, and taking action to prevent errors involving the interchange of these medications 2. Labeling all medications, medication containers (e.g., syringes, medicine cups, and basins), and other solutions on and off the sterile field 3. Reducing the likelihood of patient harms associated with the use of anticoagulation therapy
Reduce the risk of health care-associated infections (Goal 7)	1. Complying with current World Health Organization Hand Hygiene Guidelines or Centers for Disease Control and Prevention (CDC) hand hygiene guidelines 2. Managing all identified cases of unanticipated death or major permanent loss of function associated with a health care-associated infection, as sentinel events
Accurately and completely reconcile medications across the continuum of care (Goal 8)	1. There should be a process in place for comparing the patient's current medications with those ordered for the patient while under the care in a hospital 2. A complete list of the patient's medications is communicated to the next health care provider of service when a patient is referred or transferred to another setting, service, practitioner or level of care within or outside a hospital 3. The complete list of medications should also be provided to the patient on discharge
Reduce the risk of patient harm resulting from falls (Goal 9)	1. Implementing a fall reduction program and including an evaluation of the effectiveness of the program
Encourage patients' active involvement in their own care as a patient safety strategy (Goal 13)	1. Defining and communicating the means for patients and their families to report concerns about safety and encourage them to do so
Identify safety risks inherent in its patient population (Goal 15)	1. Hospitals should identify patients at risk for suicide. 2. This goal is applicable to psychiatric hospitals and patients being treated for emotional or behavioral disorders in general hospitals.
Improve recognition and response to changes in a patient's condition (Goal 16)	1. Hospitals should select a suitable method that enables health care providers to directly request additional assistance from a specially trained staff, when a patient's condition appears to be worsening.

* The number for each goal was given by the Joint Commission.
Source: Joint Commission (2007d). 2008 National Patient Safety Goals: Hospital program. Available at: http://www.jointcommission.org/PatientSafety/NationalPatientSafetyGoals/08_hap_npsgs.htm (accessed November 11, 2007).

When we are admitted to a hospital for acute inpatient care, we are seeking professionals to cure or care for us. Without many other options, we must depend on and trust our doctors and nurses because they are our "guardian angels" to save our lives. Can we assume that our doctors and nurses are doing what they can to promote the patient safety goals listed in Table 2?

However, these goals were highlighted by the Joint Commission because these patient safety issues have not been addressed thoroughly. The deficiencies in meeting these common sense patient safety aspects (e.g., unsafe care and practice) have led and may continue to lead to patient harms and complications of care during hospitalization. Our safety during hospitalization is partially in our own hands, and we do need to pay attention to the gap between the safety levels of the expected and the actual received hospital care.

International Initiatives on Patient Safety

In March 2005, the Joint Commission and Joint Commission Resources (JCR) in the United States established the Joint Commission International Center for Patient Safety (abbreviated as the Joint Commission International or JCI), which also resides in the United States. In August 2005, the World Health Organization (WHO) designated the Joint Commission and the JCI as the world's first WHO collaborating center dedicated solely to patient safety as part of WHO's major initiative—the World Alliance for Patient Safety. JCI is the operational arm for this collaboration and concentrates on worldwide attention on patient safety solutions and best practices in hospital settings to reduce safety risks to patients (Joint Commission International Center for Patient Safety, 2007a, 2007b).

In 2006, JCI developed six international patient safety goals (Joint Commission International Center for Patient Safety, 2007c), as listed in Table 3. Since January 2006, JCI has been surveying international hospitals on compliance with these goals as a way to evaluate the relevance and feasibility of international hospitals reaching a common understanding of hospital safety goals (Joint Commission International Center for Patient Safety, 2007a, 2007b).

A consensus was reached among national and international hospitals. This consensus further confirmed the importance of promoting the safety of medication administration and procedures and preventing adverse events in hospitals.

Recently, the JCI Board of Directors refined the hospital accreditation survey process for 2007 with the approved six International Patient Safety Goals and the use of tracer methodology as an evaluation method used to trace a single patient's experiences within a hospital (Joint Commission International Center for Patient Safety, 2007d; Table 3).

In April 2007, the International Steering Committee approved nine initial patient safety solutions for dissemination (Joint Commission International Center for Patient Safety, 2007e; Table 4). A patient safety solution is defined as a system design or intervention that has demonstrated the ability to prevent or mitigate patient harm stemming from the processes of regaining health. These solutions are meant to prevent health care errors that may have harmed millions of people daily through out the world (Joint Commission International Center for Patient Safety, 2007e).

Table 3. The International Patient Safety Goals
as developed by the Joint Commission International

Goal[*]	Corresponding requirement

Goal 1
Identify patients correctly
	1. Using at least two ways to identify a patient in the following three situations:
	   1.1 When giving medicines, blood, or blood products
	   1.2 When taking blood samples and other specimens for clinical testing
	   1.3 When providing any other treatments or procedures
	2. The patient's room number cannot be used to identify the patient.

Goal 2 Improve effective communication	1. Implementing a process or procedure for taking verbal or telephone orders or for the reporting of critical test results 2. This process or procedure requires a verification "read-back" of the complete order or test result by the person receiving the information. 3. It is noted that not all countries permit verbal or telephone orders.
Goal 3 Improve the safety of high-alert medications	1. Removing concentrated electrolytes from patient care units. These electrolytes include, but not limited to, potassium chloride, potassium phosphate, and sodium chloride >0.9%.
Goal 4 Eliminate wrong-site, wrong-patient, and wrong-procedure surgery	1. Using a checklist, including a "time-out" just before starting a surgical procedure, to ensure the correct patient, procedure, and body part 2. Developing a process or checklist to verify that all documents and equipment needed for surgery are on hand, correct, and functioning properly before surgery begins 3. Marking the precise site where the surgery will be performed, using a clearly understood mark, and involving the patient in doing this
Goal 5 Reduce the risk of health care-associated infections	1. Complying with generally accepted guidelines for hand hygiene
Goal 6 Reduce the risk of patient harm resulting from falls	1. Assessing and periodically reassessing each individual patient's risk for falling (e.g., the potential risk associated with the patient's medication regimen) and taking action to decrease or eliminate any identified risks

[*] The goals and the corresponding requirements for each goal are exactly the same for the 2006 and 2007 versions.

Sources: Joint Commission International Center for Patient Safety (2007c). 2006 International Patient Safety Goals. Available at: http://www.jcipatientsafety.org/15143/ (accessed November 11, 2007). Joint Commission International Center for Patient Safety (2007d). 2007 International Patient Safety Goals. Available at: http://www.jcipatientsafety.org/15137/ (accessed November 11, 2007).

Because these international patient safety goals have been endorsed by the WHO, we should also expect our hospitals to pay attention to these areas. Both the National Patient Safety goals for the hospital programs in the United States and the International Patient Safety goals were developed with the extensive participation of the Joint Commission in the United States. The patient safety goals, the corresponding requirement for each identified goal, and patient safety solutions were found to be comparable between the National Patient Safety goals and the International Patient Safety goals (Tables 2-4).

Table 4. The Joint Commission International's nine patient safety solutions

Patient safety solution	Brief rationale for the solution
Identifying look-alike medications and sound-alike medication names	Confusing drug names is one of the most common causes of medication errors. With tens of thousands of drugs currently available on the market, the potential for medication errors created by confusing brand or generic drug names and packaging is significant.
Ensuring medication accuracy at transitions in care	Medication errors happen most commonly during care transitions. Medication reconciliation is a mechanism designed to prevent medication errors at patient transition points.
Control of concentrated electrolyte solutions	All drugs, biologics, vaccines, and contrast media have a defined risk profile. The concentrated electrolyte solutions that are used for injection are especially dangerous.
Avoiding catheter and tubing misconnections	The design of tubing, catheters, and syringes currently in use may inadvertently cause patient harm through connecting the wrong syringes and tubing, and then delivering medication or fluids through an unintended wrong route.
Single use of injection devices	The reuse of injection needles may contribute to the spread of HIV, hepatitis B virus, and hepatitis C virus.
Performance of correct procedures at correct body site	The causes of performing wrong procedures or wrong-site surgeries are considered totally preventable and are largely the result of miscommunication and unavailable or incorrect information. A major contributing factor to these types of errors is the lack of a standardized preoperative process.
Patient identification	The widespread and continuing failures to correctly identify patients often leads to medication, transfusion, and testing errors. Poor patient identification may also result in wrong-person procedures and discharging infants to the wrong families.
Communication during patient hand-off or hand-over	The gaps in hand-off or hand-over communication between the patient care units, and between and among health care teams, may lead to serious breakdowns in the continuity of care, inappropriate treatment, and potential harms to patients.
Improved hand hygiene to prevent health care-associated infection	It is estimated that at any point in time, >1.4 million patients worldwide are suffering from infections acquired in hospitals. The primary preventive measure for avoiding this problem is effective hand hygiene for health care providers.

Source: Joint Commission International Center for Patient Safety (2007e). WHO collaborating center for patient safety solutions. Available at: http://www.jcipatientsafety.org/24725/ (accessed November 12, 2007).

The Movement to Promote Safe Hospital Stays

There is no doubt that the movement of promoting hospital patient safety has emerged. Patient safety in hospitals involves not only patients and their families but also hospital staff members and hospital infrastructure. The targeted patient safety issues, however, may shift over time. Published articles are usually the sources to be used as evidence to guide the directions in patient safety initiatives.

Consequently, we synthesized published research on hospital and patient safety. A consensus system was developed in this study. This consensus system can help advance knowledge in the field of patient safety in hospitals and help scholars and clinicians identify associated trends in research and studies needing to be done (Tzeng & Yin, 2007). This study is summarized below.

Synthesis of Research on Hospital and Patient Safety (1996-2007)

To further understand issues related to hospital safety, we synthesized published research to determine associated research trends for the purpose of forming a consensus system (Tzeng & Yin, 2007). This study was conducted based on the assumption that scholars, who recognized the importance of emphasizing safety in hospitals, would acknowledge this concept by including the term "safety" in the titles and abstracts of their articles.

The PubMed database was the targeted data source (US National Library of Medicine, 2007). The key words used for abstraction were "safety" and "hospital." Criteria for inclusion for the sample were: (1) written in English, (2) having an abstract, (3) included in the PubMed database, and (4) published from January 1, 1996 to March 31, 2007. The majority of records were published in peer-reviewed journals. A total of 6569 records were analyzed. This study used the content analysis method. To develop a preliminary typology, the titles and abstracts of the most recent 200 records were independently analyzed by each author. Each record then was assigned a safety code that represented the primary research focus (Tzeng & Yin, 2007).

Summary of Study Findings

The results showed that the number of studies increased steadily from 1996 to 2006. From January 1 to March 31, 2007, 305 studies were reported, which is expected to exceed a total of 1200 records for the year 2007. As shown in Table 5, the number of articles related to hospital safety has increased steadily from 1996 to 2007 (Tzeng & Yin, 2007).

Twenty-seven safety categories were identified (Table 6) and grouped into the following six dimensions: (A) safety issues related to treatment and procedures received (6 categories); (B) emphasis on adverse events and incidents (3 categories); (C) safety issues related to hospital infrastructure (6 categories); (D) safety issues related to the overall medical care system (3 categories); (E) safety concerns about hospital human resource management (5 categories); and (F) occupational hazards in hospitals (4 categories). Dimension A had the highest number of records ($n = 4224$, 64.3%) followed by dimension C ($n = 1138$, 17.3%; Tzeng, & Yin, 2007).

Table 5. Number of articles by year: 1996 to March 31, 2007

Year	No. of records
1996	354
1997	346
1998	369
1999	414
2000	438
2001	508
2002	566
2003	685
2004	722
2005	803
2006	1059
2007 (January 1 to March 31)	305
Total	**6569**

Source: Tzeng, H. M., & Yin, C. Y. (2007). No safety, no quality: Synthesis of research on hospital and patient safety (1996-2007). *Journal of Nursing Care Quality, 22*(4), 299-306.

Table 6. Descriptive information on each identified safety dimension and category: From 1996 to March 31, 2007[*]

Dimension (A-F) Safety code [ ]	No. of records	Percentage (rank)[†]
A. Safety issues related to treatment and procedures received	**4223**	**64.30% (1)**
[1] Medication choices and errors (also including chemotherapy, radiotherapy, and total parenteral nutrition)	1522	23.17 % (2)
[2] Use of sedation, pain control, or anesthesia	193	2.94% (5)
[3] Procedure (e.g., surgery, invasive or noninvasive medical treatments and procedures)	2388	36.35% (1)
[4] Allergy to medication, media, or contrast medium	11	0.17% (21)
[5] Blood transfusion (e.g., preparation, related protocols or procedures, and adverse reactions)	92	1.40% (9)
[6] Communication among physicians, nurses, and/or pharmacists (e.g., related to ongoing procedures, or medical treatment)	17	0.26% (18)
B. Emphases on adverse events and incidents	**246**	**3.74% (4)**
[7] Health care-associated infections (also called nosocomial infection; e.g., an emphasis on hospitals' infection control measures)	75	1.14% (10)
[8] Patient fall and associated injury	17	0.26% (18)
[9] Other adverse events and incidents (e.g., longer hospital stay, death, and patient complaints)	154	2.34% (7)
C. Safety issues related to hospital infrastructure	**1138**	**17.32% (2)**
[10] Physician computerized prescribing or decision support systems	181	2.76% (6)
[11] Patient identification	5	0.08% (24)
[12] Use of protocols or guidelines for improving patient outcomes (e.g., promoting a safety culture, reporting medical errors and incidents, and patient record confidentiality)	883	13.44% (3)

Dimension (A-F) Safety code [ ]	No. of records	Percentage (rank)[†]
[13] Nurse prescribing (e.g., extending nurse prescribing and nurse advice line recommendations)	2	0.03% (26)
[14] Pharmacy systems (e.g., drug inventory, dispensing errors, and medication error recovery)	33	0.50% (15)
[15] Hospital hardware, equipment, or safety-related monitoring systems	34	0.52% (14)
D. Safety issues related to the overall medical care system	**712**	**10.84% (3)**
[16] Health promotion or access to hospital services (e.g., use of the safety net hospitals and injury prevention)	619	9.42% (4)
[17] Non-health care workers' occupational hazards, injuries, or illness	37	0.56% (13)
[18] Transportation to medical facilities and related protocols (e.g., from home to hospitals and emergency departments)	56	0.85% (12)
E. Safety concerns about hospital human resource management	**108**	**1.64% (6)**
[19] Physicians' work environment (e.g., competencies and training, work hours, and stress)	26	0.40% (17)
[20] Nurses' work environment (e.g., competencies, scheduling, or nurse-to-patient ratios)	61	0.93% (11)
[21] Work environment factors associated with patient safety, mortality, and outcomes (general)[†]	13	0.20% (20)
[22] Nurse violence toward patients	2	0.03% (26)
[23] Violence toward patients (general)[†]	4	0.06% (25)
F. Occupational hazards in hospitals	**142**	**2.16% (5)**
[24] Physician exposure to biologic hazards, nonfatal occupational injuries or illness	6	0.09% (23)
[25] Nurse exposure to biologic hazards, nonfatal occupational injuries or illness	27	0.41% (16)
[26] Occupational hazards, injuries, or illness (general)[†]	101	1.54% (8)
[27] Patient or family violence toward health care providers	8	0.12% (22)
Total no. of records	**6569**	**100%**

[*] Articles included in the PubMed database and published from January 1, 1996 to March 31, 2007 were the targeted and analyzed records ($n = 6569$) for this study.

[†] Percentage and rank (1 as having the highest frequency) by 6 dimensions and by 27 safety categories were calculated based on the total number of analyzed records ($n = 6569$).

[‡] The types of healthcare professionals were not specified.

Source: Tzeng, H. M., & Yin, C. Y. (2007). No safety, no quality: Synthesis of research on hospital and patient safety (1996-2007). *Journal of Nursing Care Quality, 22*(4), 299-306.

Dimension D was less relevant to inpatient care. Dimension F was associated with the health of our health care providers. As a matter of fact, our health care providers may get sick by contracting health care-associated infections during the process of delivering patient care. For example, nurses may contract tuberculosis and other infectious disease at work and may transmit these infectious diseases to the patients under their care. No doubt, our doctors and nurses may become inpatients at some point in their lives. In addition, some injuries, such as back pain, may be related to patient handling. In summary, except for dimension D, the other five dimensions and the corresponding safety codes matter to our safety and our healing process during hospitalization.

Table 7. Frequency table on each identified safety category (indicated in code number) by year[*] (n = 6569)

Year/Dimension/Frequency

Freq. by year for each code	A. Safety issues related to treatment and procedures received (n = 4223 records, 64.30%)						B. Emphasis on adverse events and incidents (n = 246 records, 3.74%)			C. Safety issues related to hospital infrastructure (n = 1138, 17.32%)						D. Safety issues related to the overall medical care system (n = 712, 10.84%)			E. Safety concerns about hospital human resource management (n = 108, 1.64%)					F. Occupational hazards in hospitals (n = 142, 2.16%)			
Code	1	2	3	4	5	6	7	8	9	10	11	12	13	14	15	16	17	18	19	20	21	22	23	24	25	26	27
1996	89	10	123		5		2	1	6	1		54		3		48	2	1						2	2	5	
1997	93	13	124		4		2		4	6		42		1		40	1	5		1					1	9	
1998	81	14	134	1	2		2		9	9		52				50	4	1			1				2	7	1
1999	111	7	168		4		1		7	12		54				34	5	4								5	1
2000	127	14	131		9		7		16	16		56		1		39	2	4							1	13	
2001	119	23	167	1	14		4	3	9	16		72			1	56	1	4		2			1		2	11	1
2002	128	22	213		8	1	3	1	17	22		77		3		48	2	4	1	3			1		4	8	
2003	149	21	242	2	11		9	2	16	24		117		6		62	3	2	2	5	1			1	3	7	
2004	153	20	277	1	12	2	5	6	26	22	1	101	1	3		63	3	11	1	2	2			1	4	5	
2005	182	16	328	1	11	1	8		15	26	1	119		6	1	55	5	5	1	4	2	2	2		1	11	
2006	232	22	389	1	10	8	28	1	19	18	1	97	1	7	26	98	8	12	17	33	7	0	0	0	5	15	4
2007	58	11	92	2	2	5	4	3	10	9	1	42	0	3	6	26	1	3	4	11	2	0	0	2	2	5	1
Freq. by code	1522	193	2388	11	92	17	75	17	154	181	5	883	2	33	34	619	37	56	26	61	13	2	4	6	27	101	8
% by code	23.2	2.94	36.4	0.2	1.4	0.3	1.1	0.3	2.3	2.8	0.1	13.4	0.0	0.5	0.5	9.4	0.6	0.9	0.4	0.9	0.2	0.0	0.1	0.1	0.4	1.5	0.1
Rank[†]	2	5	1	21	9	18	10	18	7	6	24	3	26	15	14	4	13	12	17	11	20	26	25	23	16	8	22

For the full description corresponding to each safety code, please refer to Table 6.

[*] Articles published from January 1, 1996 to March 31, 2007 were included in the sample.

[†] The safety code with the highest frequency in the number of articles is marked as 1.

As indicated in Table 6, the most frequently studied safety issues were procedure (code 3: n = 2388, 36.4%), followed by medication (code 1: n = 1522, 23.2%), use of protocols and guidelines for improving patient outcomes (code 12: n = 883, 13.4%), health promotion and access to hospital services (e.g., use of the safety net hospitals; code 16: n = 619, 9.4%, rank = 4), use of sedation, pain control, and anesthesia (code 2: n = 193, 2.9%, rank = 5), and physician computerized prescribing and decision support systems (code 10: n = 181, 2.76%, rank = 6; Tzeng & Yin, 2007).

As seen in Table 7, in 1999, there was a significant increase in the number of articles published on medication (code 1). Since then, this safety issue has been increasingly emphasized. There also was a significant increase in 1999 in publications focused on procedure (code 3); this increased further in 2002 and is a topic that is still growing. Compared to the previous year, in 2001, there was a 50% increase in reports on the use of sedation, pain control, and anesthesia (code 2).

As for the issues related to hospital infrastructure, in 2002, there was a significant increase (about 25%) in the number of records published on physician computerized prescribing and decision support systems (code 10). Compared to the previous year, in 2003, there was a 30% increase in reports on the use of protocols and guidelines for improving patient outcomes (code 12).

From 1996 to 2007, interest has grown around safety issues related to occupational hazards for health care providers in hospitals (codes 24-27, n = 142, 2.2% in total). Since 2001, there have been more studies on safety issues related to health care providers' work environment (codes 19-21, n = 100, 1.5% in total; Tzeng & Yin, 2007).

A Comparison between Ongoing Patient Safety Initiatives and the Developed Consensus System

The six dimensions and 27 safety categories identified in this study covered the six international patient safety goals for hospitals developed by the JCI (Joint Commission International Center for Patient Safety, 2007c, 2007d; Table 3). Although the 6569 journal articles included in this study were published in English language journals, they also represented studies conducted by researchers in many countries. Because of the nature of this study, the findings could serve as a consensus on scholars' acknowledgments of the important and urgent safety matters that should be addressed by hospital system managers throughout the world (Tzeng & Yin, 2007).

Comparison with the IOM's Three-phase Timeframe
To identify emerging hot topics or reasons for shifting trends in the foci of safety research, the study findings were compared with the three-phase timeframe of the IOM's health care quality initiative (Institute of Medicine, 2007a).

The first phase (1996-1998) focused on defining problems in hospital safety as that of overuse, misuse, and underuse of health care services. Our study findings showed that the goals established by the IOM and related reports possibly influenced scholars' research foci; the number of research reports on medication (code 1) and on procedure (code 3) has increased since 1999, and an increase in studies of blood transfusion (code 5) has occurred since 2000 (Tzeng & Yin, 2007). In 2006, a total of 232 reports involved medication-related safety issues (e.g., medication errors and side effects). In 2006, the IOM published the report of *Preventing medication errors: Quality chasm series*. We expect that the trend on studying medication safety in hospitals will gain even more attention by scholars and clinicians (Tzeng & Yin, 2007).

The second phase (1999-2001) emphasized the demands to close the gap between what is known to be good quality care and what actually exists in practice. Our study findings indicated that IOM's set goals might have inspired more research reports on health care-associated infections since 2000 (code 7), patient falls and associated injuries since 2001 (code 8), and other adverse events and incidents since 2000 (code 9) (Tzeng & Yin, 2007).

The current phase of the IOM initiative, begun in 2002, focused on reforming three different overlapping levels of the health care system: (1) the environmental level, (2) the level of the health care organization, and (3) the interface between clinicians and patients. Our study findings showed that there was an increase in the number of published reports having a focus on physician computerized prescribing and decision support systems (code 10) since 2002 and on the use of protocols and guidelines for improving patient outcomes (code 12) since 2001 (Tzeng & Yin, 2007).

Comparison with Institute for Healthcare Improvement Initiatives

In December 2004, the Institute for Healthcare Improvement launched a national initiative, the "100,000 Lives Campaign." This campaign sought to engage hospitals to consistently apply six best practice interventions: (1) deployment of rapid response teams, (2) delivery of evidence-based care for acute myocardial infarction, (3) prevention of adverse drug events, (4) central line infections, (5) surgical site infections, and (6) ventilator-associated pneumonia (Institute for Healthcare Improvement, 2007d). At the end of 2006, the Institute for Healthcare Improvement initiated another campaign, "Protecting 5 Million Lives from Harm," to protect patients from 5 million incidents of medical harm over the 24 months (Institute for Healthcare Improvement, 2007e). Table 8 presents a comparison between the interventions set for the "100,000 Lives Campaign" in 2004 and the "5 Million Lives" campaign in 2006 as initiated by the Institute for Healthcare Improvement.

Table 8. A comparison between the interventions set for the "100,000 Lives Campaign" in 2004 and the "5 Million Lives Campaign" in 2006 as initiated by Institute for Healthcare Improvement

The six interventions from the "100,000 Lives Campaign"	Domain for safety issues
Delivering reliable, evidence-based care for acute myocardial infarction	Hospital infrastructure
Deploying rapid response teams	Hospital infrastructure
Preventing adverse drug events	Treatment and procedures received
Preventing central line infections	Adverse events and incidents (health care-associated infections)
Preventing surgical site infections	Adverse events and incidents (health care-associated infections)
Preventing ventilator-associated pneumonia	Adverse events and incidents (health care-associated infection)

The six interventions from the "100,000 Lives Campaign"	Domain for safety issues
The new six interventions targeted at harm from the "5 Million Lives Campaign"	
Delivering reliable, evidence-based care for congestive heart failure (to avoid readmission)	Hospital infrastructure
Getting the boards on board (to accelerate a hospital's progress toward safe care)	Hospital infrastructure
Preventing harm from high-alert medications (with a focus on anticoagulants, sedatives, narcotics, and insulin)	Treatment and procedures received
Preventing pressure ulcers	Adverse events and incidents
Reducing methicillin-resistant *Staphylococcus aureus* infection (by reliably implementing scientifically proven infection control practices)	Adverse events and incidents (health care-associated infection)
Reducing surgical complications	Adverse events and incidents

Sources: Institute for Healthcare Improvement (2007d). Overview of the 100,000 lives campaign. Available at: http://www.ihi.org/IHI/Programs/Campaign/100kCampaignOverviewArchive.htm (accessed November 12, 2007). Tzeng, H. M., & Yin, C. Y. (2007). No safety, no quality: Synthesis of research on hospital and patient safety (1996-2007). *Journal of Nursing Care Quality, 22*(4), 299-306. Institute for Healthcare Improvement (2007e). Overview of the 5 million lives campaign. Available at: http://www.ihi.org/IHI/Programs/Campaign/Campaign.htm?TabId=1 (accessed November 12, 2007).

In a comparison of the interventions set for the "100,000 Lives Campaign" and "Protecting 5 Million Lives from Harm" with the consensus system developed in our study, four interventions were related to health care-associated infections (code 7, rank = 10), two associated with medications (code 1, rank = 2), one addressed adverse events and incidents related to procedure (code 3, rank = 1), four linked to use of protocols or guidelines for improving patient outcomes (code 12, rank = 3), and one related to prevention of pressure ulcers (code 9, rank = 7). These interventions are associated with the first three most frequently studied safety issues as identified in our consensus system.

These two campaigns as initiated by the Institute for Healthcare Improvement have demonstrated the escalating concerns and committed engagements of US hospitals for achieving improvements in patient safety. Reliably using science-based guidelines to prevent harms also has been emphasized by the Institute for Healthcare Improvement. These two campaigns also indirectly supported our motive to synthesize published articles on hospital and patient safety and the importance of illustrating the associated research trends on related issues (Tzeng & Yin, 2007).

What we have Learned from this Study

An urgent need remains for research studies to identify effective means for reducing the risk of patient harm resulting from falls in hospitals. As indicated in Table 6, only 17 records were found that addressed specifically the issues of patient falls and associated injury (code 8) and 34 records focused on hospital hardware, equipment, and safety-related monitoring systems (code 15). More research should study ways to develop a safe hospital environment through improving hospital hardware and architect design (e.g., the design of patient beds and side rails, and holding bars in patient units) and revising related hospital policy (e.g., whether it is useful to raise bed side rails for the purpose of preventing patient falls; Tzeng & Yin, 2006).

To promote effective communication among patients, their families, and health care providers, more scholarly work should be devoted to develop a Web-based patient chart system embedded within a national health information infrastructure. Such a system should be capable of providing immediate access to complete patient information and decision support tools for patients, their families, and clinicians with assigned access codes for confidentiality. Easy access for patients to their own medical records may decrease misunderstandings between patients and their doctors and nurses and consequently mitigate medical disputes. Rather than being initiated by patients, a nation's health agency has the obligation to promote this concept.

As suggested by National Academy of Sciences (2004b), possible future research may focus on:

1. The respective roles of patients, health care providers, and hospitals in the prevention, early detection, and mitigation of preventable harm and errors
2. Protocols and guidelines for identifying high-risk patients
3. The utility of chart review of patient electronic records for detecting near-miss incidents

As indicated in Table 6, from 1996 to 2007, the dimension of occupational hazards in hospitals had only 2.2% of all analyzed articles, and the safety dimension related to hospital human resource management had barely over 1.5% of all analyzed articles (Tzeng & Yin, 2007). In other words, information about how to design a safe work environment to make a hospital care environment safer for patients remains limited. The health problems of health care providers (e.g., stress, fatigue, sleep deprivation, occupational injuries, and illness) and of their being imperceptible carriers of infectious diseases (e.g., tuberculosis) also may jeopardize patient safety. Research on the effects of successive work days and sustained work hours on patient safety should be encouraged (National Academy of Sciences, 2004a).

Next Step: Resolving the Gap between what is Known to be Safe Hospital Care and what Actually Exists in Practice

To close the gap between what is known to be good quality care and what actually exists in practice, the consensus system developed in our study could contribute to reframing current research directions in patient safety in hospitals. Our study findings may help scholars and clinicians identify studies needing to be done, explore trends in the research on hospital patient safety, and advance the knowledge in this area. After all, hospital delivery systems must be designed to achieve improvements in patient safety (Tzeng & Yin, 2007).

References

Institute for Healthcare Improvement (2007a). Transforming care at the bedside: Overview. Available at: http://www.ihi.org/IHI/Programs/StrategicInitiatives/TransformingCare AtTheBedside.htm (accessed November 13, 2007).

Institute for Healthcare Improvement (2007b). Transforming care at the bedside: The framework for change on medical/surgical units. Available at: http://www.ihi.org/ NR/rdonlyres/F81270CD-B8BC-47D5-B2A6- BDA550096AA9/5802/VisioTCABframework0907.pdf (accessed November 13, 2007).

Institute for Healthcare Improvement (2007c). Transforming care at the bedside: TCAB overview. Available at: http://www.ihi.org/NR/rdonlyres/BD24233D-6328-4F1E-9197- 151628F1EA35/0/TCABvideotape907.pdf (accessed November 13, 2007).

Institute for Healthcare Improvement (2007d). Overview of the 100,000 lives campaign. Available at: http://www.ihi.org/IHI/Programs/Campaign/100kCampaignOverview Archive.htm (accessed November 13, 2007).

Institute for Healthcare Improvement (2007e). Overview of the 5 million lives campaign. Available at: http://www.ihi.org/IHI/Programs/Campaign/Campaign.htm?TabId=1 (accessed November 13, 2007).

Institute of Medicine (2007a). Crossing the quality chasm: The IOM healthcare quality initiative. Available at: http://www.iom.edu/CMS/8089.aspx?printfriendly=true&redirect =0 (accessed April 12, 2007).

Institute of Medicine (2007b). Reports. Available at: http://www.iom.edu/CMS/3718. aspx (accessed April 12, 2007).

Joint Commission (2007a). Sentinel event statistics: As of June 30, 2007. Available at: http://www.jointcommission.org/NR/rdonlyres/D7836542-A372-4F93-8BD7- DDD11D43E484/0/se_stats_063007.pdf (accessed November 7, 2007).

Joint Commission (2007b). Root causes of sentinel events. Available at: http://www. jointcommission.org/NR/rdonlyres/FA465646-5F5F-4543-AC8F- E8AF6571E372/0/root_cause_se.jpg (accessed November 7, 2007).

Joint Commission (2007c). Root causes of sentinel events. Available at: http://www. jointcommission.org/NR/rdonlyres/FA465646-5F5F-4543-AC8F-E8AF6571E372/0/root_cause_se.jpg (accessed November 7, 2007).

Joint Commission (2007d). 2008 National Patient Safety Goals: Hospital program. Available at: http://www.jointcommission.org/PatientSafety/NationalPatientSafetyGoals/08_hap_npsgs.htm (accessed November 11, 2007).

Joint Commission International Center for Patient Safety (2007a). 2006 NPSG implementation expectations. Available at: http://www.jcipatientsafety.org/22406/ (accessed April 12, 2007).

Joint Commission International Center for Patient Safety (2007b). Facts about the Joint Commission International Center for Patient Safety. Available at: http://www. jointcommission.org/AboutUs/facts_jcicps.htm (accessed April 12, 2007).

Joint Commission International Center for Patient Safety (2007c). 2006 International Patient Safety Goals. Available at: http://www.jcipatientsafety.org/15143/ (accessed November 11, 2007).

Joint Commission International Center for Patient Safety (2007d). 2007 International Patient Safety Goals. Available at: http://www.jcipatientsafety.org/15137/ (accessed November 11, 2007).

Joint Commission International Center for Patient Safety (2007e). WHO collaborating center for patient safety solutions. Available at: http://www.jcipatientsafety.org/24725/ (accessed November 12, 2007).

National Academy of Sciences (2004a). Executive summary—keeping patients safe: Transforming the work environment of nurses. Available at: http://books.nap.edu/ catalog/10851.html (accessed January 19, 2008).

National Academy of Sciences (2004b). Executive summary—patient safety: Achieving a new standard for care. Available at: http://books.nap.edu/catalog/10863.html (accessed January 19, 2008).

US National Library of Medicine (2007). PubMed. Available at: http://www. ncbi.nlm.nih.gov/entrez/query.fcgi?DB=pubmed (accessed June 4, 2006 for the records published from January 1, 1996 to December 31, 2005; and accessed April 8, 2007 for the records published from January 1, 2006 to March 31, 2007).

Tzeng, H. M., & Yin, C. Y. (2006). The staff-working height and the designing-regulation height for patient beds as possible causes of patient falls. *Nursing Economics, 24*(6), 323-327, 279.

Tzeng, H. M., & Yin, C. Y. (2007). No safety, no quality: Synthesis of research on hospital and patient safety (1996-2007). *Journal of Nursing Care Quality, 22*(4), 299-306.

Problematic Patient Safety Areas in Hospitals

Hospitals Are Erratic Places

During hospital stays, patients must interact with health care providers (mainly physicians and nurses) and may work with machines and lines that are connected or attached to their bodies. Patient safety in hospital settings involves issues related to human factors (also called ergonomics). Increasing emphasis is being placed on approaches involving human factors to address patient safety concerns. These approaches are meant to enhance understanding of the interactions among humans and other elements within a hospital system to optimize human well-being and overall system performance.

A hospital system refers to the physical, cognitive, and organizational artifacts that people interact with, including: (1) a procedure, policy, or guidelines; (2) a physical environment; (3) a technology or device; or (4) a person, a team, or an organization. The interactions among people and a hospital system are the tasks (International Ergonomics Association, 2000). Physical, cognitive, and organizational ergonomic domains are often used in defining patient safety issues and generating relevant applications (Carayon, 2007; Table 1).

Hospital Accreditation: Would my Hospital Provide Safe and Quality Care?

To provide safe care, treatment, and services to patients, hospitals must implement applicable requirements as identified by the Joint Commission. Compliance with such requirements are evaluated throughout the accreditation cycle, through on-site surveys and periodic performance reviews. If a hospital does not fully comply with a requirement, it is assigned a requirement for improvement. Noncompliance with the predetermined requirements or failure to resolve a requirement for improvement would affect a hospital's accreditation status and could ultimately lead to loss of accreditation (Joint Commission, 2007a).

Table 1. Domains of ergonomics approaches to address patient safety issues

Domain	Relevant topic	Example applications to patient safety
Physical ergonomics	1. Materials handling 2. Repetitive movements 3. Safety and the health of health care providers 4. Work-related musculoskeletal disorders 5. Workplace layout	Scope: The design of a hospital's facilities and physical environment (e.g., noise, temperature, humidity, airflow, and vibration), patient room design, patient handling, alarms, etc. Example 1: The design of the patient room to facilitate and support safe patient care Example 2: The design of medication labeling so that medication labels are readable and understandable by health care providers and patients
Cognitive ergonomics	1. Decision-making 2. Human reliability 3. Human–computer interaction 4. Mental workload 5. Skilled performance 6. Work stress and training as these may related to human–system design	Scope: Analyzing human errors, the complexity of patient care, the taxonomies of medical failures, communication about unexpected errors and outcomes, etc. Example 1: Designing an adverse event reporting system. Example 2: Developing and implementing incident analysis processes
Organizational ergonomics	1. Communication 2. Cooperative work 3. Crew resource management 4. Design of working times 5. Participatory design 6. Quality management 7. Teamwork 8. Virtual organizations 9. Work design	Scope: Analyzing the job stress and burnout of the health care workers, human factor risk management in medical products, assessment of a hospital's safety culture and climate, health information management, the impact of understaffing and the poorly designed working conditions on staff's attitudes and behaviors, patient experience, the role of the families, etc. Example 1: Designing and implementing crew resource management training for surgery teams Example 2: Designing staff work schedules for reduced fatigue and enhanced performance

Source: Carayon, P. (2007). Human factors and ergonomics in health care and patient safety. In P. Carayon (Ed.), *Handbook of human factors and ergonomics in health care and patient safety* (pp. 3-20). Mahwah, NJ: Lawrence Erlbaum Associates.

Being accredited indicates that a hospital is in compliance with all standards at the time of the on-site survey or has successfully addressed all requirements for improvement in the evidence of standards compliance within 45 days following the survey. The evidence of standards compliance is a report submitted by a surveyed hospital to detail the actions that the hospital took to bring itself into compliance with a standard or clarify why this hospital believes that it was in compliance with the standard for which it received a recommendation (Joint Commission, 2007a).

This report must address compliance at the element of performance level (e.g., the specific performance expectation, and the structures or processes that must be in place for a hospital to provide safe and high-quality care, treatment, and services). This report also must include a measurement of success for all appropriate elements of performance corrections (Joint Commission, 2007a).

Regardless of the Joint Commission's rigorous accreditation processes, we must be aware that accreditation does not endorse or guarantee a hospital's quality or safety of care, nor does it prove, ensure, or testify that a hospital provides high-quality and safe care (Joint Commission, 2007a). However, the accreditation processes do motivate a hospital, its leaders, health care providers, and staff members to have their mind set for providing safe care.

Since 2002, the Joint Commission has started the mechanism of identifying the National Patient Safety Goals for the purposes of helping accredited hospitals prevent specific medical errors from occurring. These goals were selected each year by a panel of experts convened by the Joint Commission as an effective way to focus hospitals on current patient safety priorities. The Joint Commission recognized that a sound hospital system design must be intrinsic to the delivery of safe and high-quality health care. Consequently, identified patient safety goals generally focus on system-wide solutions, if appropriate. New patient safety goals are announced by July and become effective on January 1 of the following year (Joint Commission, 2007a).

As patient safety advocates, we must know whether the hospital we are using for health care services is being accredited by the Joint Commission. We often see a certificate hanging somewhere obvious in the main entrance of a hospital. If we do not see it, we should ask for it.

In addition, the hospital quality report, as issued by the Joint Commission, is available on Quality Check® at http://www.qualitycheck.org. Quality Check is a comprehensive listing of both Joint Commission-accredited hospitals and the hospitals not being accredited by the Joint Commission. Accreditation issued by the Joint Commission is recognized nationwide as a symbol of quality and safety that reflects a hospital's commitment to meeting certain performance standards (Joint Commission, 2007b). This hospital quality report is available to the public free of charge.

Unsafe Care versus Sentinel Events

The National Patient Safety Goals as initiated by the Joint Commission are the ones perceived as having deficiencies in safety practice, which resulted in sentinel events. These safety aspects of care are set yearly and may be updated due to, for example, the rising number of sentinel events. The Joint Commission routinely reviews the sentinel events reported by hospitals and other types of health care institutions (Joint Commission, 2007c).

Table 2. Additional types of sentinel events

Types of sentinel event	Brief description
Assault, rape, or homicide	1. Rape refers to any nonconsensual sexual contact involving a patient and another patient, staff member, or unknown perpetrator, while being treated on the property of the health care organization.
Infant discharge to wrong family	1. Same as the type of sentinel event
Patient abduction	1. Abduction of any patient occurring when this patient was receiving health care or treatment on the property of the health care organization
Prolonged fluoroscopy or wrong radiotherapy body region or dose	1. A prolonged fluoroscopy with cumulative dose of >1500 rads was given to a single body region 2. Any delivery of radiotherapy to the wrong body region 3. >25% above the planned radiotherapy dose was given

Suicide	1. Suicide of any patient occurring:
	  1.1 When this patient was receiving health care or treatment in a staffed, 24-hour inpatient care setting or
	  1.2 Within 72 hours of discharge.

Transfusion error	1. Any hemolytic transfusion reaction involving:
	  1.1 Administration of blood or blood products
	  1.2 Having major blood group incompatibilities.

Unanticipated neonatal death or loss of function	1. Unanticipated death of full-term infant 2. Severe neonatal hyperbilirubinemia (bilirubin >30 mg/dL).
Unintended retention of foreign body	1. A foreign object was left unintended in a patient's body after surgery or any other procedure.
Wrong-site surgery	1. Any surgery was conducted on the wrong patient or one the wrong body part.

Source: Joint Commission (2007c). About sentinel events. In Robert A. Porché, Jr. (Ed.), *Front line of defense: The role of nurses in preventing sentinel events* (2nd ed., pp. 1-20). Oakbrook Terrace, IL: Joint Commission Resources.

These sentinel events often result in an unanticipated death or major permanent loss of function or impairment in sensory, motor, physiologic, or intellectual faculties, which were not present on admission and may require continued treatment or lifestyle change. These malfunctions should not be related to the natural course of a patient's illness or underlying condition (Joint Commission, 2007c). Some other types of sentinel events are listed in Table 2.

During the period between January 2001 and July 2005, the top five sentinel events that occurred in general hospitals (Joint Commission, 2007c) were:

1. Operative or postoperative complication ($n = 397$, 17.6%)
2. Wrong-site surgery ($n = 363$, 16.0%)
3. Medication error ($n = 277$, 12.2%)
4. Delay in treatment ($n = 136$, 6.0%)
5. Falls ($n = 108$, 4.8%)

Table 3. The most frequently cited root causes, potential problems, and possible solutions for nurses working in acute inpatient care units

Root cause of sentinel events	Potential problems	Possible solutions

Available of information	1. In the process of delivering inpatient care, the availability of information is crucial, such as:
	   1.1 The expectations of each health care provider's role and performed tasks
	   1.2 Patients' potential problems that could lead to sentinel events
	   1.3 Patient's special needs, specific care, and treatment
		1. Information should be readily accessible.
		2. Possible strategies for providing an information-rich environment include:
		   2.1 Using biomedical monitoring to provide ongoing information on patients' status for patients with complex, critical problems
		   2.2 Using graphical and visual data display to develop optimal care plans
		   2.3 Building local epidemiologic knowledge to be used to guide clinical decision- making

Communication	1. Communication failures may occur among health care providers, between providers and patients and their family members. 2. The colleagues of the health care providers may fear negative consequences if they point out real or potential problems on, for example, medication orders. 3. Patients and their family members may not speak up if they believe an error is imminent or has occurred.	1. The colleagues of the health care providers need to understand their roles in reminding each other to help prevent medication errors, wrong-site surgery, or health care-associated infections. 2. Patients and their family members need to speak up to help reduce or prevent errors, harms, and sentinel events.

Competency or credentialing	1. Hospital leaders must ensure the competency, knowledge, and skills of their health care providers to effectively provide safe care and meet the needs of patients.	1. Registered nurses must be equipped with the knowledge and skills of:
		   1.1 Systematic and continuing assessment
		   1.2 Monitoring of patients' changes in health status as related to their age, received treatments and medications, and their baseline assessment data

Table 3. The most frequently cited root causes, potential problems, and possible solutions for nurses working in acute inpatient care units

Root cause of sentinel events	Potential problems	Possible solutions

Continuum of care	1. Transitions in care are points of risk, when transferring a patient from one patient unit to another (e.g., from an intensive care unit to a medical patient care unit).	1. Hospitals need to develop the mechanisms to manage transitions smoothly and ensure that all important data are communicated between health care providers.
		2. A checklist for hand-off communication, this checklist may include:
		  2.1 A summary of the patient's current health status, including the resuscitation status (e.g., do not resuscitate), the nutritional and dietary status (e.g., the time the patient last received nourishment), etc.
		  2.2 A problem list and a to-do list for the receiving staff
		  2.3 A list of the patient's allergies
		  2.4 The medications the patient is receiving
		  2.5 Procedures and treatments performed recently and their results
		  2.6 A list of recent laboratory results
		  2.7 The patient's unique needs or request (e.g., religious and cultural issues that may not be known to most staff)

Environmental safety and security	1. Environmental safety and security are crucial for health care providers to perform their jobs safely and to protect patients, their family members, and visitors.	1. Health care providers, patients, and their families may easily tell the failures in environmental safety and security.
		  1.1 If there is any concern, it is important for health care providers to report to their administrators in a timely manner.
		  1.2 Patients and their families should also voice their concerns to their nurses and hospital administrators.
		2. Interventions are available to increase safety and security, such as:
		  2.1 Installing emergency signaling, alarms, and monitoring systems
		  2.2 Installing security devices (e.g., metal detectors to prevent armed persons from entering the hospital, and good lighting in hallways
		  2.3 A safe, patient-centered design of hospital patient rooms

Root cause of sentinel events	Potential problems	Possible solutions

Leadership	1. For health care providers to function effectively, strong leadership support is demanded.
	2. The style and skills of leaders (e.g., nurse managers in patient care units) can influence the success with which root causes are managed to promote safe care.
	3. Participation of health care providers in problem identification and resolution is key to prevent future sentinel events.
		1. The transformational leadership style is preferred for hospitals.
		   1.1 A leader with this leadership style tends to focus on care safety and quality as the shared goals and provides the leadership needed for nurses to participate actively in error reduction, reduction of near misses, and prevention of sentinel events.
		2. In contrast, the transactional leadership style may be overloaded with opportunities for errors, sentinel events, and near misses.
		   2.1 A leader with this leadership style may tend to show less consideration for patient safety and care needs.
		   2.2 Often, the relationships between leaders and subordinates depend on maintaining the bargain (e.g., staff members' preferences for work schedules) and focusing on individual interests.

Organizational culture	1. A hospital's culture determines how this hospital will approach sentinel events.
	2. A pathologic culture may emphasize blame and compliance with rigid procedures.
	   2.1 Such an environment is not encouraging to error and risk reduction and prevention.
	   2.2 The hospital with a pathologic culture and its managers may view individual health care providers who make errors as having deficient cognitive or analytic abilities, or as being lazy, careless, negligent, or unconcerned.
	   2.3 Corrective actions on these individuals may involve counseling about the proper actions, disciplinary measures, threats and re-education or retraining.
	   2.4 Often, dialogue and disagreement are not viewed as helpful, and creativity is often reserved.
		1. A hospital needs to achieve a balance that enables identification and resolution of system and process problems as related to the occurrence of sentinel events or errors, but also addresses problems with specific health care providers as appropriate.
		2. A hospital and its managers should not use punishment as their risk-reduction strategy nor only view individuals as responsible for errors.

Table 3. Continued

Root cause of sentinel events	Potential problems	Possible solutions

Orientation and training	1. Orientation lays the foundation for the provision of safe care. Insufficient orientation and training may lead to sentinel events.
	2. Health care providers need to know:
	  2.1 What is expected of them
	  2.2 How they fit into their working unit and its culture
	  2.3 The needs of the populations served
	  2.4 How to modify care and services to individual patients' needs
		1. Standardized processes and protocols need to be developed for each provider role that clearly defines expectations and how to accomplish various tasks for that role.
		2. Staffing orientation is given at each patient care unit and related education activities will be continued as on-the-job training.
		3. The training information needs to be provided in a manner that is relevant to the learning styles of the employees.
		4. Regularly scheduled meetings will help promote clear communication and build team spirit.

Patient assessment	1. Proper assessment requires considerable knowledge and observation skills. 2. Patient assessment involves assessment of the physical, behavioral, religious, and cultural needs and characteristics, including patients and their family members. 3. Ongoing assessment and validation of impression gained during initial assessment is essential to observe patients' responses to care and treatment.	1. Patient assessment is ongoing. Nurses need to conduct proper assessment before, during, and after surgical and other procedures and medication administration. 2. Patient assessment may help identify risk factors for sentinel events and prevent them, if actions are taken appropriately in a timely manner.
Plan of care	1. Failing to institute a plan of care may contribute a sentinel event. 2. A plan of care needs to be comprehensive and based on thorough assessment of the patient's physical and behavioral status.	1. A comprehensive plan of care should have evidence of anticipation of the patient's needs and problems to help promote safe care. 2. The care plan should include an assessment of the patient's environment and any safety devices. 3. Ongoing reassessment and adjustment of the care plan is crucial.
Procedural compliance	1. Low compliance with a particular procedure may result in errors or harms. 2. Low compliance may indicate a need for additional on-the-job education and training. 3. The procedure itself or related processes and operational systems may be the problem.	1. Procedural compliance is a foundation of safe care. 2. Procedures provide standard approaches to the ways of providing care. 3. Two example solutions follow: 3.1 The use of a checklist for the preoperative verification process in surgery. Such checklist would provide a standard way:

Root cause of sentinel events	Potential problems	Possible solutions

		3.1.1 To ensure that appropriate documents are available
		 3.1.2 To verify and document the correct patient identity, operative side and site, and patient position
		 3.2. The use of a standardized hand-off communication among nurses and between nurses and physicians
		     3.2.1. Hand-off communications should provide accurate, clear, and complete information about a patient's care and treatment, current condition, and recent or anticipated changes.
		     3.2.2. The organization of a standardized hand-off communication may use the situation, background, assessment, and recommendation technique.
		 When it is needed and appropriate, repeat-back mechanisms may be used for verification purposes.

Staffing	1. Inadequate staffing may affect patient safety and result in negative clinical outcomes, including increased incidences of failing to restore a patient's condition to the previous status (also called failure to rescue). 2. Scheduling can be another concern (e.g., the distribution of nursing workforce during shifts, on weekdays and weekends, during holiday and vacation periods, and during breaks). 3. Long work hours may contribute to an increase in the number of errors made by nurses.	1. Solutions to staffing problems are linked to: 1.1 Health care cost 1.2 The location, type, and culture of the hospital 1.3 Qualifications of the potential nurse pool in the community 1.4 Patient populations served 1.5 The patient turnover rate (e.g., the number of patient admissions and discharges during a shift) 1.6 The amount of non-nursing duties performed by nurses (e.g., obtaining supplies, performing housekeeping tasks, and delivering meal trays) 1.7 The amount of indirect nursing care duties performed (e.g., filling out the documentation and paperwork required by the hospital) 1.8 The flexibility of the staff

Source: Joint Commission (2007c). About sentinel events. In Robert A. Porché, Jr. (Ed.), *Front line of defense: The role of nurses in preventing sentinel events* (2nd ed., pp. 1-20). Oakbrook Terrace, IL: Joint Commission Resources.

When a sentinel event is identified in a hospital, this hospital is expected to conduct a timely, thorough, and credible root cause analysis on this event. This hospital must develop an action plan to implement quality improvement actions to reduce future occurrence of the same type of sentinel events and to monitor the effectiveness of the improvements. Table 3 illustrates the most frequently cited root causes, possible problems, and potential solutions for each root cause.

Risk Factors for Unsafe Care and Sentinel Events in Acute Inpatient Care Units

We want to be patient advocates to promote inpatient care safety because we want to heal. Patient advocates are not able to intervene before they know what kind of risk factors they should watch for.

The risk factors for sentinel events and preventable hospital harms and errors may be classified into two categories of intrinsic and extrinsic risk factors. More detailed definitions on intrinsic and extrinsic risk factors follow (Joint Commission, 2005; Tzeng & Yin, 2008a, 2008b):

1. *Intrinsic risk factors.* These factors are integral to each individual patient and may be associated with age-related changes. Using inpatient falls as an example, the intrinsic risk factors may include previous falls, reduced vision, unsteady gait, musculoskeletal system deficits, mental status deficits, acute illness, and chronic illness.

2. *Extrinsic risk factors.* These factors are external to each individual patient and associated with the immediate physical environment surrounding a patient. We also use inpatient falls as an example. The extrinsic risk factors for falls may include side effects of medications, lack of supporting equipment surrounding the bathtub and toilet, poor design of furnishings (e.g., heights of beds and chairs), slippery floors, poor illumination, inappropriate footwear, improper use of devices (e.g., bedside rails), and inadequate assistive devices (e.g., lifting devices, walkers, and wheelchairs).

The extrinsic risk factors for harms and errors are generally more concrete than the intrinsic risk factors. Patients may detect, observe, or assess the extrinsic risk factors for unsafe care because most of these unsafe concerns are linked to the safety of the care environment (e.g., the design of patient rooms and equipment) and observable processes of care deliveries (e.g., medication administration to patients at bedside, answering call lights, and transferring patients).

As a matter of fact, health care providers often overlook the extrinsic risk factors for harm or sentinel events because they are used to the working environment. For example, health care providers and hospital managers often take for granted the existing work setting and patient rooms, as long as the layout of patient rooms does not hamper deliveries of patient care, treatments, or procedures. Hospital leaders and health care providers often forget that a hospital can be a dangerous place for patients because of its unfamiliar physical environment (e.g., being different from our home settings) and changes in patients' medical conditions.

For the intrinsic risk factors, what we as patients can do is to tell our doctors and nurses about any changes in our physical condition. We may need to constantly remind our doctors and nurses our previous medical history (e.g., allergies) and special needs (e.g., poor vision). We do need to speak up if we have any concerns about our health status.

To be patient advocates, we first need to identify which unsafe patient care areas we should be alert to. Hopefully, by actively participating in our own care, we will heal and regain our prehospitalization health status to the extent possible.

Unsafe Patient Care Areas
within Inpatient Care Units

Based on the patient safety dimensions and issues in hospitals as developed in our previous study (Tzeng & Yin, 2007), we made a comparison with the types of sentinel events and the 2008 National Patient Safety Goals for hospital programs as identified by the Joint Commission. As indicated in Table 4, most of the patient safety issues related to treatment and procedures (dimension A), adverse events and incidents (dimension B), and hospital infrastructure (dimension C) in our consensus system were also addressed by the Joint Commission in the sentinel event reports and included in the 2008 National Patient Safety Goals.

Table 4. A comparison table across the patient safety dimensions in hospitals as identified in Tzeng and Yin's study (2007), types of sentinel events, and the 2008 National Patient Safety Goals for hospital programs

Dimension (A-F)/Safety code [ ]*	Type of sentinel events†	2008 National Patient Safety Goals‡
A. Safety issues related to treatment and procedures received		
[1] Medication choices and errors (also including chemotherapy, radiotherapy, and total parenteral nutrition)	1. Medication error	(Goal 3) Improve the safety of using medications (Goal 8) Accurately and completely reconcile medications across the continuum of care
[2] Use of sedation, pain control, or anesthesia	1. Anesthesia-related event	
[3] Procedure (e.g., surgery, invasive or noninvasive medical treatments and procedures)	1. Operative or postoperative complication 2. Unintended retention of foreign body 3. Ventilator-associated death or injury 4. Wrong-site surgery	

Table 4. Continued

Dimension (A-F)/Safety code [ ]*	Type of sentinel events†	2008 National Patient Safety Goals‡
[4] Allergy to medication, media, or contrast medium	1. Medication error 2. Operative or postoperative complication	(Goal 3) Improve the safety of using medications
[5] Blood transfusion (e.g., preparation, related protocols or procedures, and adverse reactions)	1. Transfusion error	
[6] Communication among physicians, nurses, and/or pharmacists (e.g., related to ongoing procedures, or medical treatment)	1. Wrong-site surgery 2. Delay in treatment	(Goal 2) Improve the effectiveness of communication among caregivers
B. Emphasis on adverse events and incidents		
[7] Health care-associated infections (also called nosocomial infection) (e.g., emphasis on a hospital's infection control measures)	1. Infection-related event	(Goal 7) Reduce the risk of health care-associated infections
[8] Patient fall and associated injury	1. Patient fall	(Goal 9) Reduce the risk of patient harm resulting from falls
[9] Other adverse events and incidents (e.g., longer hospital stay, death, and patient complaints)	1. Assault, rape, or homicide 2. Delay in treatment 3. Maternal death 4. Perinatal death or loss of function 5. Suicide	
C. Safety issues related to hospital infrastructure		
[10] Physician computerized prescribing or decision support systems	1. Medication error.	(Goal 3) Improve the safety of using medications
[11] Patient identification	1. Medication error 2. Transfusion error 3. Wrong-site surgery	(Goal 1) Improve the accuracy of patient identification
[12] Use of protocols or guidelines for improving patient outcomes (e.g., promoting a safety culture, reporting medical errors and incidents, and patient record confidentiality)	1. Infant discharge to wrong family 2. Patient death or injury in restraints 3. Patient elopement or abduction	(Goal 16) Improve recognition and response to changes in a patient's condition (Goal 15) Organization identifies safety risks inherent in its patient population
[13] Nurse prescribing (e.g., extending nurse prescribing and nurse advice line recommendations)	1. Medication error	(Goal 3) Improve the safety of using medications.
[14] Pharmacy systems (e.g., drug inventory, dispensing errors, and medication error recovery)	1. Medication error	(Goal 3) Improve the safety of using medications

Dimension (A-F)/Safety code [ ]*	Type of sentinel events[†]	2008 National Patient Safety Goals[‡]
[15] Hospital hardware, equipment, or safety-related monitoring systems	1. Fire 2. Medical equipment-related 3. Utility systems-related event	
D. Safety issues related to the overall medical care system		
[16] Health promotion, or access to hospital services (e.g., use of the safety net hospitals and injury prevention)		
[17] Non-health care workers' occupational hazards, injuries, or illness		
[18] Transportation to medical facilities and related protocols (e.g., from home to hospitals and emergency departments)		
E. Safety concerns about hospital human resource management		
[19] Physicians' work environment (e.g., competencies and training, work hours, and stress)		
[20] Nurses' work environment (e.g., competencies, scheduling, or nurse-to-patient ratios)		
[21] Work environment factors associated with patient safety, mortality and outcomes (general)		
[22] Nurse violence toward patients		
[23] Violence toward patients (general)		
F. Occupational hazards in hospitals		
[24] Physician exposure to biologic hazards, nonfatal occupational injuries or illness		(Goal 7) Reduce the risk of health care-associated infections
[25] Nurse exposure to biologic hazards, nonfatal occupational injuries or illness		(Goal 7) Reduce the risk of health care-associated infections
[26] Occupational hazards, injuries, or illness (general)		(Goal 7) Reduce the risk of health care-associated infections
[27] Patient or family violence toward health care providers		

Sources:
* Tzeng, H. M., & Yin, C. Y. (2007). No safety, no quality: Synthesis of research on hospital and patient safety (1996-2007). *Journal of Nursing Care Quality, 22*(4), 299-306.
† Joint Commission (2007d). Sentinel event statistics: As of June 30, 2007. Available at: http://www.jointcommission.org/NR/rdonlyres/D7836542-A372-4F93-8BD7-DDD11D43E484/0/se_stats_063007.pdf (accessed November 7, 2007).
‡ Joint Commission (2007e). 2008 National Patient Safety Goals: Hospital program. Available at: http://www.jointcommission.org/PatientSafety/NationalPatientSafetyGoals/08_hap_npsgs.htm (accessed November 11, 2007).

Dimension D, safety issues related to the overall medical care system, were not closely linked to patient care deliveries in acute, inpatient care units. As for dimension E (safety concerns about hospital human resource management) and dimension F (occupational hazards in hospitals), some of the safety issues included in these dimensions were associated with the root causes of the reported sentinel events (Table 3) and mentioned in the *2008 Comprehensive Accreditation Manual for Hospitals: The Official Handbook* (abbreviated as 2008 CAMH; Joint Commission, 2007a).

The 2008 CAMH listed a total of 14 priority focus areas. These areas are related to the structure, process, and operational systems within a hospital that may have a significant impact on the safety of care provided (Joint Commission, 2007a; Table 5).

Table 5. The 14 priority areas in the Joint Commission's accreditation process for hospitals

Priority area	Brief description	Subprocesses

Assessment and care for patients	1. This area comprises the execution of a series of processes, including:
	  1.1 Assessment
	  1.2 Planning care and treatment
	  1.3 Provision of care
	  1.4 Ongoing reassessment of care
	  1.5 Discharge planning, referral for continuing care, or discontinuation of care services
		1. Screening
		2. Assessment
		3. Reassessment
		4. Planning care and treatment
		5. Provision of care and treatment
		6. Discharge planning or discontinuation of services

Communication	1. This area involves the process by which information is exchanged between individual health care providers, patient care units, departments, or health care institutions. 2. Effective communication ensures permeating every aspect of a health care organization from the provision of care to performance improvement.	1. The communication between health care providers and patients 2. Patient and family education 3. Staff communication and collaboration 4. Information dissemination 5. Multidisciplinary teamwork
Credentialed practitioners	1. Health care professionals, whose qualifications to provide patient care services have been verified and assessed, will then result in the granting of clinical privileges. 2. These professionals include licensed independent practitioners (e.g., physicians) and others, who are permitted to provide patient care services under the direction of a sponsoring physician.	

Priority area	Brief description	Subprocesses

Equipment use	1. This area incorporates the selection, delivery, setup, and maintenance of equipment to meet patient and staff needs. The fixed equipment is excluded.
	2. Equipment use includes efforts of:
	  2.1 Planning and selecting
	  2.2 Maintaining, testing, and inspecting
	  2.3 Educating and providing instructions
	  2.4 Delivering and setting up the equipment
	  2.5 Preventing risks related to equipment or supplies
		1. Selection
		2. Maintenance strategies
		3. Periodic evaluation
		4. Orientation and training

Infection control	1. This area involves the surveillance and identification, prevention, and control of infections among patients and their families, physicians, nurses, other health care providers, volunteers, students, and visitors. 2. Infection control is a system-wide, integrated process that is applied to all the working areas and health care services within the hospital.	1. Surveillance and identification 2. Prevention and control 3. Reporting 4. Measurement
Information management	1. This area is an interdisciplinary field concerning the timely and accurate creation, data collection, storage, retrieval, transmission, analyses, control, dissemination, and use of data. 2. Written and verbal information, supporting information technology, and information services are all included in the area of information management.	1. Planning 2. Procurement 3. Implementation 4. Collection 5. Recording 6. Protection 7. Aggregation 8. Interpretation 9. Storage and retrieval 10. Data integrity 11. Information dissemination

Medication management	1. This area includes the systems and processes a hospital uses to provide medications to patients, who receive care in this hospital.
	2. Medication management requires:
	  2.1 Coordinated efforts of multidisciplinary health care providers
	  2.2 Constantly improving the processes of selecting, procuring, storing, ordering, transcribing, preparing, dispensing, administering, self-administering (by patients themselves) and monitoring the effect of medications throughout the patients' continuum of care.
	3. This area also involves patient education and family education as appropriate about each medication, its administration, and potential side effects.
		1. Selection
		2. Procurement
		3. Storage
		4. Prescribing or ordering
		5. Preparing
		6. Dispensing
		7. Administration
		8. Monitoring

Table 5. Continued

Priority area	Brief description	Subprocesses
Organizational structure	1. A hospital's structure refers to the framework for a hospital to carry out its vision and mission.	1. Management requirements 2. Corporate by-laws and governing body plans 3. Organization management 4. Compliance 5. Planning 6. Business ethics 7. Contracted services
Orientation and training	1. Whereas orientation is a one-time process, training is a continuous one. 2. Orientation refers to the process of educating newly hired staff in hospitals to hospital-wide, departmental, and job-specific competencies before they provide direct patient care services. 3. Training is the process of developing and implementing certain programs that foster staff development and continued learning and address skill deficiencies. 4. Training may help to ensure staff retention.	1. Hospital-wide orientation 2. Departmental, program and service orientation 3. Job-specific orientation 4. Training and on-the-job ongoing education
Patient safety	1. This area entails proactively identifying the potential and actual risks to patient safety, identifying the underlying causes of the potential risks, and making the necessary improvements to reduce these risks. 2. A hospital also needs to establish processes to respond to sentinel events, identify risks through root cause analyses, and make necessary improvements. 3. This area also involves system-wide approaches, which are driven by the hospital's leadership, including performance improvement and risk management. 4. Effective reduction of errors and unintended adverse outcomes requires a hospital in which patients, their family members, health care providers, and leaders can identify and manage actual and potential risks to patient safety.	1. Planning and designing health care services 2. Directing health care services 3. Integrating and coordinating care 4. Error reduction and prevention 5. Use of sentinel event alerts 6. Adopting the Joint Commission's National Patient Safety Goals 7. Clinical practice guidelines 8. Active patient involvement in their care

Priority area	Brief description	Subprocesses

Physical environment	1. A hospital's physical environment should be safe, accessible, functional, supportive, and effective for patients and their families, visitors, health care providers, and the other staff.
	2. This area involves:
	  2.1 Managing physical design
	  2.2 Construction and redesign
	  2.3 Maintenance and testing
	  2.4 Planning and improvement
	  2.5 Risk prevention (e.g., utilities, fire protection, security, privacy, storage, and hazardous materials and waste)
		1. Physical design
		2. Construction and redesign
		3. Maintenance and testing
		4. Planning and improvement
		5. Risk prevention

Quality improvement activities	1. Quality improvement efforts involve identifying, measuring, implementing, monitoring, analyzing, planning, and maintaining processes to ensure these processes function effectively.
	2. Quality improvement activities include, for example:
	  2.1 Designing a new service
	  2.2 Experimenting with new ways of carrying out a function
	  2.3 Creating flow charts for a clinical process
	  2.4 Collecting and analyzing data about performance measures or patient outcomes
		1. Identifying quality issues
		2. Establishing quality improvement priorities
		3. Developing quality measures
		4. Collecting data to evaluate status on structures, processes, and outcomes
		5. Analyzing and interpreting data
		6. Making and implementing recommendations
		7. Monitoring and sustaining performance improvement

Patients' rights and the ethics for the hospital and health care providers	1. This area addresses issues including, such as:
	  1.1 Patient privacy
	  1.2 Confidentiality and protection of patient health information
	  1.3 Advance directives
	  1.4 Organ procurement
	  1.5 Use of restraints
	  1.6 Informed consent for procedures
	  1.7 Patients' rights to participate in their own care decisions
		1. Patient rights
		2. A hospital's ethics pertaining to patient care
		3. A hospital's responsibility
		4. Consideration of patients
		5. Care sensitivity
		6. Informing patients and their family members

Staffing	1. Staffing involves assessing those defined competencies and allocating the human resources necessary for patient safety and improved patient outcomes. 2. Effective staffing includes providing the optimal number of competent health care providers with the appropriate skill mix to meet the patients' needs.	1. Competency 2. Skill mix 3. Number of staff

Source: Joint Commission (2007a). *2008 comprehensive accreditation manual for hospitals: The official handbook* (pp. ACC-19-ACC-23). Oakbrook Terrace, IL: Joint Commission Resources.

After incorporating the patient safety concerns instituted by the Joint Commission, the Joint Commission International, and Institute for Healthcare Improvement, we identified 12 patient safety areas commonly seen in acute inpatient care units and address these areas in this book:

1. Inpatient falls
2. Health care-associated pressure ulcers
3. Serious injury or death in physical restraints or seclusion
4. Inpatient suicide
5. Medication errors
6. Transfusion errors
7. Wrong-site surgery
8. Treatment delays
9. Operative and postoperative errors and complications
10. Health care-associated infections
11. Impact of hospital human resource management on patient outcomes
12. Unsafe design of patient rooms

Regardless how hard we try, the gap in medical knowledge between our physicians and nurses and us is huge and cannot be overcome. Even if we have professional health training, we may still have difficulties in understanding all the medications and procedures we are receiving. We certainly can try our best to learn about our treatments and procedures by asking our doctors, nurses, or pharmacists.

Working with our Nurses to Promote a Safer Hospital Stay

Registered nurses provide about 57% of our care in acute inpatient care units (Rutherford, 2007). To promote a safer hospital stay, we should work closely with our nurses to identify potential risk to our safety and prevent any occurrence of preventable hospital harms and errors. The World Health Professions Alliance (2002) claimed that the enhancement of patient safety (e.g., preventing the occurrence of adverse events) may engage in a wide range of possible actions involving:

1. Human resource management (e.g., recruitment, training, and retention of nurses, physicians, and pharmacists)
2. Performance improvement
3. Environmental safety and risk management (e.g., safe environment of care, equipment safety, infection control, safe use of medications, and safe clinical practice)

**Table 6. Patient safety actions as recommended by the
World Health Professions Alliance**

Dimension	Actions
Patients	Patients should: 1. Inform their health care providers of all medications that they have been taken, and their medical conditions. 2. Ask questions to clarify medical information given by their health care providers. 3. Increase understanding about their own health conditions, medications, and health care provision. 4. Make sure to get the results of any tests or procedures. 5. Report medical errors or adverse events to the proper authorities.
Governmental or federal health agencies	Governmental or federal health agencies should: 1. Establish national reporting systems to record, analyze, and learn from adverse incidents. 2. Promote an overall culture of reporting adverse incidents. 3. Emphasize safety as a prime concern in health care system performance and quality management. 4. Implement mechanisms for ensuring that, where adverse events or unsafe practice lessons are identified, the necessary changes are put into practice and the progress is tracked. 5. Develop evidence-based policies that will improve health care. 6. Build up mechanisms to recognize the characteristics of health care institutions that offer a benchmark for excellence in patient safety (e.g., hospital accreditation).
Hospitals and other health care facilities	Hospitals should: 1. Maintain adequate human resource levels. 2. If an adverse event occurred, focus on improving the operational systems of delivering care, instead of blaming individual health care providers. 3. Establish rigorous infection control guidelines or protocols. 4. Standardize treatment policies and protocols to avoid confusion and reliance on memory (relying on memory is known to be fallacious and responsible for many errors). 5. Avoid similar-sounding and look-alike names and packages of medications.
Health care providers	Health care providers (physicians, nurses, and pharmacists) should: 1. Take an active role in assessing the safety and quality of care in practice. 2. Improve communication with patients and other health care providers. 3. Inform patients of potential risks in their care. 4. Work together to improve practice-related systems. 5. Report adverse events to the appropriate authorities. 6. Strengthen the collaboration aspects of drug treatment plans.

Source: World Health Professions Alliance (2002). Health professionals call for priority on patient safety (press release April 29, 2002). Available at: http://www.whpa.org/factptsafety.htm (accessed November 24, 2007).

The World Health Professions Alliance (2002) also recommended several possible actions to patients, hospitals, health care providers, and governmental or federal agencies for the same goal of promoting patient safety during hospital stays (Table 6). In reality, no single magic solution can resolve all the risk factors of preventable hospital harms and errors within our patient room during hospitalization. However, patient advocates may intervene most effectively in any unsafe care occurring in patient rooms, where patients spend most of their time during the entire hospital stay.

References

Carayon, P. (2007). Human factors and ergonomics in health care and patient safety. In P. Carayon, (Ed.), *Handbook of human factors and ergonomics in health care and patient safety* (pp. 3-20). Mahwah, NJ: Lawrence Erlbaum Associates.

International Ergonomics Association (2000). What is ergonomics? Available at: http://www.iea.cc/browse.php?contID=what_is_ergonomics (accessed November 9, 2007).

Joint Commission (2005). Defining the problem of falls. In I. J. Smith (Ed.), *Reducing the risk of falls in your health care organization* (pp. 13-27). Oakbrook Terrace, IL: Joint Commission on Accreditation of Healthcare Organizations.

Joint Commission (2007a). *2008 comprehensive accreditation manual for hospitals: The official handbook.* Oakbrook Terrace, IL: Joint Commission Resources.

Joint Commission (2007b). Quality Check® What can this site do for me? Available at: http://www.jointcommission.org/qualitycheck/qc_what.htm (accessed November 15, 2007).

Joint Commission (2007c). About sentinel events. In R. A. Porché, Jr. (Ed.), *Front line of defense: The role of nurses in preventing sentinel events* (2nd ed., pp. 1-20). Oakbrook Terrace, IL: Joint Commission Resources.

Joint Commission (2007d). Sentinel event statistics: As of June 30, 2007. Available at: http://www.jointcommission.org/NR/rdonlyres/D7836542-A372-4F93-8BD7-DDD11D43E484/0/se_stats_063007.pdf (accessed November 7, 2007).

Joint Commission (2007e). 2008 National Patient Safety Goals: Hospital program. Available at: http://www.jointcommission.org/PatientSafety/NationalPatientSafetyGoals/08_hap_npsgs.htm (accessed November 11, 2007).

Rutherford, P. (2007). Transforming care at the bedside. Available at: http://www.ihi.org/NR/rdonlyres/BD24233D-6328-4F1E-9197-151628F1EA35/0/TCABvideotape907.pdf (accessed November 24, 2007).

Tzeng, H. M., & Yin, C. Y. (2007). No safety, no quality: Synthesis of research on hospital and patient safety (1996-2007). *Journal of Nursing Care Quality, 22*(4), 299-306.

Tzeng, H. M., & Yin, C. Y. (2008a). Nurses' solutions to prevent inpatient falls in hospital patient rooms. *Nursing Economics, 26*(3) (in press; May/June, 2008).

Tzeng, H. M., & Yin, C. Y. (2008b). The extrinsic risk factors for inpatient falls in hospital patient rooms. *Journal of Nursing Care Quality, 23*(3) (in press; July-September 2008).

World Health Professions Alliance (2002). Health professionals call for priority on patient safety (press release April 29, 2002). Available at: http://www.whpa.org/factptsafety.htm (accessed November 24, 2007).

Section II:
Preventing Harms and Errors

Inpatient Falls

Learning from a Patient Case

Two days after a surgical procedure, a hospitalized man, Mr. A, began to experience increased weakness, unsteady balance, and absent-mindedness. Nurse B, Mr. A's nurse on the 3:00 P.M. to 11:00 P.M. shift, reassessed his condition and changed the fall prevention program. However, before Nurse B left the surgical inpatient care unit, Nurse B failed to document the changes on Mr. A's care plan and did not verbally communicate this change to the responsible nurse, Nurse C, on the next shift.

Because Nurse C on the 11:00 P.M. to 7:00 A.M. shift did not receive the information about the change on Mr. A' health status, Nurse C helped Mr. A into a chair for breakfast and left him unattended. When the breakfast tray was brought into the room an hour later, Mr. A was found sitting on the bathroom floor bleeding from a large head wound (Joint Commission, 2007a).

Learning from a Legal Case Summary

On May 23, 2002, appellee Mrs. X was admitted to Hospital A to undergo laparoscopic gastric bypass surgery. After surgery, Mrs. X developed acute respiratory distress syndrome and was placed on a ventilator and was in a medically induced coma for approximately 4 weeks. During the period of the induced coma, she remained in a supine position in a surgical intensive care unit.

On June 24, 2002, while being weaned off the ventilator and in preparation for bringing her out of the coma, Mrs. X was transferred to a regular inpatient unit.

After bringing Mrs. X out of the coma, on June 25, 2002, Mrs. X's bed was raised to a seating position for the first time since her surgery. Within a minute after the bed was put in the seating position, she gradually slid toward the floor and eventually fell out of her bed onto the floor. Mrs. X sustained injuries to her right shoulder, arm, and hand.

Nurse Y was Mrs. X's nurse on the date and shift when the fall occurred. Before the fall occurred, Nurse Y documented the mental status of Mrs. X as not being oriented times three ('oriented times three' refers to that a patient is awake, alert, and fully oriented). In other words, Mrs. X did not know who she was, where she was, and the approximate time or date.

Mr. X testified that he watched his wife fall and he was too far away to prevent the fall from happening. Mr. X also mentioned that Nurse Y had raised the bed and then turned away.

After deliberation, the jury returned a verdict in favor of Mr. and Mrs. X. The jury awarded Mrs. X $1,000,000 for past noneconomic loss for her pain and suffering, embarrassment and humiliation, disfigurement, and loss of life's pleasures; $3,000,000 for future noneconomic losses; and $30,000 per year for future medical and related expenses from and including 2006 until 2038. The jury also awarded Mr. X $50,000 for past noneconomic losses.

Source: NexisLexis®Academic: Federal & State Cases (Case number: 005216; February 6, 2007, decided) (accessed on December 3, 2007).

Learning from a Legal Case Summary

On February 13, 1997, Ms. V, a 14-year-old girl, went to visit her grandmother, Mrs. M, in the intensive care unit at Hospital P. Ms. V sustained personal injuries due to a slip and fall in her grandmother's patient room. Ms. V suspected that she slipped and fell on urine because Nurse A negligently failed to connect Mrs. M's Foley catheter tube.

Nurse A testified that she did not see any liquid on the floor of Mrs. M's room when making her earlier rounds at 6 P.M. She had a good, lighted view of the floor and noticed no liquid on the floor. The fall was reported to her by Ms. V and two other relatives at 6:18 P.M. After the accident, Nurse A saw a small amount of urine had leaked onto the floor.

Because of the aforementioned fall accident and as a direct and proximate cause, Ms. V sustained an acute umbosacral strain, acute hip strain, and contusions to her hip, left foot, and left toe. She was treated by Dr. E, a board certified orthopedic surgeon, at Hospital P's emergency room at no charge. Later, Ms. V returned to Dr. E's office several times for continuous treatments. On October 16, Ms. V's physical examination showed that she was doing fairly well and was finally discharged, about 8 months after her accident of February 13, 1997.

The court determined that Ms. V should be awarded general damages of $7000 and medical bill of $710.

Source: NexisLexis®Academic: Federal & State Cases (Case number: 99-CA-3116; November 15, 2000, decided) (accessed on January 12, 2008).

A Success Story

The Director of Nursing Practice Programs at the M. D. Anderson Cancer Center at the University of Texas in Houston looked at the characteristics of patients who fell in a surgical inpatient care unit and found that many patients who had undergone a particular gastrointestinal surgery were falling. Because these patients can develop diarrhea after surgery, nurses at this unit found that putting a bedside commode near the bed reduced fall incidents.

Hourly safety checks were also instituted so that nurses would check on their responsible patients and offer assistance with toileting or any other activities that require patients to move. Safety checks have become part of this hospital's policies for all patients (Institute for Healthcare Improvement, 2007).

Knowing about Inpatient Falls

Based on the data collected during the period between July 1998 and March 2000, if an acute hospital had a fall injury rate of 6.6%, these fall incidents with injuries may report a median of 7.5-day increase in total length of stay and a median increase of $5317 in total lost revenues to hospitals. It was estimated that the average cost per fall, including falls with and without injury, would be $351 (Bates et al., 1995; Boswell et al., 2001; Granek et al., 1987). We further used the inflation calculator provided on the Web site of the US Department of Labor Bureau of Labor Statistics (2007) to calculate the estimated cost of falls to hospitals in 2007. As given by the inflation calculator, $100 in 2000 has the same buying power as $121.07 in 2007. It was estimated that, for hospitals, the projected cost per fall with injury in 2007 would be at least $6437 and the average cost per fall would be $425.

Other than the cost of falls to hospitals, additional cost may arise to individual patients (e.g., lost of working days and income). The cost of falls to our society should also be justified by considering the upward trends in the national health expenditures per capita. The expenditure per capita has increased from $2813 in 1990 to $7498 (projected) in 2007, which would be 16.2% of the US gross domestic product (Henry J. Kaiser Family Foundation, 2007). In fact, the cost of falls that occur during hospitalization is an important patient safety issue for governmental health agencies, federal insurance programs (e.g., Medicare), private health insurance companies, hospitals, and individuals with and without health insurance coverage.

Patient falls have been a challenging safety and care quality issue in acute care settings, where an aging patient population and persons with physical and cognitive limitations are exposed to unfamiliar and potentially hazardous surroundings. At some point during patients' hospital stays, they are at their most vulnerable. This may be when they first come in for treatment with acute, life-threatening medical conditions, or immediately after treatments, procedures, or surgeries (Reiling, 2006).

Hospitals have devoted quality improvement and research efforts to prevent falls, but patient falls nonetheless consistently comprise the largest single category of reported incidents in hospitals (Joint Commission, 2005a). Fall prevention programs (e.g., using fall risk assessment tools to evaluate patients' risks for falls) apparently do not effectively reduce inpatient fall rates. A patient-centered facility design should be able to promote patient safety. A safety-driven design with a goal to prevent inpatient fall-related injuries should be a hospital design principle.

Nurses assume the primary responsibility and are liable when a patient falls in the inpatient care unit. Inpatient fall incidents could be most improved through nurse-led safety strategies or interventions. However, we still often hear that people we know fell out of the hospital patient beds, broke their bones, or died shortly after the fall incident. Most of these kinds of stories involved the elderly during their hospital stays.

Epidemiology of Hospital Inpatient Falls

As for the locations at time of fall, Krauss and associates (2007) showed that 79.5% of falls occurred in patient rooms, 11% in patient bathrooms, and 9.5% in hallways, examination or treatment rooms, or by the nurses' stations. In the United States, the four most reported activities at time of fall were (Hitcho, et al., 2004):

1. 19.1% occurred during ambulation
2. 10.9% when getting out of bed
3. 9.3% while sitting down or standing up
4. 4.4% while using the bedside commode or toilet

The physical environment seems to have a significant impact on patient safety during hospital stays. However, most hospitals are not explicitly designed to enhance patient safety (Reiling, 2006). Hignett and Masud (2006) used an ergonomic system perspective to analyze inpatient falls. They concluded that from a patient-centered perspective, the first hazard interaction was the layout and equipment of a patient room.

For example, one of our previous studies found that the staff working height of hospital occupied beds and the height of patient beds in low position in acute patient care units were much higher than the average height of beds designed for residential use. The height of patient beds seems to be an overlooked cause of patient falls (Tzeng & Yin, 2006). Another study (Tzeng & Yin, 2008a) conducted at a US medical center demonstrated that the average staff working height measurement taken on weekends was significantly higher than that taken on weekdays. The average height of beds for patients on fall precautions was significantly higher than for those not on fall precautions.

These findings affirmed the conclusion of Hignett and Masud (2006) that the first hazard to inpatients after being admitted into an inpatient care unit was the improper layout and equipment of a patient room. Nurses and the other health care providers, who have direct contact with patients, may also contribute to falls by failing to lower patient beds after completing their tasks. In the next section, risk factors for falls are described in detail.

Risk Factors and Possible Solutions

Individual Risk Factors for Falls

Individual risk factors for falls can be categorized as either intrinsic or extrinsic to the patient's system (Joint Commissions, 2005a). Intrinsic risk factors are integral to the patient's system and may be associated with age-related changes, including previous falls, reduced vision, unsteady gait, musculoskeletal system deficits, mental status deficits, acute illness, and chronic illness. Extrinsic risk factors are external to the patient's system and related to the physical environment, including medication, lack of support equipment by bathtubs and toilets, design of furnishings, condition of floors, poor illumination, inappropriate footwear, improper use of devices, and inadequate assistive devices (Joint Commissions, 2005a). The Joint Commission (2006a, 2007b) also listed the commonly seen intrinsic and extrinsic risk factors for falls (Table 1).

Table 1. The commonly seen intrinsic and extrinsic risk factors for inpatient falls

Being intrinsic or extrinsic to the patient	Factor
Intrinsic risk factors	1. Demographic characteristics and history 1.1 Age 1.2 Fear of falling 1.3 Gender 1.4 History of previous falls 1.5 Length of stay in the current hospitalization 2. Diagnoses and condition 2.1 Acute illnesses (e.g., rapid onset of symptoms associated with seizures, and febrile conditions) 2.2 Ambulatory aids 2.3 Cardiac arrhythmias 2.4 Chronic illnesses (e.g., conditions such as arthritis, cataracts, glaucoma, and diabetes) 2.5 Confusion 2.6 Dehydration 2.7 Delirium 2.8 Dementia 2.9 Depression 2.10 Disorientation 2.11 Dizziness 2.12 Elimination status (e.g., incontinence of bowel or bladder) 2.13 History of fractures 2.14 Impaired memory 2.15 Inability to understand 2.16 Lower extremity strength 2.17 Musculoskeletal conditions (e.g., myopathy and deformities) 2.18 Orthostatic hypotension 2.19 Parkinson's disease 2.20 Reduced vision, visual and auditory impairments 2.21 Stroke 2.22 Transient ischemic attacks 2.23 Unsteady or problems with mobility and gait

Table 1. Continued

Being intrinsic or extrinsic to the patient	Factor

	3. Other factors
	   3.1 Confined to a chair
	   3.2 Having an IV therapy or heparin lock
	   3.3 Postoperative

Extrinsic risk factors	1. Medications
	   1.1 Analgesics
	   1.2 Antiarrhythmics
	   1.3 Antidepressants
	   1.4 Antihypertensives
	   1.5 Benzodiazepines
	   1.6 Diuretics
	   1.7 Hypnotics
	   1.8 Hypoglycemics
	   1.9 Laxatives and cathartics
	   1.10 Neuroleptics
	   1.11 Nonsteroidal anti-inflammatory agents
	   1.12 Polypharmacy (multiple medications)
	   1.13 Psychotropics
	   1.14 Sedatives
	   1.15 Tranquilizers
	   1.16 Vasodilators
	2. Environmental factors
	   2.1 Being confined to a chair
	   2.2 Improper use of restraint devices (e.g., bed rails)
	   2.3 Inadequate assistive devices (e.g., walkers, wheelchairs, and lifting devices)
	   2.4 Inappropriate type and condition of footwear (e.g., ill-fitting shoes or incompatible soles)
	   2.5 Poor illumination conditions (e.g., intensity or glare issues)
	   2.6 The condition of the ground surfaces (e.g., wet ground surfaces)
	   2.7 The design of furnishings (e.g., height of chairs and beds)
	   2.8 The shower areas and toilets (e.g., equipment without support or grab bars)

Sources: Joint Commission (2006a). Goal 9: Reduce the risk of patient harm result from falls. In A. Grayson. (Ed.), *Meeting the Joint Commission's 2007 National Patient Safety Goals* (pp. 75-94). Oakbrook Terrace, IL: Joint Commission. Joint Commission (2007b). *Patient safety pocket guide* (2nd ed., pp. 1-14). Oakbrook Terrace, IL: Joint Commission.

The Morse Fall Scale (Morse, 1997) is one of the most widely used risk assessment tools used by nurses at the time of the patient admission. This tool was created to assess a patient's intrinsic risk factors for falling. Poor scores on this assessment tool may trigger either further assessments or changes in the patient's care plans and interventions aimed to reduce the risks of falling. The risk factors for falls included in the Morse Fall Scale are (Morse, 1997):

1. History of falling (immediate or within 3 months)
2. Secondary diagnosis (e.g., having more than one medical diagnosis listed on the patient chart)
3. The proficiency level in using ambulatory aids (e.g., wheelchair, walker, cane, or crutch)

4. Having IV therapy or a heparin lock inserted
5. Weak or impaired gait characteristics
6. Patient's self-assessment of ability to ambulate (e.g., being oriented to own ability versus forgetting one's own limitations)

In one of our studies (Tzeng & Yin, 2008b), we identified the extrinsic risk factors for inpatient falls from incident reports and from the transcriptions of interviews with nurses and nursing attendants, who worked in an acute, adult medical unit of a Michigan medical center. The attributional theory of success and failure (Weiner, 1986; Weiner et al., 1979) and a three-dimensional typology (including patient room setting and design, hospital equipment, and manpower concerns) were used together to elicit data. In this study, inpatient falls, a complicated phenomenon, were conceptualized as a failure in nursing practice.

Weiner and associates' locus-stability classification scheme (a 2-by-2 categorization scheme; internal and external control orientations by having stability or not) was used to characterize the perceived causes of achievement-related context (success or failure; Weiner, 1986; Weiner et al., 1979; Table 2). For example, a success or failure at an examination may be perceived as being dependent on the university's grading policy, a relatively fixed external criterion (context 3: objective task characteristics), and on lucky or unlucky guessing during the examination, a fluctuating external cause (context 4: chance). Aptitude is perceived as a constant capacity (context 1), whereas such a causal factor as temporary exertion (context 2) is perceived as more inconsistent and changing from one time internal to the next.

Table 2. The locus-stability classification scheme in the attributional theory of success and failure

A 2-by-2 categorization scheme for the perceived causes of achievement outcome[*]		
	Internal	External
Stable	Context 1: Aptitude (e.g., skills)	Context 3: Objective task characteristics (e.g., hospital policies and staffing)
Unstable	Context 2: Temporary exertion (e.g., efforts)	Context 4: Chance (e.g., bad luck)

[*] This scheme was modified from the one used by Weiner and associates (Weiner, 1986; Weiner et al., 1979).

Sources: Weiner, B. (1986). *An attributional theory of motivation and emotion.* New York, NY: Springer-Verlag New York. Weiner, B., Frieze, I. H., Kukla, A., Reed, L., Rest, S., & Rosenbaun, R. M. (1979). *Perceiving the causes of success and failure.* Morristown, NJ: General Learning Press.

As indicated in Table 3, 16 extrinsic fall risk contributors were abstracted from the structured form section of the fall incident reports; 4 were related to patient room designs and settings, 3 were linked to hospital equipment, and 9 were related to staffing and manpower concerns. Breakdown of the communication between the patient and nurse (n = 14, 17.0%) was the most often chosen risk factor, followed by misplaced equipment lines or tubes (n = 10, 12.8%). Falls most often occurred between 3:00 A.M. and 7:00 A.M. (n = 29, 27.9%), followed by 3:00 P.M. to 7:00 P.M. (n = 25, 24%). Table 4 summarizes the findings from nurse and nursing attendant interviews. As a study limitation, these results should be interpreted cautiously. According to the attributional theory of success and failure, respondents tend to attribute the causes of failure to external control causes, which may be stable or unstable characteristics (Tzeng & Yin, 2008b).

Table 3. The extrinsic risk factors for inpatient fall abstracted from a total of 104 fall incident reports

Locus X stability classification* and dimensions [A, B, C]† Descriptive information	n (%)	Internal versus external	Stable versus unstable	Dimension
The descriptive analyses on the structured-form portion of the fall incident reports				
Extrinsic contributing factors to falls				
(n = 78; multiple options may be chosen)				
Patient–nurse communication breakdown	14 (17.9)	Internal	Unstable	C
Equipment lines or tubes misplaced	10 (12.8)	External	Unstable	B
Patients needed more staff assistance	7 (9.0)	External	Unstable	C
Bed rails were down	7 (9.0)	External	Unstable	C
Patients slipped or tripped	6 (7.7)	External	Stable	A
Patients were unattended	6 (7.7)	External	Unstable	C
Using sedative medications	6 (7.7)	External	Unstable	C
Lack of personal safety measures	5 (6.4)	External	Stable	A
Wet floor or ground	4 (5.1)	External	Unstable	A
Inadequate assistive device (e.g., walker)	4(5.1)	External	Stable	B
Footwear inappropriate	2 (2.5)	External	Unstable	B
Heavy workload (e.g., acuity level)	2 (2.5)	External	Unstable	C
Family visitor behavior inappropriate	2 (2.5)	External	Unstable	C
Unsafe physical environmental design	1 (1.3)	External	Stable	A
Staff transfer technique inappropriate	1 (1.3)	Internal	Stable	C
Junior staff (<1 yr)	1 (1.3)	Internal	Stable	C
Shift during which the fall occurred				C
3-7 A.M.	29 (27.9)			
3-7 P.M.	25 (24.0)			
7-11 A.M.	20 (19.2)			
11 A.M.-3 P.M.	11 (10.6)			
7-11 P.M.	10 (9.6)			
11 P.M.-3 A.M.	9 (8.7)			
Fall safety precautions at the time of the fall (n = 760; multiple options may be chosen)				
Call light in reach	84 (11.1)			A
Bed in low position	72 (9.5)			A
Fall precautions implemented	65 (8.6)			C
Free of environmental hazards	59 (7.8)			A
Clear path to bathroom	56 (7.4)			A
Bed brakes locked	55 (7.2)			A
Fall care plan completed	54 (7.1)			C
Nonskid footwear on	47 (6.2)			B
Bed table in reach	46 (6.1)			A
Personal items in reach	46 (6.1)			A

Locus X stability classification* and dimensions [A, B, C]† Descriptive information	n (%)	Internal versus external	Stable versus unstable	Dimension
Phone in reach	40 (5.3)			A
Light or night light on	37 (4.9)			A
Staff assisted patient with ambulation	22 (2.9)			C
Sitter was with patient	13 (1.7)			C
Timed toileting plan	12 (1.6)			C
Urinal or bedpan in reach	11 (1.4)			A
Family invited to stay with patient	10 (1.3)			C
Staff supervised during ambulation	9 (1.2)			C
Timed observation plan	7 (0.9)			C
Sitter requested, but not available	6 (0.8)			C
Bed alarm was on	5 (0.7)			A
Family assisted patient with ambulation	4 (0.5)			C
The content analyses on the narrative portion of the fall incident reports				
Accompanying family at the time of fall				
Patient's wife	4 (3.8)			C
Visitor other than wife or husband	4 (3.8)			C
Patient's husband	2 (1.9)			C
Not indicated	94 (90.4)			—
Accompanying staff at the time of fall				
Sitter	8 (7.7)			C
Nurse or nursing attendant	7 (6.7)			C
Physical therapist	4 (3.8)			C
Not indicated	85 (81.7)			—
Patient's activity at the time of fall				
Not indicated in the narrative	38 (36.5)			—
Getting out of the bed	20 (19.2)			A
On the way from the bed to the bathroom	10 (9.6)			A
Slipped off the toilet	10 (9.6)			A
Getting back to the bed	5 (4.8)			A
On the way from the bathroom to the bed	5 (4.8)			A
Moving from the bed to the bedside commode or wheelchair	4 (3.8)			A
Moving from the bedside commode or wheelchair back to the patient bed	4 (3.8)			A
Fell from the room chair	4 (3.8)			A
Slipped from the bed edge	3 (2.9)			A
On the way from the patient room bathroom to the bedside chair	1 (1.0)			A

* Attributions to failures were categorized from the viewpoints of the nurses who completed the fall incident reports. All attributions were marked as being external versus internal and being stable versus unstable.

† The proposed typology was used to elicit data that include three dimensions: (A) patient room setting and design, (B) hospital equipment, and (C) staffing and manpower concerns.

Source: Tzeng, H. M., & Yin, C. Y. (2008b). The extrinsic risk factors for inpatient falls in hospital patient rooms. *Journal of Nursing Care Quality, 23*(3) (in press; July 2008).

Table 4. The extrinsic risk factors for inpatient falls elicited from the interview transcriptions of nine nurses and four nursing attendants

Locus X stability classification[*] Dimensions [A, B, C][†]	Internal versus external	Stable versus unstable
A. Patient room design and settings		
Room design		
1. Limited room space	External	Stable
2. Distance and path from the bed to the bathroom	External	Stable
3. Limited storage space for patients' personal items	External	Stable
4. Patients may trip on the dip at the bathroom door, not handicapped accessible	External	Stable
5. Unused equipment left in the rooms	External	Unstable
The ceiling lift system		
1. The ceiling lift does not go to the bathroom, only around the bed	External	Stable
2. Insufficient slings and bars to go with the ceiling lift system	External	Stable
3. Nurses rarely use the ceiling lift	Internal	Unstable
Patient bed		
1. Bed in low position, still too high and needing a stool for getting in and out	External	Stable
2. Patients unable to adjust the bed height for the whole bed (only able to adjust the heights of the head and foot sections)	External	Stable
3. Specialty beds too high and unable to lower due to thick mattress	External	Stable
4. Hard to hear the beeping sound from the bed alarm if it went off	External	Stable
5. Bed maintenance, insufficient and missing safety measures (e.g., seatbelts)	External	Unstable
6. Bed rails not being used appropriately	External	Unstable
7. Nurses not familiar with bed functions	Internal	Stable
8. Bed height, not kept in low position	Internal	Unstable
9. Bed pressure alarm not being used regularly	Internal	Unstable
Bedside chair		
1. Chairs too low, hard for ingress and egress	External	Stable
2. Stability, lacking rubber stoppers	External	Stable
3. Chairs and recliners for families, insufficient	External	Stable
4. Chair maintenance, insufficient	External	Unstable
Bathroom and toilet		
1. Shower room, insufficient space	External	Stable
2. Bathroom space, lacking shelf or organizer to store needed equipment	External	Stable
3. Toilet seat height too low, hard for ingress and egress	External	Stable
4. Grab bars insufficient to generate pushup force to get up from toilet	External	Stable
5. No fan to take the moisture out and to keep the bathroom floor dry	External	Stable
6. Wet shower seats, slippery and lack traction	External	Stable
7. Wet shower floor, slippery and lack traction	External	Stable
8. Water does not drain to the drain after shower; water drains out to the room	External	Stable
9. Diaper/brief design, difficult to take off or put on and to keep balance before and after toileting	External	Stable
10. Housekeeping, not cleaned in time	External	Unstable

Locus X stability classification[*] Dimensions [A, B, C][†]	Internal versus external	Stable versus unstable
Grab bars		
1. No grab bars in patient rooms for patients to hold onto on the way from the bed to the bathroom	External	Stable
2. Lacking sufficient grab bars in the bathroom for patients to hold onto	External	Stable
3. Grab bars in the bathroom, lacking traction	External	Stable
The call light system		
1. After call lights go off, no signal to tell whether a nurse or nursing attendant is in a specific patient room	External	Stable
2. Visually impaired patients unable to locate the call light button on the control panel	External	Stable
3. The beeping sounds from staff's pagers, which indicate patients have called for help, easily ignored	Internal	Unstable
Lighting		
1. Insufficient floor lighting at night	External	Stable
2. Night light maintenance, broken night light bulbs not replaced in time	External	Unstable
3. Nurses have to take initiative to turn on the nightlights/floor lights after dark	Internal	Unstable
B. Hospital equipment		
Bedside commode		
1. Sturdiness of bedside commodes	External	Stable
2. Lacking sufficient backrest and armrest support	External	Stable
3. Insufficient number of bedside commodes	External	Stable
Miscellaneous equipment		
1. Raised toilet seats, not readily available in the unit	External	Stable
2. Better IV poles needed; hard to manage all the tubing	External	Stable
3. Walkers, canes, and sliding boards not readily available in the unit when patients are in need	External	Stable
4. The arms of the wheelchairs not removable, which may result in difficulty in transferring patients	External	Stable
5. The portable lifting system not readily available in the unit when it is needed	External	Stable
C. Staffing and manpower concerns		
Nursing manpower		
1. Patient assignments not in close proximity	External	Unstable
2. Insufficient nursing attendants	External	Unstable
3. Nurses have difficulty knowing patient care priorities	Internal	Stable
4. Misconception about the purpose of call lights so that responses can be delayed because patients may need nothing important	Internal	Stable
5. Nurses' efforts on implementing fall precaution program	Internal	Unstable
6. Difficulty in implementing timed observation plan and toileting plan	Internal	Unstable
7. Call lights not answered in time or being ignored by nurses	Internal	Unstable
8. Assistance after toileting delayed	Internal	Unstable
9. During shift changes or just after shift changes, call lights tend not to be answered	Internal	Unstable
10. Teamwork and responsibility sharing between nurses and nursing attendants	Internal	Unstable
11. Nursing attendants' efforts on taking initiative to check on their patients	Internal	Unstable

Table 4. Continued

Locus X stability classification[*] Dimensions [A, B, C][†]	Internal versus external	Stable versus unstable
Patient and family education on fall prevention		
1. Fall precaution programs and related care plans not thoroughly implemented	Internal	Unstable
2. Fall precaution programs perceived by nurses as routine and useless in preventing falls	Internal	Unstable
Using sitters in preventing falls		
1. Sitters' knowledge about and ability on fall precaution actions vary	External	Stable
2. Sitters' efforts in promoting patient safety vary	External	Unstable
3. Hand-off information on the condition of the high-risk patient among sitters between shifts insufficient	External	Unstable
Families		
1. Family involvement in care varies and unpopular	External	Unstable
2. Families' knowledge about and ability on fall precaution actions, insufficient	External	Unstable

[*] Attributions of failure were categorized from the viewpoints of the interviewed nurses and nursing attendants. All attributions were marked as being external versus internal and being stable versus unstable.

[†] The proposed typology was used to elicit data that include three dimensions: (A) patient room design and settings, (B) hospital equipment, and (C) staffing and manpower concerns.

Source: Tzeng, H. M., & Yin, C. Y. (2008b). The extrinsic risk factors for inpatient falls in hospital patient rooms. *Journal of Nursing Care Quality*, 23(3) (in press; July 2008).

Possible Solutions to Resolve the Risk Factors for Falling

In the 2008 National Patient Safety Goals for hospitals, Goal 9 was to reduce the risk of patient harm resulting from falls (Joint Commission, 2007c, 2007d). Hospitals are expected to implement a fall reduction program and include an evaluation of the effectiveness of the fall program (e.g., decreased number of falls and decreased number and severity of fall-related injuries).

As appropriate to the patient population served, a fall reduction program may include risk assessment of individual patients and periodic reassessment of individual patients and of the environment of care. A well-documented program should include risk reduction strategies, on-the-job training, involving patients and their families in fall precaution education, and a better design of the care environment. The development and implementation of transfer protocols should be included, when relevant (Joint Commission, 2007c, 2007d).

As indicated in the 2008 International Patient Safety Goals for hospitals, Goal 6 was meant to reduce the risk of patient harm resulting from falls (Joint Commission International, 2007). Hospitals are urged to develop an approach to reduce the risks of patient harm resulting from falls. A collaborative process among hospital leaders and health care providers (e.g., physicians, nurses, pharmacists, etc.) should be used to develop hospital policies and procedures that address reducing the risk of patient harm resulting from falls during hospital stays.

In addition, hospitals must implement a process for the initial assessment of patients for fall risk and reassessment of patients when indicated by a change in condition, treatment, or medications. Fall prevention measures should be implemented to reduce fall risk for those assessed to be at risk (Joint Commission International, 2007).

Based on the root cause analyses of the reported sentinel events on the falls that occurred during 1995-2005, the Joint Commission (2007a) identified five major root causes for falls and the corresponding prevention strategies (Table 5). These prevention strategies involve primarily nurses, but require support of hospital leaders in the areas of the safety of the care environment.

Table 5. The major root causes of the reported sentinel events related to patient falls and the corresponding prevention strategies for nurses

Root cause	Prevention strategy

Inadequate communication among health care providers
1. Insufficient communication and transfer of patient information between nurses and among health care providers may result in falls and aggregate patients' fall risk.
2. Omitting communication of important patient information and lacking consistent communication of the risk of falls may contribute to falls.
3. Poorly coordinated communication in patient needs for care plan revision between nurses is a concern.
	1. Nurses should help ensure effective communication.
	  1.1 A standardized approach to what needs to be communicated during hand-off communications can help make it difficult to omit and easy to include important information during shift changes.
	  1.2 During hand-off communication, nurses must have an opportunity to ask and respond to questions.
	  1.3 Communication must occur among all levels and all disciplines of health care providers and staff as needed, including administrators, administrative staff, and environment-of-care staff.
	2. Documentation in the traditional or paperless clinical records is essential and should be enhanced by a verbal report whenever possible.
	  2.1 Nurses have to ensure changes to patients' care plans as soon as the needs and approaches have been established.
	  2.2 The risk of falling can be identified in care plan documents by color-coded dot or other measures (e.g., a means of flagging records for the electronic care plans).
	  2.3 A color-coding system for patients at high risk for falls should be coordinated within the hospital (e.g., wristbands, a sign used over the head of the patient bed, on the chart, and at the entrance to the patient room).

Inadequate assessment and reassessment	1. Nurses must thoroughly assess and reassess each patient for fall risk.
	  1.1 Nurses must conduct initial assessment when admitting patients to the unit and reassess their responsible patients for fall risk as part of the nursing assessment process, as often as needed.
	  1.2 Comprehensive initial assessment and reassessment enable nurses to suggest and implement a proactive approach to fall prevention as part of the care planning and provision processes.
	  1.3 Assessment of each patient for fall risk should be part of the interdisciplinary assessment process.

Table 5. Continued

Root cause	Prevention strategy
	2. Nurses must consider all prescriptions, over-the-counter medications, supplements, medication allergies, and history of substance abuse as part of the assessment and reassessment processes.

2. Nurses must consider all prescriptions, over-the-counter medications, supplements, medication allergies, and history of substance abuse as part of the assessment and reassessment processes.

    2.1   It is essential to communicate with patients about the medications, which they are receiving or taking, and the effect noted (e.g., therapeutic, unintended, or adverse effects).

    2.2   Nurses must pay attention to the medications that may lead to delirium and increased risk of falling. These medications include but are not limited to:

        2.2.1   Alcohol

        2.2.2   Anticholinergics

        2.2.3   Antidepressants

        2.2.4   Antihypertensives

        2.2.5   Central nervous system depressants

        2.2.6   Corticosteroids

        2.2.7   Diuretics

        2.2.8   Hypoglycemics

        2.2.9   Narcotics

3. Nurses may use a combination of assessment techniques to help conduct an assessment as thoroughly as possible, including observation and communication with the patients and their family visitors.

    3.1   Simply asking patients whether help is needed in walking across the room may not provide accurate information and may not be sufficient.

    3.2   Nurses must understand patients' feelings about asking for help and their rationales of not asking for help.

    3.3   Some patients may be unaware of their need for help because of medications or a cognitive impairment or change or both.

        3.3.1   Some patients may be embarrassed about their need for help (e.g., toileting at the bathroom).

        3.3.2   Some patients may feel that they are adding additional burdens to already busy nurses.

        3.3.3   Some patients may simply have a strong desire to remain independent.

4. Nurses must assess patients according to the hospital's established criteria.

    4.1   Hospital leaders and nurses must adopt or develop appropriate assessment tools for patients at risk of falling for adult and pediatric populations. Assessment tools (e.g., the Morse Fall Scale) help raise awareness of the fall risk.

    4.2   According to the hospital's established criteria, nurses need to use the fall assessment tools several times during their shifts, if their patients become confused as a result of new medication or disruptions in daily routine.

Root cause	Prevention strategy

	5. Nurses must inform family members about factors that increase the risk of falling and inquire about the presence of any such factors. Patients and their families need to be educated about fall prevention strategies.
	  5.1 For example, physical therapists may provide techniques to improve strength and balance, and nurses can reinforce this education.
	6. Nurses need to reassess patients regularly to detect increased fall risk and ensure success of interventions.
	  6.1 Situations that may create the need for vigilant monitoring include but are not limited to:
	    6.1.1 Changes in medications (e.g., possible new side effects)
	    6.1.2 Changes in behaviors indicating impaired judgment
	    6.1.3 Changes in the laboratory values
	    6.1.4 After patients have had a procedure involving anesthesia
	7. Nurses should increase the awareness of the diseases processes related to dementia and provide appropriate care to patients with dementia and those experiencing sundowning.
	  7.1 In unfamiliar surroundings (e.g., being hospitalized), patients with dementia may experience an increased level of confusion at dusk and during the night (also called sundowning).
	  7.2 Sundowning may also occur in patients without dementia.
	  7.3 Nurses may need to justify their patients' care plans if there is a need to increase fall prevention measures at this time of day.

Inadequate care planning and provision	1. Nurses should tailor fall prevention strategies to the patients' unique needs.
	  1.1 Depending on the design and equipment available in hospitals, nurses may adopt any of the following fall prevention strategies, including:
	    1.1.1 Placing patient beds in the lowest position
	    1.1.2 Offering walkers or assistance devices as needed
	    1.1.3 Placing a large mat beside the bed
	    1.1.4 Setting up fall alarms on patients' beds or chairs (also called pressure alarms)
	    1.1.5 Having patients wear hip protectors to prevent hip factures
	  1.2 Nurses may need to offer frequent toileting for cognitively impaired patients and those who are taking diuretics. Nurses may suggest that physicians adjust medications, if needed.
	2. Nurses should ensure providing timeliness of care.
	  2.1 Anticipation of patients' needs is one of the keys to timely care (e.g., the needs for toileting, food and liquid, or pain control medication).
	  2.2 One strategic approach is to decrease the amount of time taken to answer call lights.
	3. Nurses should eliminate restraint use when possible.
	  3.1 The use of restraints will not reduce fall incidences and may increase the risk of harm or causing harm.

Table 5. Continued

Root cause	Prevention strategy
	3.2 The use of restraints may also cause adverse psychological and emotional effects (e.g., sensory deprivation, loss of dignity, feeling of dependence, frustration, and embarrassment).
	3.3 However, a half rail in the up position at the head of the bed may help prevent patients rolling out of the bed.
Inadequate staffing, orientation, training, and supervision	1. Nurses need to understand the physiology of falls. A fall is often the result of coming together of the effects of multiple minor challenges to the delicate balance that keep patients upright.
	2. Nurses must be familiar with identified risk factors for falling.
	3. Nurses must be competent to address population- and age-specific patient needs and identify conditions that place people at risk for falling, including cognitive impairments and gait instability.
	4. Nurses must know which patient is at risk for falling and implement the fall prevention program as needed.
	4.1 Thorough assessment and reassessment and the use of appropriate intervention techniques are important in identifying patients at risk of falling.
	4.2 Effective communication between nurses on patients' fall risks, fall prevention strategies, and changes in their conditions are essential to fall prevention.
	5. Nurses need to inform their supervisor about the unsafe staffing situations. Without adequate staffing, patients may receive less assistance when needed.
	6. Nursing leaders may consider the use of sitters as one of the alternatives for patients who need constant observation.
	6.1 Sitters can provide one-to-one observation for high-risk patients.
	6.2 Nurses should retain the responsibility for ongoing assessment.
Unsafe environment of care	1. Hospital leaders must ensure planning for a safe environment.
	1.1 Safety efforts should include having trained staff make regular environmental rounds to check for possible hazards that may contribute to falls.
	1.2 Hospitals should institute an environmental checklist to identify fall risks.
	2. Nurses have a key role in ensuring a safe care environment, including the aspects of:
	2.1 Appropriate temperature in patient rooms
	2.2 Being free of odors and having adequate air ventilation in patient rooms
	2.3 Having an acceptable noise level in patient rooms
	2.4 Lighting in patient rooms and hallways sufficient without glaring
	2.5 Floors in patient rooms and hallways clean, dry, and free of clutter
	2.6 Patient rooms free of hazards (e.g., electrical cords out of the way)
	2.7 Bedside tables (also called over-bed tables) available and within reach of the patients

Root cause	Prevention strategy
	2.8 Call light system in working order and accessible to each patient
	2.9 Bed wheels locked
	2.10 Closet and shelf space in patient rooms accessible to patients
	2.11 Patients' personal items within reach
	2.12 The hand rails or grab bars present and secure in bathroom
	2.13 Equipment in good repair (e.g., lift device, wheelchairs, or walkers)
	3. Nurses should encourage patients to use nonskid footwear.
	4. Nurses need to be particularly alert to unsafe bathrooms (e.g., wet floor).
	5. Be trained and knowledgeable about the hospital's preventive maintenance program and vigilant about the equipment needs and concerns.
	5.1 Nurses need to be familiar with how to check for the safety considerations of the equipment used by patients.
	5.2 If needed, nurses must notify their supervisors or appropriate personnel for maintenance of unsafe equipment.

Source: Joint Commission (2007a). Preventing falls. In R. A. Porché, Jr. (Ed.), *Front line of defense: The role of nurses in preventing sentinel events* (2nd ed., pp. 73-86). Oakbrook Terrace, IL: Joint Commission.

In one of our previous studies (Tzeng & Yin, 2008c), we also explored possible ways to address the extrinsic risk factors for inpatient falls in patient rooms, based on interviews with nurses. Table 6 compares the intervention strategies to prevent inpatient falls as identified by the Joint Commission (left column) and those abstracted from the nurse interview transcriptions (right column). The five major dimensions of fall causes as identified by the Joint Commission (2005b) were used to structure the content analysis findings. Twenty-four solutions were identified from the nurse interviews.

Table 6. A comparison between the intervention strategies toward preventing patient falls as identified by the Joint Commission and the ones abstracted from the nurse interview transcriptions

Five dimensions of fall causes as identified by the Joint Commission intervention strategy toward preventing patient falls	
Joint Commission's perspective	Nurses' perspective
A. Inadequate communication	
1. Ensure continual observation of the patient.	1. **Patient assignments for each nurse should be in fairly close proximity if possible:** "Maybe we should group patients at high risk for falls closer together or group work assignments closer together so responsible nurses can hear the bed alarms."
	2. **Use sitters to provide constant observation for high-risk patients.**
	3. **Use family visitors to care for confused patients:** "If you have elderly patients who are confused easily and if they had a family member in there at all times or most of the time, they would not be as confused because they would have someone there who frequently orients them and knows their baseline."

Table 6. Continued

Five dimensions of fall causes as identified by the Joint Commission intervention strategy toward preventing patient falls	
Joint Commission's perspective	**Nurses' perspective**
2. Ensure care is provided in a coordinated manner.	1. **Share responsibility between nurses and nursing attendants to ensure continual observation:** "It's difficult to implement a timed observation plan and a timed toileting plan." "It's the nurse's responsibility to make rounds to make sure that the patients are doing okay and their needs are met." "When some patients are on fall precaution, nurses stress and literally beat into patients' heads to use the call light when they want to go to the bathroom. Patients use the call light, and they are waiting 5, 10, 15 minutes and nobody comes in. These patients are going to get up and go to the bathroom by themselves. I would not blame them. I mean, who is going to wait that long for somebody to come answer the call light and take them to the bathroom?"
3. Communicate changes in the patient's condition and behaviors during shift changes.	1. **Improve information hand-off about the conditions of the high-risk patients among sitters between shifts:** "It's the nurses' and nursing attendants' responsibility to orient sitters."
4. Reassess and revise the care plan of the patient who is at risk for falls, if needed.	—
B. Inadequate staff orientation and training	
1. All caregivers must be competent in addressing age-specific care needs and identifying cognitive impairments, gait instability, or other conditions that place patients at risk for falls.	—
2. All staff must be competent in fall reduction program elements, if any, before providing care to recipients who are at risk for falls.	—
C. Inadequate assessment and reassessment	
1. Use observation techniques and communicate with the individual or family for specific health concerns. Educate the patient and family visitors about fall prevention strategies.	1. **Let patients know the importance of calling nurses for help:** "To prevent falls, I let patients know the importance of calling for assistance. I tell my patients: Please bother me, that's my job and you should ask for my help so that I can help you get well. Then, you can go home quicker and do what you would like to do." "I understand that you are used to doing everything by yourself, but if you fall you could suffer greater injuries than what you were originally here for. You could potentially be here for a longer time." 2. **Fall precaution programs and related care plans should be implemented thoroughly:** "I've heard some nurses tell the patients that they are on fall precaution. Nurses put a sign over the bed. What this means is the patient can't get out of bed without help. They put the wrist band on, slap the brochure on the desk, and then they walk out. Fall precaution is being done as a formality."

Five dimensions of fall causes as identified by the Joint Commission intervention strategy toward preventing patient falls	
Joint Commission's perspective	**Nurses' perspective**
	3. **Request family visitors to accompany their high-risk patient:** "We explain to the families that this patient might get up out of the bed and might fall. We can't get anybody to sit with them or we would. Could you possibly come in? Or, is there any family member who could sit with the patient at least half the night? Or any portion of the night? And most families are very cooperative." "I think the families are there more just to make sure things are getting done."
2. Develop a care plan to address the specific condition of the patient.	—
3. Increase caregivers' awareness of processes related to dementia and provide appropriate care to patients with dementia.	—
4. Allow caregivers sufficient time to assess and reassess a patient's risk of falling.	—
5. Consider all prescription and over-the-counter drugs and supplements the patient is taking.	—
6. Frequently monitor the patient's condition for changes.	—
7. Thoroughly assess and reassess a patient's risk of falling.	—
8. Consider the physical environment and all the possibilities of a fall.	—
D. Unsafe environment of care	
1. Improve environmental assessment by staff.	1. **Use low beds:** "As I know, the beds in the children's hospital are about a foot to a foot and half off the ground. Low beds would be very useful in the adult hospital." "We hope that the bed is as low as the floor." "Most falls are by the bedside." 2. **Use the bed pressure alarm as needed.** 3. **The bed pressure alarm system needs improvement in sending alerts to nurses:** "It's hard to hear the beeping sound from the bed alarm when it goes off." "If the beds are equipped with alarms and if we could tie bed alarms into our pagers, we might be able to get there fast enough to prevent a fall." "The bed pressure alarm is not connected to the responsible nurse's and nursing attendant's pagers and is not connected to any blinking lights, just sound; it should be connected to pagers or call light signals." "Another nearby hospital connects call lights with speakers into staff's wireless phones so nurses or nurse aides can talk to patients before entering patient rooms."

Table 6. Continued

Five dimensions of fall causes as identified by the Joint Commission intervention strategy toward preventing patient falls	
Joint Commission's perspective	**Nurses' perspective**
	4. **Install grab bars or hand rails in patient rooms, bathrooms, and hallways for patients to hold onto:** "It might be wise as well to have a handlebar-like type thing along all the sides of the rooms. Inside the rooms right along the main walkway just have a handlebar that somebody can just hold onto as they walk." "A lot of times, people fall because of losing balance and not having something to hold onto like a grab bar or walker." 5. **Provide needed hospital equipment (e.g., walkers and canes):** "No walker or cane is readily available in the units. Patients can bring their own walker or cane." "The portable lifting system is not readily available in the unit when it is needed." 6. **Need better designed hospital equipment (e.g., IV poles, wheelchairs, bedside commodes, and bedside chairs):** "An IV pole that is designed to better manage all the tubing, oxygen tank, and the Foley or draining bag may be helpful. When patients are in the bathroom, if they are on oxygen, they may not have it with them in the bathroom. They could be oxygen deprived at that point and losing a lot of energy because of that. They do not always have a long enough line, and they do not always ask for a tank. And some think they can make it on their own without an oxygen tank. A long enough line for oxygen or another option is needed to decrease related falls in the bathroom." "The arms of some wheelchairs come out; this type of wheelchair is more convenient for transferring patients." "When using the bedside commode, someone has to keep the patient company and prevent slipping off the commode." "We must use the right size bedside commode for big patients." "Chair depth, difficulty for ingress and egress, too low." "Patients may fall back in the chairs." "Some chairs may be comfortable for families, but can also be hard for patients to sit on." "The bedside chairs lack stability and need rubber stoppers on legs to give legs some type of traction to prevent falls." 7. **Redesign patient rooms: Shorten the travel distance between the patient bed and the bathroom in semiprivate rooms:** "A lot of falls occur between the bed further from the bathroom and the bathroom." "To prevent this, we put the patients at high risk of falling by the bathroom, because they have two beds, one bed is by the bathroom, one is by the window." "The bathroom should be between the two beds for semiprivate rooms; on the wall close to the footboard." "If possible, semiprivate rooms should have two bathrooms, one for each patient." 8. **Use the ceiling lift system to prevent inpatient falls:** "The ceiling lift system should go from the patient bed to the bathroom." "Having review sessions about how to use hospital equipment, like the ceiling lift system, may increase the use frequency and safe transfers, and result in fewer personnel needs."
2. Have specially trained staff make regular environmental rounds to check for possible hazards.	—
3. Ensure that the temperature of patient rooms is comfortable.	—
4. Ensure that the ventilation of patient rooms is adequate.	—

Five dimensions of fall causes as identified by the Joint Commission intervention strategy toward preventing patient falls	
Joint Commission's perspective	**Nurses' perspective**
5. Ensure that the bedside table is available to the patient and the bed wheels are locked.	—
6. Ensure that closet and shelf spaces are accessible.	—
7. Ensure that the noise level is acceptable.	—
8. Ensure that the equipment (e.g., walkers, wheelchairs, lift devices) are in good repair.	—
9. Ensure that lighting is adequate and minimizes glare.	1. **Improve the floor and night lighting system:** "The control panel for night lights is located next to the door. Hard to tell and recognized by patients or families." "Nurses working night shifts should turn on the night lights as a routine. Maybe we need to use an autonomic lighting system that will turn on when the environment is too dark." 2. **Improve the maintenance of floor and night lights:** "Broken night light bulbs are not replaced in time."
10. Ensure that hand rails in the toilet area are present and secure.	1. **Improve bathroom setting and design:** "Grab bars next to the toilets lack traction and are not sufficient to generate pushup force to get off the toilet." "Shower seats and floors are slippery and lack traction." "Bathrooms need some space or shelf to store unneeded or needed equipment, like toilet hats and graduated cylinders to measure urine." "I think our toilets are not handicap toilets at all. They are very low. When I actually sit on the toilet, my knees sit at less than a 90° angle. Some of our taller patients have the same problem. So, if our toilets were more of a handicap-type toilet, it may be easier, especially for the elderly, to get up. We're using a bedside commode to put that over the toilet seat, so that our patients don't have to sit down as far." "Raised toilet seats are not readily available." "We need autonomic sinks with preadjusted water temperature and volume." 2. **Bathroom housekeeping:** "Bathrooms need to be cleaned after use as soon as possible." 3. **Better diaper design to ease taking off and pulling up:** "The diapers we are using are difficult to take off and pull up. Patients have hard time taking off the diaper and keeping their balance without assistance before using toilet."
11. Ensure that the call light system is in working order and accessible to the patient.	1. **Improve the call light system:** "Visually impaired patients cannot locate the call light button on the control panel." "After call lights go off, there is no signal to tell whether a nurse or nursing attendant is in a specific patient room." "I hope there will be a sensor and light by the patient room door to indicate whether any staff is in the rooms." "The call light system should also have the talk function from the nurses' station or the individual nurse's or attendant's phone set or pager."
12. Ensure that the floors of patient rooms are free of clutter and hazards, clean and dry, and free of odors.	1. **Increase room space and storage space to prevent tripping:** "Private rooms are too small, and semiprivate patient rooms are too crowded. More room space is needed for private rooms." "Unneeded equipment is often left in the rooms (e.g., bedside commode and extra IV poles, extra chairs). This equipment should be removed from patient rooms." "Each patient room needs more storage space for patients' belongings."

Table 6. Continued

Five dimensions of fall causes as identified by the Joint Commission intervention strategy toward preventing patient falls	
Joint Commission's perspective	**Nurses' perspective**
E. Inadequate care planning and provision	
1. Perform a thorough medication assessment of each individual patient on admission, and document medication allergies and drug reactions that may increase fall risk.	—
2. Ensure a multifactorial, interdisciplinary approach to assessment and reassessment.	—
3. Communicate and document the patient's condition across the continuum of care and disciplines as a team approach.	1. **Improve teamwork and responsibility sharing between nurses and nursing attendants:** "Aides think that nurses are lazy and nurses think it's an aide's job specifically to answer the call lights. No teamwork between nurses and nurse aides as far as I can tell." "It's the nurses' responsibility to go and make rounds to make sure that the patients are doing okay and their needs are met. Nurses should not depend on the sitter."
4. Assess the condition of all walking aids and equipment.	—
5. Fall reduction strategies should be highly individualized.	—

Sources: Joint Commission (2005b). Strategies for addressing the root causes of falls. In I. J. Smith (Ed.), *Reducing the risk of falls in your health care organization* (pp. 29-50). Oakbrook Terrace, IL: Joint Commission. Tzeng, H. M., & Yin, C. Y. (2008c). Nurses' solutions to prevent inpatient falls in hospital patient rooms. *Nursing Economics, 26*(3) (in press; May 2008).

Previous studies also showed that the height of the hospital patient beds may be an overlooked cause of patient falls (Tzeng & Yin, 2006, 2008a). As shown in a study conducted in a medical center located in Michigan (Tzeng & Yin, 2008a), nurses have a tendency to keep patient beds higher during the weekend than on weekdays. It is possible that in an effort to prevent high-risk patients from falling, nursing staff consciously or unconsciously kept the beds in higher positions, possibly as a means of restraint, which does not require a physician's order (Tzeng & Yin, 2008a).

If the patient beds are too high for the patients even when the beds are in the lowest position, nurses may teach patients to use the prone position (Figure 1) to get out of bed, instead of using the traditional sitting-standing position (Figure 2). Adopting the prone position to get out of bed (Figure 1) may lead to fewer bed-related falls and fall-related injuries. The prone position may not be appropriate for patients who recently had major chest or abdominal surgery and for patients with other conditions (Tzeng & Yin, 2008d).

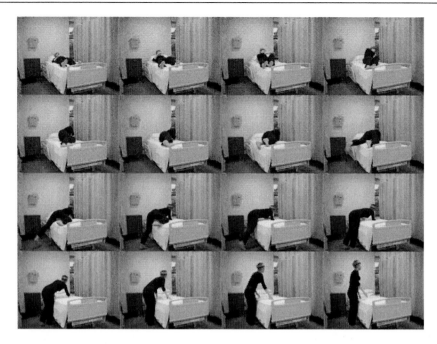

Figure 1. The prone position was used to get out of the bed. The bed was 27 inches in height and 34.5 inches in width. Examine the images from the first row, far left upper corner (the first image) to the first row, far right upper corner, the second row far left image to the second row far right image, the third row far left one to the third row far right one, then the fourth row far left one to the fourth row far right one (the last image). The subject in these images is 5 feet 6 inches tall.

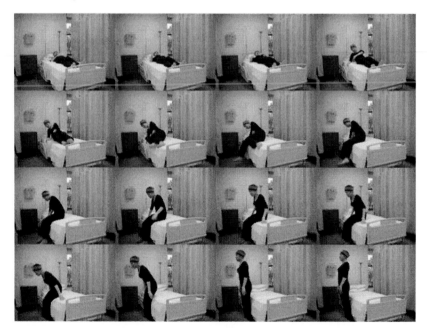

Figure 2. The traditional sitting-standing position was used to get out of the bed. The patient bed was 27 inches in height and 34.5 inches in width. Examine the images from the first row, far left upper corner (the first image) to the first row, far right upper corner, the second row far left image to the second row far right image, the third row far left one to the third- ow far right one, then the fourth row far left one to the fourth row far right one (the last image). The subject in these images is 5 feet 6 inches tall.

Family involvement in inpatient care is increasingly emphasized to provide safe and error-free care (Remen, 2006). As indicated in the National Patient Safety Goals for 2008, the Joint Commission (2007c) emphasized the need to define and communicate ways for patients and their families to report concerns about safety and encourage them to do so. As the first step, hospitals and clinicians should encourage family members to visit their loved ones frequently. However, the qualifications and roles of family members and the economic burdens to families have not been well addressed (Tzeng & Yin, 2007).

We counted the number of visitors for each patient on two weekdays and two weekend days at three predetermined time points on each day in two medical units and one pediatric unit of a Michigan hospital. We found that family involvement is popular for hospitalized sick children (about 70%). Only about 24% of adult patients had at least one family visitor, however. Staying in a private room did not correlate with having more frequent family visits than staying in a semiprivate room. We also found that family members may not always be able to assist with inpatient care and cannot effectively prevent inpatient falls. More than 35% of the family members who were watching patients were unable to prevent falls (Tzeng & Yin, 2007; Tzeng et al., 2007). In other words, regardless of having constant observation from family visitors or sitters, nurses must assume the primary responsibility for fall prevention because preventing inpatient falls demands professional skills and knowledge.

Critical Tips to Prevent Inpatient Falls and Fall-related Injuries

Promoting a Safe Care Environment

Hospitals, indeed, have been improving the settings of patient rooms. In the process of hospital accreditation, hospitals are expected to provide a safe, supportive, and effective environment for patients, their families, health care providers, and other staff members and individuals. As indicated in the section of Management of the Environment of Care *2008 Comprehensive Accreditation Manual for Hospitals: The Official Handbook*, it is important for hospitals to ensure that the physical care environment is functional and promotes healing and caring (Joint Commission, 2007d).

For example, the interior spaces should include closet and drawer space for storing personal property and other items provided for use by patients. The furnishings and equipment should be maintained to be safe and in good repair and reflect the patients' needs and levels of ability. Areas used by patients should be safe, clean, functional, and comfortable. Lighting should be suitable for care and treatment. Ventilation systems must provide for acceptable levels of temperature and humidity and eliminate odors (Joint Commission, 2007d).

Eliminating the Extrinsic Risk Factors to Falls

Crucially, a safety-driven design with a goal to prevent inpatient fall-related injuries should be a hospital design principle by, for example, eliminating the extrinsic risk factors associated with inpatient falls. Nurses must work with their managers to eliminate the extrinsic risk factors for falls. As indicated in Table 6 (Tzeng & Yin, 2008c), the identified solutions from nurse interview transcripts, as empirical evidence, may help nursing leaders and nurses form the rationale to have their hospital leaders accept their ideas.

Some of these intervention ideas indicated in Table 6 seem obvious. However, hospital leaders seem to fail to notice and, if they notice, fail to address these identified extrinsic risk factors for falls (e.g., the design of hospital patient bed and bathroom). We believe that ensuring the safety of the care environment is the most urgent strategy to prevent falls and that hospital and nursing leaders can work together to decrease falls and fall-related injuries. A safe care environment should be designed from the patients' viewpoint and for promoting safe hospital stays.

We had an opportunity to hear a nursing professor's hospitalization experience. We visited her at her home, the third day after her discharge, just after Christmas in 2007. She shared her experience and insights after being hospitalized in a medical center for 7 days for acute medical problems. This was her first hospitalization. She claimed that she was unable to lower her electric bed to safely get out of the bed, because she was unable to reach the control button, which was located at the footboard.

She told us that the bed was too narrow for her to reposition herself and so uncomfortable that she sweated heavily all the time. Also, she was so desperate that she was unable to lower the bed rails herself, while lying on the bed. She felt restrained and powerless to maintain her autonomy and safety. As a recently hospitalized patient, she expressed her desperate feelings and realized that most of the inpatients may also struggle with the same issues of the poor design of hospital patient beds. About 2 weeks later, she told us that this hospitalization experience was so awful that she even did not want to recall it.

Often, intervention strategies that have been implemented or suggested in inpatient settings seem to overlook clinical nurses' perspectives toward interventions to prevent falls. To guarantee successful implementation, the fall prevention programs must be endorsed by both hospitals and nurses. Table 7 lists our suggestions and critical tips to prevent inpatient falls for hospital and nurse leaders and nurses. Table 8 includes our suggestions and critical tips to prevent inpatient falls for our patients, their families, and patient advocates.

We want to save our bones (no fractures). We must say no to inpatient falls and fall-related injuries.

Table 7. Preventing falls: Critical tips for hospital and nursing leaders, and nurses, who work in acute inpatient care units

Dimension	Tip

The safety of the care environment	1. The design of patient rooms should be as close to a home environment as possible, including beds and mattress, chairs, toilet, and shower areas.
	   1.1 When designing the layout of a patient room, hospitals must put themselves in patients' positions and assume that hospitalized patients are frail.
	2. Hospitals should purchase and use only low patient beds. Health care providers should ensure that patient beds are in low position to prevent fall-related injuries.
	   2.1 Hospitals should purchase patient beds that can go as low as possible. Hospital patient beds should be no higher than home beds.
	   2.2 The height of the patient beds at the lowest position, including the mattress, should not be higher than 6-8 inches from the floor to the top of the mattress.
	   2.3 The patient beds should allow patients to control the overall height of the beds, though only the lowering down button is suggested. The control panel should be reachable by patients themselves.
	   2.4 The height of beds should be maintained in the lowest position. Nurses and physicians may raise the patient bed when delivering care or treatment or doing procedures. After completing the tasks, nurses and physicians must lower down the bed to its lowest position.
	3. Hospitals should purchase and use patient beds with a safe width.
	   3.1 A standard patient bed should be 39-45 inches (3.5 feet) in width (being comparable to the twin/single size for home beds; 39 inches) to avoid patients falling off the beds when turning.
	      3.1.1 The size of the hospital beds available in the US market is 34.5-36 inches in width. We suggest that a safe bed width of 45 inches is needed to allow patients to turn freely without fear.
	      3.1.2 Fear of falling may result in decreased self-initiated repositioning or changing positions, which may further lead to dysfunction and an increased possibility of developing pressure ulcers.
	4. Hospitals should install continuous grab bars or hand rails in patient rooms, bathrooms, and hallways for patients to hold onto.
	   4.1 Hospitals should install continuous grab bars on every wall of the patient room to provide supports for patients when they travel from the bed to the bathroom or on the hallway.
	   4.2 These grab bars or hand rails should be able to bear the weight of a patient up to 400 pounds.
	   4.3 High-low horizontal grab bars or hand rails should be mounted with heights of 26 inches (low) and 36 inches (high) above the floor in all areas commonly used by patients.
	   4.4 The grab bars in bathrooms should have special considerations.
	      4.4.1 The grab bars surrounding the toilet should be sufficient enough to generate push-up force for getting off the toilet.
	      4.4.2 The grab bars in the shower areas should not be slippery when they are wet and soapy.
	5. Hospitals should improve the floor and night lighting systems with a routine maintenance plan.
	6. Hospitals should provide free assistive devices for patients to use in a timely fashion, as appropriate (including wheelchairs, walkers, and canes).
	7. Nurses must ensure that the patient room and the bathroom within the patient room are clean, dry, and tidy.
	8. Bed rails are considered as restraint use. Nurses should use bed rails according to the hospital's policies related to restraint use.

Dimension	Tip

Communication to patients and families	1. When communicating with patients, nurses must put themselves in patients' positions. If a family member is willing to assist in inpatient care (e.g., transferring and ambulating), the responsible nurse must provide educational information about fall prevention to both families and patients.
	    1.1 Nurses must communicate or educate patients and their families in an understandable format and using the language preferred.
	    1.2 Nurses must repeat the educational information as often as needed because family visitors may take turns.
	2. Hospitals should provide interpreters to assist with the education or translate materials.

Staffing	1. Patient assignments for each nurse should be in fairly close proximity if possible.
	2. Nurses need to inform their supervisor about the unsafe staffing situations.
	    2.1 Without adequate staffing, patients may receive less assistance when needed.
	    2.2 However, it is not suggested to use sitters or family members (to provide constant observation) to replace or supplement nurses' functions in monitoring.
	3. Nurses should tailor fall prevention strategies to the patients' unique needs. Nurses may need to offer frequent toileting for cognitively impaired patients and patients who are taking diuretics.
	4. Nurses should ensure providing timeliness of care. Anticipation of patients' needs is one of the keys to timely care (e.g., the needs for toileting, food and liquid, or pain control medication). One strategic approach is to decrease the amount of time taken to answer call lights.
	5. Hospitals should use the response time for answering call lights as one of the nursing care quality measures to ensure the promptness of meeting patients' needs.

Communication among health care providers	1. Nursing leaders and nurses should help ensure effective communication, especially on the conditions of the patients at high risk for falls, when the staff shifts change.
	    1.1 A standardized approach to what needs to be communicated during hand-off communications can help make it difficult to omit and easy to include important information during shift changes.
	    1.2 During hand-off communication, nurses must have an opportunity to ask and respond to questions.
	2. Documentation in the traditional or paperless clinical records is essential and should be enhanced by a verbal report whenever possible.

Table 8. Preventing falls: Critical tips for patients and families

Dimension	Tip

Know our physical capability	1. We must know our own limits and do not bully beyond our physical capability.
	    1.1 We must ask our nurses (at least once a day) what they think about our physical limit. Our nurses may have a very different perspective from ours. When we are hospitalized, we are sick and can be very frail.
	    1.2 We may not aware that we may need help, for example, to use the bathroom, because of our medications or a cognitive change.
	    1.3 We may be embarrassed about our need for help.
	    1.4 We may feel that we are creating an additional burden to already busy nurses.
	    1.5 We may simply have a strong desire to remain independent.
	    1.6 If our physical condition does not allow us to move without assistance, we must use call lights and wait for assistance.
	    1.7

Table 8. Continued

Dimension	Tip

	2. We must tell our nurses, if we sense any changes in our condition as related to new medications, treatments, or procedures (e.g., postoperatively).
	 3. Families should know their own limits in helping their hospitalized loved ones.
	     3.1 Assisting patients requires not just strength but also skills to safely transfer patients and prevent hurting ourselves in the process (e.g., back injury).
	     3.2 When patients have a need to move or make a transfer, we must call nurses for assistance. Families may participate in transferring patients, if appropriate.

Demand a safe care environment	1. Our patient room is an unfamiliar environment and is not our home. We have to be extremely cautious when getting out of bed, using the toilet, and taking a shower. 1.1 For example, our bed may be too high and too narrow for us. We must be especially cautious when moving around after dark and when waking up in the middle of night for toileting. 2. We should make a request to our nurses for housekeeping. We should have a clean and dry patient room and bathroom. 3. We must ask our nurses to remove unused equipment from our patient room. 4. We should ask for safer and steadier furniture (e.g., chairs and beds) and equipment (e.g., bedside commodes and wheelchairs), if needed.

Bring our own assistive devices to be used during hospitalization	1. We should always bring our own assistive devices and use our own assistive devices during hospitalization (e.g., walkers, and canes).
	     1.1 Not all the hospital-provided equipment suits our needs.
	     1.2 We should bring the ones we have been using and that have been adjusted to meet our needs.
	 2. We should always bring our own nonslip footwear, when admitted to the hospital. Most hospitals do not provide nonslip footwear.
	 3. We should bring our own glasses for nearsightedness or farsightedness. We need to see well to avoid falling.

References

Bates, D. W., Pruess, K., Souney, P., & Platt, R. (1995). Serious falls in hospitalized patients: correlates and resource utilization. *American Journal of Medicine, 99*(2), 137-143.

Boswell, D. J., Ramsey, J., Smith, M. A., & Wagers, B. (2001). The cost-effectiveness of a patient-sitter program in an acute care hospital: A test of the impact of sitters on the incidence of falls and patient satisfaction. *Quality Management in Health Care, 10*(1), 10-16.

Granek, E., Baker, S. P., Abbey, H., Robinson, E., Myers, A. H., Samkoff, J. S., & Klein, L. E. (1987). Medications and diagnoses in relation to falls in a long-term care facility. *Journal of the American Geriatrics Society, 35*(6), 503-511.

Henry J. Kaiser Family Foundation (2007). Trends in health care costs and spending. Available at: http://www.kff.org/insurance/7692.cfm (accessed October 27, 2007).

Hignett, S., & Masud, T. (2006). A review of environmental hazards associated with in-patient falls. *Ergonomics, 49*(5), 605-616.

Hitcho, E. B., Krauss, M. J., Birge, S., Claiborne Dunagan, W., Fischer, I., Johnson, S., Nast, P. A., Costantinou, E., & Fraser, V. J. (2004). Characteristics and circumstances of falls in a hospital setting: A prospective analysis. *Journal of General Internal Medicine, 19*(7), 732-329.

Institute for Healthcare Improvement (2007). 2007 progress report: Status quon't. Available at: http://www.ihi.org/NR/rdonlyres/858C562A-A535-4344-9573-3AACD1E01CA1/0/ 2007ProgressReportFINAL.pdf (accessed November 26, 2007).

Joint Commission (2005a). Defining the problem of falls. In I. J. Smith (Ed.), *Reducing the risk of falls in your health care organization* (pp. 13-27). Oakbrook Terrace, IL: Joint Commission.

Joint Commission (2005b). Strategies for addressing the root causes of falls. In I. J. Smith (Ed.), *Reducing the risk of falls in your health care organization* (pp. 29-50). Oakbrook Terrace, IL: Joint Commission.

Joint Commission (2006a). Goal 9: Reduce the risk of patient harm result from falls. In A. Grayson. (Ed.), *Meeting the Joint Commission's 2007 National Patient Safety Goals* (pp. 75-94). Oakbrook Terrace, IL: Joint Commission.

Joint Commission (2007a). Preventing falls. In R. A. Porché, Jr. (Ed.), *Front line of defense: The role of nurses in preventing sentinel events* (2nd ed., pp. 73-86). Oakbrook Terrace, IL: Joint Commission.

Joint Commission (2007b). *Patient safety pocket guide* (2nd ed., pp. 1-14). Oakbrook Terrace, IL: Joint Commission.

Joint Commission (2007c). 2008 National Patient Safety Goals: Hospital programs (manual chapter). Available at: http://www.jointcommission.org/NR/rdonlyres/82B717D8-B16A-4442-AD00-CE3188C2F00A/0/08_HAP_NPSGs_Master.pdf (accessed November 26, 2007)

Joint Commission (2007d). *2008 Comprehensive accreditation manual for hospitals: The official handbook.* Oakbrook Terrace, IL: Joint Commission Resources.

Joint Commission International (2007). *Joint Commission International accreditation standards for hospitals* (3rd ed.). Oakbrook Terrace, Illinois: Joint Commission International.

Krauss, M. J., Nguyen, S. L., Dunagan, W. C., Birge, S., Costantinou, E., Johnson, S., Caleca, B., & Fraser, V. J. (2007). Circumstances of patient falls and injuries in 9 hospitals in a midwestern healthcare system. *Infection Control and Hospital Epidemiology, 28*(5), 544-550.

Morse, J. M. (1997). *Preventing patient falls.* Thousand Oaks, CA: Sage Publicaitons.

Reiling, J. (2006). Safe design of healthcare facilities. *Quality & Safety in Health Care, 15*(Suppl 1), i34-i40.

Remen, R. N. (2006). Including your patients in a culture of safety. In M. McGreevey (Ed.), *Patients as partners: How to involve patients and families in their own care* (pp. 7-31). Oakbrook Terrace, IL: Joint Commission.

Tzeng, H. M., & Yin, C. Y. (2006). The staff-working height and the designing-regulation height for patient beds as possible causes of patient falls. *Nursing Economics, 24*(6), 323-327, 279.

Tzeng, H. M., & Yin, C. Y. (2007). Using family visitors, sitters, or volunteers to prevent inpatient falls. *Journal of Nursing Administration, 37*(7-8), 329-334.

Tzeng, H. M., & Yin, C.Y. (2008a). Heights of occupied patient beds: A possible risk factor to in-patient falls. *Journal of Clinical Nursing* (in press; 2008).

Tzeng, H. M., & Yin, C. Y. (2008b). The extrinsic risk factors for inpatient falls in hospital patient rooms. *Journal of Nursing Care Quality, 23*(3) (in press; July 2008).

Tzeng, H. M., & Yin, C. Y. (2008c). Nurses' solutions to prevent inpatient falls in hospital patient rooms. *Nursing Economics, 26*(3) (in press; May/June 2008).

Tzeng, H. M., & Yin, C. Y. (2008d). Innovation in patient safety: A new task design in reducing patient falls. *Journal of Nursing Care Quality, 23*(1), 34-42.

Tzeng, H. M., Yin, C. Y., Tsai, S. L., Lin, S., & Yin, T. J. (2007). Patient falls and open visiting hours: A case study in a Taiwanese medical center. *Journal of Nursing Care Quality, 22*(2), 145-151.

US Department of Labor Bureau of Labor Statistics (2007). Consumer price indexes: Inflation calculator. Available at: http://www.bls.gov/cpi/#data (accessed October 27, 2007).

Weiner, B. (1986). *An attributional theory of motivation and emotion*. New York, NY: Springer-Verlag New York.

Weiner, B., Frieze, I. H., Kukla, A., Reed, L., Rest, S., & Rosenbaun, R. M. (1979). *Perceiving the causes of success and failure*. Morristown, NJ: General Learning Press.

Chapter 2.2.

Health Care-associated Pressure Ulcers

Learning from a Legal Case Summary

After several fainting episodes, Mrs. X, a 78-year-old woman, was admitted to the intensive care unit at Hospital A on January 7, 1999. Mrs. X had been suffering from multiple health problems, including atrial fibrillation, anemia, gastrointestinal bleeding, and hematuria. Ten days after staying in the intensive care unit of Hospital A, Mrs. X developed a bedsore on her coccyx area. This bedsore expanded ultimately into a wound measuring 6 by 10 inches.

On February 17, 1999, Mrs. X was transferred to a rehabilitation facility and her bedsore began to heal. She died on March 30, 1999. The death certificate attributed the cause of death to respiratory failure. However, no autopsy was performed.

An expert testified that Mrs. X was not repositioned, was not properly hydrated, and did not have proper nutrition based on the fact that she lost 30 pounds in 1 month. The treatment for the wound was improper. Another expert indicated that the cause of Mrs. X's death was sepsis arising from the bedsore; blood tests revealed a certain bacteria in the Mrs. X's bloodstream.

The trial judge found negligence and omissions by the nursing staff and physicians of Hospital A in failing to adequately turn Mrs. X and in failing to provide proper hydration. These two negligent acts were immediate contributing causes of the skin breakdown, bedsore development, and the death of Mrs. X.

Due to the size of the wound and the pain and suffering of Mrs. X, the court awarded Mrs. X's estate $1,000,000 in damages. The fault was apportioned to 50% at Hospital A and 50% at the responsible physicians.

Source: NexisLexis®Academic: Federal & State Cases (Case number: 2004-CA-02208-SCT; September 13, 2007, decided) (accessed on December 3, 2007).

A Success Story

Francis Medical Center in Peoria, Illinois implemented a comprehensive pressure ulcer prevention program, 'Save-Our-Skin.' Save-Our-Skin combined three efforts, including:

1. Training programs with visual reminders (e.g., stickers on the charts of at-risk patients)
2. Regular reporting incidents
3. Sharing of incidence data across inpatient adult units about the prevalence of pressure ulcers

A Save-Our-Skin skin care team met monthly with the unit manager of every adult unit and provided additional support or training in problematic areas. This effort had successfully reduced the incidence of hospital-acquired pressure ulcers from 9.4% in 2001 to 1.6% in December 2006. (Institute for Healthcare Improvement, 2007a).

A Success Story

Owensboro Medical Health System in Owensboro, Kentucky, implemented an innovative pressure ulcer prevention program to ensure admission assessment and implementation of prevention strategies for all admitted patients. This program included three parts:

1. Hospital-wide training
2. Changes in documentation processes
3. The use of pressure-relieving surfaces for patients at highest risk

Two strategies were instituted to assist nursing staff in the continuous prevention processes:

1. Placing turn-clock posters in each high-risk patient's room
2. Setting nursing staff's beepers to alarm every 2 hours to remind them to reposition high-risk patients

The pressure ulcer incidence rates in acute care units dropped 93% (from 20.59% in March 2004 to 1.43% in June 2006) in just over 2 years of implementing this prevention program (Institute for Healthcare Improvement, 2007b).

A Success Story

Pressure sores are a leading cause of delayed discharges. At Kaiser Roseville, nursing attendants carried in their pockets a small card with drawings of the human body to review when they do bed baths. If nursing attendants see reddened areas on a patient, they circle that area on the card. Then, the responsible nurse validates the finding and flags the change in skin integrity in the doctor's progress notes of this patient.

This intervention was a simple idea that turned into a powerful tool to detect existing pressure ulcers and prevent deterioration of stage 1 pressure ulcers. This card was called the "skin integrity card" (Institute for Healthcare Improvement, 2007d).

Knowing about Pressure Ulcers

Health care-associated pressure ulcers continue to be a concern in all clinical settings. Pressure ulcers are also called decubitus ulcers or bedsores. A pressure ulcer refers to any skin lesion caused by unrelieved pressure resulting in damage of underlying tissue and usually occurs over bony prominences (Institute for Healthcare Improvement, 2007b).

Immobility for any reasons contributes to the risk of health care-associated pressure ulcers. The elderly, wheelchair users, and patients who are bedridden are most at risk. Patients living with incontinence (especially women) are also at risk for developing pressure ulcers. A prolonged exposure to moisture can cause breakdown of skin tissues. Patients with medical conditions (e.g., diabetes and arterial diseases) can have an increased risk because the supply of blood and oxygen to body tissues may be restricted (Judy-waterlow.co.uk, 2007b).

We thought that the initial formation of any health care-associated pressure ulcers is primarily due to immobility, which results in moisture being continuously contained between a certain skin area and an airtight surface. Due to deconditioning as a result of immobility during hospital stays or the previously existing health conditions, some patients may be unable to turn themselves freely. These patients may need assistance to help them change positions on beds or chairs.

Even when we are sleeping, we subconsciously change or readjust our lying positions constantly. The purpose of repositioning is to let the skin areas breathe and dry because they have direct and airtight contacts with the covers of the mattress. Without sufficient air ventilation to let the specific area of skin breathe, these skin areas can be soaked by the moisture and increased heat.

The incidence rates of pressure ulcers vary by the types of health care institution. The incidence rates range from 0.4% to 38% in acute care settings and from 2.2% to 23.9% in long-term care institutions. In acute care settings, the estimated pressure ulcer prevalence (the percentage of patients with pressure ulcers at any point in time) is 15%, and the incidence rate (the rate at which new cases occur in a patient population over a given time period) is about 7% (Institute for Healthcare Improvement, 2007b; Joint Commission, 2006a; Lyder, 2003).

It is estimated that each year, 1.3-3 million adults develop pressure ulcers in the United States and about 2.5 million patients are treated for pressure ulcers in US acute hospitals. The cost of treatment varies from $500 to $40,000 per ulcer (Institute for Healthcare Improvement, 2007b; Joint Commission, 2006a).

Stages of Pressure Ulcers

The National Pressure Ulcer Advisory Panel Pressure Ulcer Staging System (National Pressure Ulcer Advisory Panel, 1989, 1993) classified pressure ulcers into four stages:

1. Stage 1: The ulcer shows as a defined area of persistent redness in lightly pigmented skin, whereas in darker skin tones, the ulcer may appear with persistent red, blue, or purple colors. The lesion may include changes in one or more of the following:
2. Skin temperature (warmness or coolness)
3. Tissue consistency (firm or boggy feel)
4. Sensation (pain and itching)
5. Stage 2: The ulcer appears as partial-thickness skin loss, involving epidermis, dermis, or both. This stage of ulcer is superficial and presents clinically as an abrasion, blister, or shallow crater.
6. Stage 3: The ulcer shows full-thickness skin loss, which involves damage to or necrosis of subcutaneous tissue. The damage may reach down to, but not through, underlying fascia. This stage of ulcer appears clinically as a deep crater or hole with or without damaging of adjacent tissue.
7. Stage 4: The ulcer appears as full-thickness skin loss with extensive destruction, tissue necrosis, or damage to muscle, bone, or supporting structures (e.g., tendon, joint, and capsule). In this stage, the lesion extends beyond deep fascia into tendon, bone, muscle, or joint.

Most pressure ulcers can be prevented. Deterioration at the early stage of pressure ulcers can be halted. However, among some patients, skin breakdown reflects the advanced state of debilitation, including, for example, a progressive underlying disease, chronic infections, or malnourishment (Joint Commission, 2006a).

Risk Factors and Possible Solutions

In the 2008 National Patient Safety Goals, Goal 14 was meant to prevent health care-associated pressure ulcers (Joint Commission, 2007b). Health care institutions and providers are expected to assess and periodically reassess each patient's risk for developing pressure ulcers and take needed actions to address any identified risks. Although this goal was meant for long-term care facilities, the same goal should be applicable to acute hospitals.

**Table 1. The commonly seen intrinsic and extrinsic risk factors
for health care-associated pressure ulcers**

Dimension	Factor
Intrinsic risk factors	1. Intrinsic factors can influence the architecture and integrity of the skin and supporting structures (particularly collagen and elastin) and diminish the ability of soft tissues to absorb and tolerate mechanical load.
	2. Associated risk factors include
	2.1 Age
	2.2 Skin condition
	2.3 Low body weight
	2.4 Immobility
	2.5 Incontinence
	2.6 Poor nutritional status or malnutrition
	2.7 Poor fluid status or dehydration
	2.8 Febrile illnesses
	2.9 Altered mental status
	2.10 Decreased sensation
	2.11 Low arteriolar pressure
Extrinsic risk factors	1. Skin moisture
	1.1 Exposure of the skin to moisture (e.g., bathing, perspiration, amniotic fluid, and incontinence as urine and fecal are acidic) can lead to maceration and rashes and weaken the natural barrier of the epidermis.
	1.2 Moisture causes softening of the stratum corneum (the outermost layer of epidermis), which makes the skin tissues more susceptible to shear and friction.
	1.3 Certain skin areas are more vulnerable to pressure ulcer formation than others, bony prominences in particular (e.g., heels, sacrum, buttocks, hips, and elbows).
	2. Pressure
	2.1 When the pressure between the support surface and the body prominence is increased, the blood flow to skin stops. This situation can result in non-bleachable erythema, including ischemia, acidosis, toxin accumulation, or hemorrhage into interstitium. If the pressure continues, necrosis and cell death can occur.
	2.2 A pressure is more easily distributed in superficial tissues. The skin areas closest to the bone often sustain maximal damage.
	2.3 The possibility of developing pressure ulcers is inversely related to the frequency of repositioning. For the patients who are unable to reposition themselves, repositioning every 2 hours is a standard of care.
	3. Friction
	3.1 Friction can weaken the natural barrier of the epidermis as a result of movement over a rough surface. For example, friction of skin against bedding can occur when moving patients.
	3.2 Friction causes removal of stratum corneum and damage to underlying, more delicate layers.
	4. Shear
	4.1 Shearing results when the outer layers of the skin slide along a rough or sticky surface. Shearing pulls and potentially tears the underlying tissues.
	4.2 In other words, shear occurs when friction holds skin in place, but gravity pulls the axial skeleton down. Consequently, shear results in stretching of perforating arterioles and compromise of perfusion of dermal layers.

Sources: Bergstrom, N., Braden, B. J., Laguzza, A., & Holman, V. (1987). The Braden scale for predicting pressure score risk. *Nursing Research, 36*(4), 205-210. Judy-waterlow.co.uk (2007a). Pressure ulcers: Causes. Available at: http://www.judy-waterlow.co.uk/pressure-sore-causes.htm (accessed November 26, 2007). Koretz, B., & Eslami, M. (2007). Pressure ulcers. Available at: http://www.ucop.edu/agrp/docs/la_ulcers.pdf (accessed December 1, 2007).

The Joint Commission (2007a) suggested that the use of clinical practice guidelines can effectively identify patients at risk for pressure ulcers and define early intervention for prevention of pressure ulcers. A systematic risk assessment tool (such as the Braden Scale or Norton Scale) was recommended, which may help improve assessment and identification of at-risk patients.

Table 2. The suggested tips from the Joint Commission to help prevent pressure ulcers

Dimension	Tip
Hospital design	1. Controlling environmental factors to prevent moisture skin
Hospital equipment	1. Using available pressure-reducing devices for beds and chairs

Nurse skills and efforts	1. Repositioning
	    1.1 Turning patients at least every 2 hours with effective devices (e.g., pillows or foam wedges) and not using ring cushions or donut-type devices
	    1.2 When a patient is positioned on his or her side, positioning the patient at an angle, rather than directly on the trochanter (a bony prominences toward the near end of the thigh bone)
	    1.3 Free-float the heels
	    1.4 When patients are sitting in chairs, repositioning patients at least hourly, or instructing patients to shift weight every 15 minutes if they are able to do so themselves
	    1.5 Using proper positioning, transferring, and turning techniques
	    1.6 Lifting, never dragging, patients
	    1.7 Limiting elevation of the head of the bed when possible
	2. Maintaining skin integrity and preventing further skin breakdown
	    2.1 Regularly examining each individual patient's skin condition
	    2.2 Providing meticulous skin care and routinely cleansing skin when soiled
	    2.3 Minimizing skin moisture, due to incontinence, drainage, and perspiration
	    2.4 Using lubricants, protective films, or padding to prevent friction and shear injuries
	    2.5 Avoiding massage of the skin over bony prominences because massage can damage underlying tissues
	    2.6 Applying barriers to prevent further skin breakdown
	    2.7 Nurses and physicians recognizing that pressure ulcers may develop from surgical equipment and braces used in the operating room
	3. Monitoring nutritional status and promoting range of motion
	    3.1 Assessing each individual patient's nutritional status
	    3.2 Maintaining each individual patent's activity level, mobility, and range of motion

Source: Joint Commission (2007a). *Patient safety pocket guide* (2nd ed., pp. 97-104). Oakbrook Terrace, IL: Joint Commission.

The Braden Scale assesses six areas of pressure ulcer risk, including: (1) sensory perception, (2) moisture, (3) activity, (4) mobility, (5) nutrition, and (6) friction and shear. The Norton Scale has five areas of pressure ulcer risk, including: (1) physical condition, (2) mental condition, (3) activity, (4) mobility, and (5) incontinence (Joint Commission, 2007a).

The National Pressure Ulcer Advisory Panel (1992) also emphasized that pressure ulcer risk assessment demands a comprehensive approach, including: (1) skin assessment, (2) evaluation of immobility, (3) inactivity, (4) nutritional factors, (5) fecal and urinary incontinence, and (6) decreased sensory perception. Table 1 summarizes the extrinsic and intrinsic risk factors for developing health care-associated pressure ulcers.

The Joint Commission (2006a) stated that an effective plan for the prediction, prevention, and early treatment of pressure ulcers should include:

1. Recognizing at-risk patients and the specific factors that place them at risk
2. Identifying a prevention program that is specific to each at-risk patient
3. Maintaining and improving tissues tolerance to pressure
4. Protecting against the adverse effects of external mechanical forces
5. Meeting the patient's nutritional support needs
6. Reducing the incidence of pressure ulcers through on-the-job education programs to health care providers

As for possible solutions to pressure ulcers, the Joint Commission (2006a) identified three major prevention strategies: (1) skin inspection periodically, skin cleansing, care for dry skin, use of moisture barriers, and massage; (2) improvement in the techniques of positioning, transferring, and turning to reduce skin injury caused by friction and shear forces; and (3) continued focus on increasing or maintaining patient activity or mobility. The Joint Commission (2007a) further suggested several approaches to help prevent pressure ulcers (Table 2).

For preventing pressure ulcers, the Institution for Healthcare Improvement (2007b, 2007c) suggested two major steps: (1) identifying patients at risk and (2) reliably implementing prevention strategies for all patients identified as being at risk. The six essential elements of pressure ulcer prevention are summarized in Table 3.

Table 3. The six essential steps of pressure ulcer prevention as suggested by the Institute for Healthcare Improvement

Step	Strategy to implement each step

Step 1. Conducting an initial pressure ulcer assessment at admission for all patients	1. The admission assessment (the initial pressure ulcer risk assessment) should include both a risk assessment of developing pressure ulcers and a skin assessment to detect existing pressure ulcers.
	 2. Reassessment should be done periodically based on each patient's condition.
	 3. Using a validated risk assessment tool is essential for accurate, prompt identification of at-risk patients and timely implementation of pressure ulcer prevention strategies.
	 4. Hospitals can adopt the following strategies to ensure compliance with the assessment and identification of any patient at risk for pressure ulcers:
	   4.1 Improving processes to ensure that the initial risk assessment is conducted within 4 hours of admission for all patients
	   4.2 Including a visual cue on each admission documentation record for the completion of a total skin assessment and the initial risk assessment
	   4.3 Adopting the use of a standard risk assessment tool (e.g., the Braden Scale)

Table 3. Continued

Step	Strategy to implement each step
	4.4 Using multiple methods to visually cue nursing staff as to which patients are at risk of developing pressure ulcers
	4.5 Building shared pride in progress among nursing staff (e.g., posting 'days since last pressure ulcer' data)
Step 2. Reassessing risk for all patients daily	1. The complexity and acuity of hospitalized patients require daily reassessment of the potential for developing pressure ulcers. For example changes in a patient's mobility, continence, or nutrition may alter the risk of developing pressure ulcers.
	2. Assessing the risk for developing pressure ulcers daily provides nursing staff the opportunity to adjust prevention strategies.
	3. Hospitals can adopt the following strategies to ensure daily reassessment of patients at risk for pressure ulcers:
	3.1 Adapting documentation tools to prompt daily risk assessment, recording findings, and initiating prevention strategies as needed (e.g., including the risk assessment in daily clinical notes)
	3.2 Educating all levels of staff about potential risk factors for developing pressure ulcers and the process for implementing prevention strategies
	3.3 Adopting the use of a standard risk assessment tool for nursing staff to easily identify the degree of risk and the needed prevention strategies

Note: The Institution for Healthcare Improvement suggested implementing steps 3-6 for all patients identified as being at risk for developing pressure ulcers.

Step	Strategy to implement each step
Step 3. Inspecting skin integrity for all patients daily	1. Skin integrity may deteriorate in hours among hospitalized patients. Risk levels for developing pressure ulcers can change rapidly in acutely ill patients. Daily skin inspection is crucial to prevent further skin deterioration.
	2. Patients who are identified as being at high risk should have a daily inspection of all skin surfaces, from head to toe.
	3. Nursing staff should give special attention to areas at high risk for developing pressure ulcers, including the sacrum, back, buttocks, heels, and elbows.
	4. Hospitals can adopt the following strategies to ensure daily inspection of the skin:
	4.1 Adapting documentation tools to prompt daily skin inspection, recording findings, and initiating prevention strategies as needed (e.g., including the skin inspection in daily clinical notes)
	4.2 Educating all levels of nursing staff to inspect the skin integrity any time they are assisting patients (e.g., when assisting or transferring patient to the chair or while bathing the patient)
	4.3 If any changes in skin integrity are seen, notifying the responsible nursing staff, so that appropriate interventions can be initiated
Step 4. Managing moisture by keeping the patient dry and moisturize skin	1. It is well recognized that wet skin is conducive to the development of rashes and tends to break down more easily.
	2. Skin should be cleansed when soiled and at routine intervals. Skin should be cleansed with use of a mild cleansing agent that minimizes irritation and dryness of the skin.
	3. Applying moisturizers to dry skin has been shown to be effective in preventing pressure ulcers.
	4. Skin care should emphasize minimizing exposure of the skin to moisture because of incontinence, perspiration, or would drainage.
	5. If needed, under-pads, which are made of materials that absorb moisture and present a quick-drying surface to the skin, may be used.
	6. Applying topical agents, which act as moisture barriers and moisturize the skin, may be helpful.

Step	Strategy to implement each step
	7. Hospitals can adopt the following strategies to ensure effective management of moisture:
	7.1 Designing a process for periodic activities (e.g., offering toileting, assessing for wet skin, applying barrier agents, offering fluid, and repositioning) and looking for opportunity to combine these routine activities in a protocol (e.g., the pressure ulcer prevention protocol). This way, nursing staff can complete multiple tasks while in the room every 2 hours and document findings all at once.
	7.2 Providing sufficient supplies at the bedside of each at-risk patient who is incontinent
	7.3 Limiting the use of disposable briefs or containment clothes if possible. Hospitals should provide under-pads made of materials that pull the moisture away from the skin.
	7.4 Providing premoistened, disposable barrier wipes to help cleanse, moisturize, and deodorize. Such wipes can protect patients from perineal dermatitis because of incontinence.
Step 5. Optimizing nutrition and hydration	1. A review of nutritional status and an assessment of hydration are needed, including impaired intake, low body weight or unintentional weight loss since being hospitalized, and dehydration. 2. If significant nutritional needs are identified, a registered clinical dietitian should be consulted for further assessment and feasible nutritional interventions. 3. Hospitals can adopt the following strategies to optimize nutrition and hydration: 3.1 Nursing staff assisting patients with meals, snacks, and hydration 3.2 Making efforts to allow patient preferences when medically appropriate 3.3 Documenting the amount of nutritional intake. 3.4 Notifying the responsible physician or the dietitian if a patient does not have adequate intake 3.5 Offering water to every patient who needs assistance to shift position 3.6 Designing an integrated process to include related tasks such as: (1) offering toileting, (2) assessing for needs of cleanliness, (3) changing wet surfaces, and (4) offering water
Step 6. Minimizing pressure	1. Patients with limited mobility are especially at risk for developing pressure ulcers. Relieving pressures, especially over bony prominences, is essential. 2. For patients with or without limited mobility, nursing staff should make every effort to redistribute the pressure on the skin by: (1) repositioning patients every 2 hours or (2) using pressure-relieving surfaces (or both). 3. Hospitals can adopt the following strategies to minimize pressure: 3.1 Adopting tools (e.g., placing a reminder above the head of the bed) placed inside the patient room to remind nursing staff to reposition the patient every 2 hours 3.2 Using unit- or hospital-wide musical cues to remind nursing staff to turn all at-risk patients for developing pressure ulcers at 2-hour intervals (e.g., setting nursing staff's beepers to sound every 2 hours) 3.3 Using correct positioning and transferring techniques to minimize friction and shear injury 3.4 Using pressure redistribution mattresses or overlays to assist with minimizing pressure as appropriate

Sources: Institute for Healthcare Improvement (2007b). Getting started kit: Prevent pressure ulcers (how-to guide). Available at: http://www.ihi.org/NR/rdonlyres/5ABABB51-93B3-4D88-AE19-BE88B7D96858/0/PressureUlcerHowtoGuide.doc (accessed December 1, 2007).

Institute for Healthcare Improvement (2007c). What you need to know about pressure sores: A fact sheet for patients and their family members. Available at: http://www.ihi.org/NR/rdonlyres/F2EF9AB3-BB0F-4D3D-A99A-83AC7E0FB0D3/5862/WhatyouneedtoknowPU_1022.pdf (accessed December 2, 2007).

The Institution for Healthcare Improvement (2007c) also recommended some ways that family members can help prevent pressure ulcers by asking the nurses and physicians the following three questions:

1. Is our hospitalized loved one at risk for developing pressure ulcers?
2. What types of food and how much water should our hospitalized loved one eat and drink a day?
3. What are nurses and physicians doing to decrease pressure on our hospitalized loved one's skin?

The National Pressure Ulcer Advisory Panel (1992) emphasized that the responsibility for preventing the development of pressure ulcers is shared by physicians, nurses, enterostomal therapy nurses, physical and occupational therapists, nutritionists, pharmacists, administrators, patients, and their families. The suggested educational programs for health professionals and the information for patients and their families are summarized in **Table 4**.

Table 4. The educational program for health care professionals and the one for patients and their families as suggested by the National Pressure Ulcer Advisory Panel

Targeted audience	Program
Health care professionals	1. Knowing characteristics of normal and healthy skin 2. Understanding the characteristics of skin tissue deformation and the performance of skin tissue under mechanical loading 3. Being knowledgeable about the etiology and staging of pressure ulcers 4. Adopting research-based risk assessment tools as appropriate for specific patient populations 5. Being familiar with the elements of skin assessment 6. Understanding the risk factors for developing pressure ulcers 7. Learning the role of nutrition in pressure ulcer prevention 8. Using proper techniques for positioning and repositioning patients 9. Understanding the indications and limitations of pressure-reducing devices and support surfaces 10. Being familiar with the indications and limitations of friction reducing products 11. Documenting the findings of skin assessment and implemented skin care programs
Patients and their families	1. Understanding the etiology of pressure ulcers 2. Conducting skin inspection daily 3. Learning ways to protect skin integrity 4. Performing proper, safe cleansing techniques, and using appropriate agents 5. Learning ways to reduce pressure ulcer risk 6. Knowing the role of nutrition in preventing the development of pressure ulcers 7. Understanding the importance and needs for repositioning or position changes 8. Learning and using proper and correct positioning techniques 9. Using pillows or other pressure reducing devices as needed and as appropriate 10. Being aware of the importance of reporting changes in skin integrity and health status to responsible health care professionals (e.g., physicians and nurses)

Source: National Pressure Ulcer Advisory Panel (1992). Statement on pressure ulcer prevention: Forward. Available at: http://www.npuap.org/positn1.htm (accessed December 1, 2007).

Critical Tips to Prevent Health Care-associated Pressure Ulcers

Most pressure ulcers can be prevented and deterioration at the early stage of pressure ulcers can be halted. As we have observed in practice, the initial formation of any health care-associated pressure ulcers is primarily due to immobility, which results in moisture continuously contained between a certain skin area and an airtight surface. Without sufficient air ventilation to let the specific area of skin breathe, these skin areas can be soaked by the moisture and increased temperature or heat between the skin areas and the airtight surfaces.

Below is a story about a nursing professor's hospitalization experience.

A nurse, who is in her early sixties and independent, shared with us her experience and insights after being hospitalized in an acute inpatient unit for a week for her acute medical problems. She claimed that she sweat a lot during her hospital stay. After her pajamas and bed sheet were soaked by perspiration, her bed became really uncomfortable, even though the mattress was covered by a cotton bed sheet. She emphasized that the room temperature was fine with her.

She told us that she was trying to constantly reposition herself to decrease the heat between her back and the airtight bed surface. However, it did not make much difference. In addition, the bed was so small she found it difficult to turn and find a comfortable position. As a recently hospitalized patient, she expressed her desperation and realized that most inpatients may also experience the same discomfort resulting from the heat between the skin area and the airtight surface and the soaked bed sheet due to perspiration.

Based on our observation, we developed critical elements to prevent pressure ulcer development. Table 5 includes the tips for hospital and nursing leaders and nurses who work in acute inpatient care units to prevent the development of pressure ulcers. Tips were categorized into four domains: (1) hospital design, (2) hospital equipment and supplies, (3) nursing staff's skills and efforts, and (4) integrated care delivery. Figure 1 shows a patient repositioning herself on a patient bed in 34.5 inches in width; Figure 2 illustrates the same patient changing her position on a patient bed 34.5 inches wide with two half-size side rails up.

Table 5. Preventing the development of pressure ulcers: Critical tips for hospital and nursing leaders and nurses who work in acute inpatient care units

Dimension	Tip

Hospital design	1. Increasing the width of patient beds to 45 inches
	     1.1 Patients may tend not to reposition themselves when lying in bed because of the limited width of patient beds. We suggest that a safe bed width of 45 inches is needed to allow patients to turn freely without fear.
	     1.2 The current size of the hospital beds available in the US market ranges from 34.5 to 36 inches in width, which is too narrow and may prevents patients from turning when lying on bed (Figures 1 and 2).

Table 5. Continued

Dimension	Tip
	1.3 The patient beds should be at least 39 inches in width (comparable to the twin/single size for home beds) to avoid the fear of falling off the beds when patients are turning. However, we suggest a safe bed width of 45 inches.
	1.4 When purchasing new hospital inpatient beds, hospital and nursing leaders should consider a bed width of 45 inches.
Hospital equipment and supplies	1. Using summer sleeping and chair mats to relieve skin moisture for all patients
	1.1 As an innovative strategy for pressure ulcer prevention, hospitals should supply one summer sleeping mat to each inpatient (e.g., bamboo sleeping mats). The summer sleeping mat can relieve skin moisture and the heat between skin areas and the top of the mattress.
	1.1.1 The summer sleeping mat should be placed in between the mattress cover and the cotton bed sheet.
	1.1.2 If the under-pad is used, place the under-pad on the top of the cotton bed sheet.
	1.1.3 If the summer sleeping mat is soiled, have the laundry department clean it with water and detergent and air dry it. Then, return the cleaned mat to the same patient.
	1.1.4 The summer sleeping mat should be used for the same patient for the purpose of infection control. The patient may take it home at the time of discharge.
	1.2 Hospitals should also provide summer chair mats (e.g., bamboo chair mats) to relieve skin moisture and the heat between the skin and the sitting area. This feature should be standard equipment and placed on the top of the cushion of each bedside chair. Patients should sit directly on the top of the summer chair mats.
	2. Supplying high-quality under-pads
	2.1 Hospital must provide appropriate under-pads for patients who are incontinent. Nurses should limit the use of disposable briefs or containment clothes if possible.
	2.2 Under-pads should be made of materials that absorb moisture and present a quick-drying surface to the skin.
Nursing staff's skills and efforts	1. With or without the assistance from nursing attendants or family visitors, the responsible nurses must ensure that the pressure ulcer prevention programs for at-risk patients as documented in the care plans are implemented thoroughly (e.g., daily skin assessment and routine skin care).
	2. If families are willing to participate in patient care (e.g., bathing, cleansing when soiled, and repositioning patients), the responsible nurse must provide educational information about pressure ulcer prevention to families and patients. Nurses must repeat the educational information as often as needed as family visitors may take turns.
	3. Nurses are expected to perform the following tasks:
	3.1 Repositioning patients at least every 2 hours
	3.1.1 If patients are able to shift positions themselves, nurses must encourage them to do so as often as possible.
	3.1.2 If patients have limited mobility, nurses should reposition patients at least every 2 hours.
	3.1.3 It is important for nurses to work with physical therapists to help patients retain their activity level, mobility, and range of motion.

Dimension	Tip
	3.1.4 Nurses must use proper positioning, transferring, and turning techniques to avoid friction and shear injuries.
	3.2 Maintaining skin integrity and preventing further skin breakdown. The following three tasks may be conducted by the responsible nurse, the assigned nursing attendant, or the families:
	3.2.1 Nurses must examine each individual patient's skin condition daily when providing daily meticulous skin care.
	3.2.2 Nurses must make ensure that patients' skin is being routinely cleansed and the soiled bed sheets or clothes are changed in a timely manner.
	3.2.3 Nurses may use lubricants, protective films, or padding to prevent friction and shear injuries.
	3.3 Monitoring patients' nutritional status
	3.3.1 Nurses should assess patients' nutritional status by recording the amount of their intake (e.g., meals and snacks).
	3.3.2 If needed, the responsible nurse, the assigned nursing attendant, or families (if any) have to assist in feeding patients.
Integrated care delivery	1. Physicians should ensure that patients' needs are met in time (e.g., treatment for skin lesions and requests for the consults from dietitians and physical therapists).
	2. If a pressure ulcer occurs, physicians and nurses should adopt pressure-reducing devices as appropriate for beds and bedside chairs.
	3. Physical therapy should be a routine service for patients who have limited mobility or are bedridden. Maintaining and retaining the activity level as before admitting to the hospital as much as possible are important.

Table 6 presents tips for patients and their families to be part of the efforts to prevent the development of pressure ulcers during hospital stays.

Table 6. Preventing the development of pressure ulcers during hospital stays:
Critical tips for patients and their families

Dimension	Tip
Patient	If I am not well enough to do any of the actions indicated below, I should ask a family or friend to help.
Patient	1. If I am able to shift positions myself, I should reposition myself as often as possible when lying on bed or sitting on chair.
	2. I should retain my mobility by getting out of bed and ambulating often.
	2.1 Retaining my mobility is very important to keep my skin healthy.
	2.2 After lying on bed for a while, I may experience weak muscle strength and dizziness. I must ask for assistance before making a move, if I am instructed by my nurse to do so to prevent falls. Retaining independence and mobility does not mean that I need to risk falling.
	2.3 I should bring my own assistive device to the hospital (e.g., walker and cane), because my own device has been set for my own use. If I experience a need to use an assistive device for walking and I do have my own assistive device with me or do not have one, I should talk to our doctor or nurse and ask for one. A physical therapist may come to assess me for the need for assistive devices.
	3. I should remind my nurses to examine my skin condition daily for me.
	4. I must report to my nurse if I have pain or itchy feelings on any part of my skin areas. I should ask my nurse to check these areas for me.

Table 6. Continued

Dimension	Tip
	5. If I am unable to clean myself, I should ask my nurse or my family to help me. It is also one of my nurse's responsibilities to provide daily skin care and routinely cleanse my skin due to incontinence, drainage, and perspiration.
	6. I should ask my nurse for available equipment and supplies to relieve my skin moisture (e.g., a summer sleeping or chair mats to relieve skin moisture).
	6.1 I may bring my own summer sleeping mat to be used during my hospital stay.
	6.2 Families need to make sure that the patient is comfortable whey lying in bed. Discomfort may indicate, for example, overheated skin areas and soiled bed sheets.
	7. I should ask my nurse to use high-quality under-pads, if needed.
	7.1 Hospitals must provide appropriate under-pads for incontinent patients. Under-pads should be made of materials that absorb moisture and present a quick-drying surface to the skin.
	7.2 If I have to purchase under-pads for my own use, I should ask for the kind made of materials that absorb moisture and present a quick-drying surface to the skin.
Families	1. If we, as families, are willing to assist and participate in the care of our hospitalized loved one in the efforts to prevent pressure ulcers (e.g., bathing, cleansing when soiled, and repositioning), we must ask the responsible nurse to provide related educational information about pressure ulcer prevention.
	2. First of all, we must know what nurses are expected to do to prevent the development of pressure ulcers. We may participate in any of the following tasks, only if we feel comfortable doing so.
	2.1 Repositioning the patient at least every 2 hours
	2.2 Using proper positioning, transferring, and turning techniques to avoid friction and shear injuries
	2.3 Maintaining skin integrity and preventing further skin breakdown by:
	2.3.1 Examining the patient's skin condition daily when providing daily meticulous skin care
	2.3.2 Routinely cleansing skin due to incontinence, drainage, and perspiration
	2.3.3 Using lubricants, protective films, or padding to prevent friction and shear injuries
	2.4 Monitoring the patient's nutritional status and intake

More Information about Summer Sleeping Mats

Providing summer sleeping mats to all inpatients is our innovative approach to preventing pressure ulcers in inpatients. The cotton bed sheet may absorb perspiration, but it is unable to promote air ventilation between the skin and the mattress. The purpose of using summer sleeping mats between the airtight mattress cover and the cotton bed sheet is to relieve the skin moisture and the increased heat between the skin area and the supporting surface it contacts. Summer sleeping mats have been commonly used in many areas, especially in the tropical regions (e.g., Hawaii, Asian, and Africa).

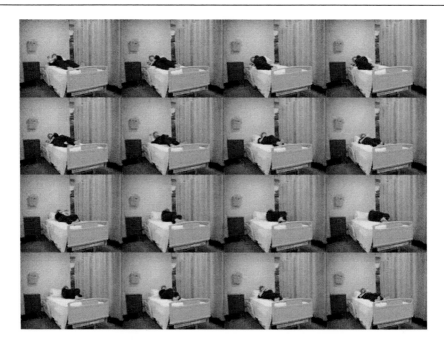

Figure 1. Repositioning on a hospital patient bed. The bed was 34.5 inches in width. None of the four half-size bed rails was raised. Examine the images from the first row, far left upper corner (the first image) to the first row, far right upper corner, the second row far left image to the second row far right image, the third row far left one to the third row far right one, then the fourth row far left one to the fourth row far right one (the last image). The subject was about 5 feet and 6 inches tall and weighed 140 pounds.

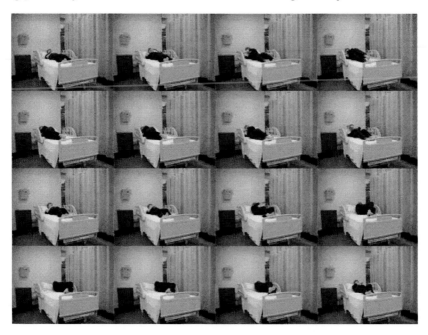

Figure 2. Repositioning on a hospital patient bed. The patient bed was 34.5 inches in width, and two of the four half-size bed rails were raised. Examine the images from the first row, far left upper corner (the first image) to the first row, far right upper corner, the second row far left image to the second row far right image, the third row far left one to the third row far right one, then the fourth row far left one to the fourth-row far right one (the last image). The subject was about 5 feet and 6 inches tall and weighed 140 pounds.

Summer sleeping mats made of bamboo or any other natural materials are recommended. Bamboo sleep mats use 100% natural bamboo as the weaving material. The nature of bamboo is cool, lightweight, and absorbent. The advantage of the bamboo matting is that it is smooth, soft and cool. The raw material is cooked in ways to be mildew and worm resistant and to resist corrosion (e.g., Fujian Summer Health Bamboo Products Co., Ltd., 2007; NingBo Brother Bamboo Ware Co., Ltd., 2007). With a good bamboo sleeping mat, when patients lie down on the mat, their body temperature will cool down quickly. Also, patients do not feel cold and their hair will not be nipped on it.

The Chinese or Japanese market stores in the United States often carry bamboo sleeping mats or some other types of summer sleeping mats. Products with similar effects for purchase in the United States can also be found online. For example, Lauhala Mats are made of Hala trees, and cost $18.99 each for a size of 4 feet by 8 feet (Bamboo and Tikis, 2007).

Bamboo sleeping mats should be used for all patients and placed between the mattress (usually covered by airtight and waterproof fabric) and the cotton bed sheet to provide a ventilating, cool, and comfortable sleeping surface. Using bamboo sleeping mats can prevent accumulated moisture on skin areas and decrease the heat between the skin and the surface with direct contact. To increase the comfort level, the cotton bed sheet may be used, but it is not always needed depending on the patient's preferences. To remove stains or body fluids, the bamboo sleeping mats are washable and air dry quickly. For infection control purposes, even after disinfection, each patient should only use his or her own summer sleeping mat.

References

Bamboo and Tikis (2007). Lauhala mat. Available at: http://shop.1asecure.com/prod.cfm?ProdID=272756&StID=4633 (accessed December 2, 2007).

Bergstrom, N., Braden, B. J., Laguzza, A., & Holman, V. (1987). The Braden scale for predicting pressure score risk. *Nursing Research, 36*(4), 205-210.

Fujian Summer Health Bamboo Products Co., Ltd. (2007). Summer sleeping bamboo mat. Available at: http://naturebamboos.ec51.com/product/Summer_sleeping_bamboo_mat_190298.html (accessed December 2, 2007).

Institute for Healthcare Improvement (2007a). Relieve the pressure and reduce harm (published on May 21, 2007). Available at: http://www.ihi.org/IHI/Topics/PatientSafety/SafetyGeneral/ImprovementStories/FSRelievethePressureandReduceHarm.htm (accessed November 26, 2007).

Institute for Healthcare Improvement (2007b). Getting started kit: Prevent pressure ulcers (how-to guide). Available at: http://www.ihi.org/NR/rdonlyres/5ABABB51-93B3-4D88-AE19-BE88B7D96858/0/PressureUlcerHowtoGuide.doc (accessed December 1, 2007).

Institute for Healthcare Improvement (2007c). What you need to know about pressure sores: A fact sheet for patients and their family members. Available at: http://www.ihi.org/NR/rdonlyres/F2EF9AB3-BB0F-4D3D-A99A-83AC7E0FB0D3/5862/WhatyouneedtoknowPU_1022.pdf (accessed December 2, 2007).

Institute for Healthcare Improvement (2007d). Transforming care at the bedside: Sparking innovation and excitement on the hospital unit. Available at: http://www. ihi.org/IHI/Topics/MedicalSurgicalCare/MedicalSurgicalCareGeneral/ImprovementStori es/TransformingCareattheBedsideinitiativePrototypephase.htm (accessed December 2, 2007).

Joint Commission (2006a). Goal 14: Prevent health care-associated pressure ulcers (decubitus ulcers). In A. Grayson. (Ed.), *Meeting the Joint Commission's 2007 National Patient Safety Goals* (pp. 125-126). Oakbrook Terrace, IL: Joint Commission.

Joint Commission (2007a). *Patient safety pocket guide* (2nd ed., pp. 97-104). Oakbrook Terrace, IL: Joint Commission.

Joint Commission (2007b). Facts about the 2008 National Safety Goals. Available at: http://www.jointcommission.org/PatientSafety/NationalPatientSafetyGoals/08_npsg_fact s.htm (accessed December 1, 2007).

Judy-waterlow.co.uk (2007a). Pressure ulcers: Causes. Available at: http://www.judy-waterlow.co.uk/pressure-sore-causes.htm (accessed November 26, 2007).

Judy-waterlow.co.uk (2007b). Pressure ulcers: Prevention. Available at: http://www.judy-waterlow.co.uk/pressure-sore-prevention.htm (accessed November 26, 2007).

Koretz, B., & Eslami, M. (2007). Pressure ulcers. Available at: http://www.ucop.edu/ agrp/docs/la_ulcers.pdf (accessed December 1, 2007).

Lyder, C. H. (2003). Pressure ulcer prevention and management. *JAMA, 289*(2), 223-226.

National Pressure Ulcer Advisory Panel (1989). 1989 NPUAP pressure ulcer stages. Available at: http://www.npuap.org/positn6.htm (accessed December 1, 2007).

National Pressure Ulcer Advisory Panel (1992). Statement on pressure ulcer prevention: Forward. Available at: http://www.npuap.org/positn1.htm (accessed December 1, 2007).

National Pressure Ulcer Advisory Panel (1993). Stage 1 assessment in darkly pigmented skin. Available at: http://www.npuap.org/positn6.htm (accessed December 1, 2007).

NingBo Brother Bamboo Ware Co., Ltd. (2007). Summer sleeping bamboo mat and bamboo sleeping mat. http://xiongdi.en.alibaba.com/product/50151427/52170725/Summer_ Sleeping_Bamboo_Mats/Summer_sleeping_bamboo_mat.html and http://xiongdi.en. alibaba.com/product/50151427/50763924/Summer_Sleeping_Bamboo_Mats/Bamboo_Sl eeping_Mat.html (accessed December 2, 2007).

Serious Injury or Death in Physical Restraints or Seclusion

Learning from a Patient Case

A temporary nurse, who normally worked in the newborn nursery, was assigned to work in a surgical unit where most of the patients were older than 75. He was unfamiliar with the effects of anesthesia on the elderly and lacked knowledge on proper selection and application of physical restraints and related practice policies or guidelines.

On the first day, after working on this surgical unit for less than an hour, he saw a postsurgical patient attempting to climb over his bed rails. This patient was recovering from a routine appendectomy. This nurse grabbed the first type of physical restraint he found (a vest) and applied it to this patient, without calling this patient's doctor for a restraint order. This nurse also failed to report the use of the vest to the charge nurse. Then, he continued the care and treatments for the other patients.

About 45 minutes later when this patient's son arrived the patient room to visit his father, the patient's son found his father hanging from the vest restraint, which was attached to the bed rail. This patient was blue and cold and had only a weak pulse. The nurse was notified and attempted to revive this patient. This patient was put on a mechanical ventilator and was admitted to the intensive care unit. Unfortunately, he died 1 hour later (Joint Commission, 2007b).

Learning from a Patient Case

Mr. A, a patient who was receiving care in a behavioral health care unit (also called a psychiatric unit), experienced severe delirium, hallucinations, and tremors. Mr. A began to exhibit dangerous behaviors.

Later on, Mr. A's responsible nurse, Nurse B, started making an arrangement to transfer Mr. A to an acute medical care unit, due to Mr. A's medical problems. However, Nurse B was very concerned about Mr. A's safety and the safety of the other patients and staff. Despite those concerns, Mr. A was transferred to an acute medical care unit for treatment of his medical problems.

When Mr. A was in the acute medical unit, Nurse C, the responsible nurse, tried a variety of alternatives to restraint use, but each alternative was unsuccessful in calming down Mr. A. Several nurses then together placed Mr. A in four-point restraints in the only available private room, which was located far from the nurses' station.

Unfortunately, staff was in short supply that evening, and no nursing staff was available to remain with Mr. A and provide constant observation. The charge nurse intended to return every 5 minutes for observation. However, other urgent situations developed in this unit. The charge nurse and Nurse C did not return to Mr. A's room to check on him for almost 1 hour.

Just then, Nurse C found that Mr. A was unresponsive after having a heart attack. Mr. A also had huge ridges on all four extremities (Joint Commission, 2007b).

Learning from a Legal Case Summary

On August 1, 1995, Patient R, an 86-year-old man, was admitted into an inpatient care unit in Hospital S because of heart problems. Patient R also suffered from confusion and disorientation.

On August 3, 1995, Patient R was observed attempting to get out of his bed and was then moved to a patient room near the nurses' station. At the same time, Patient R was restrained with a vest restraint, which is a cloth device designed to limit a patient's ability to get out of bed. Due to his heart problems, Patient R was also monitored by a telemetry technician at a remote site.

According to the telemetry technician on duty the night of August 4, 1995, Patient R made a total of four requests after 11:00 P.M. asking for a nurse's assistance. The responsible nursing staff did not respond to any of these four requests. At 12:01 A.M., August 5, 1995, the telemetry monitor on Patient R showed that Patient R was suffering from ventricular fibrillation. The nurses' station was notified and a nurse immediately ran to Patient R's room.

Patient R was found beside his bed. The vest restraint was wrapped around Patient R's neck and he was caught on the bed. The nurse cut the vest away immediately and tried to revive Patient R. Patient R was pronounced dead at 12:40 A.M. The medical examiner concluded that Patient R had died of asphyxia by hanging.

The daughters and the estate of Patient R filed a malpractice suit against Hospital S, alleging that the nursing staff's negligence resulted in the death of Patient R while he was a patient in Hospital S. The jury found that damages in the amount of $3,310,000 should be awarded to Patient R's daughters and the estate. The judgment and the amount of award were affirmed in the court of appeals.

Source: NexisLexis®Academic: Federal & State Cases (Case number: 13-00-341-CV; December 20, 2001, decided) (accessed on December 4, 2007).

Knowing about physical restraints and seclusion

Physical restraint refers to physically restricting a patient's freedom of physical activity, normal access to his or her body, and movement, by using physical devices such as wrist restraints, jacket vests, and physical procedures (e.g., therapeutic or protective holds). Figure 1 shows a patient with wrist restraints; Figure 2 illustrates the use of both wrist and vest restraints.

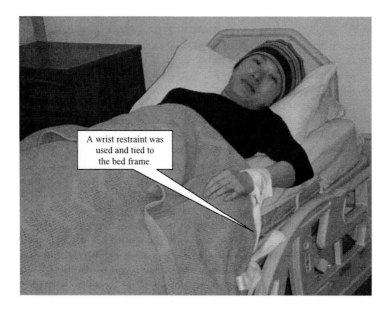

Figure 1. A patient with only the wrist restraint being used.

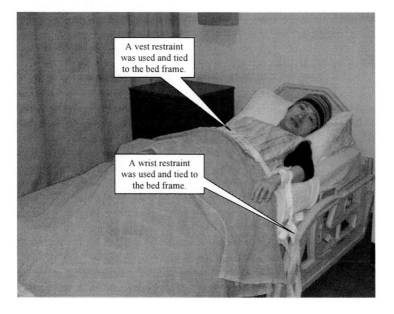

Figure 2. A patient in both the wrist and vest restrains.

Efforts to prevent aggression, agitation, confusion, and wandering often lead to restraint use. Violence by patients against others represents a safety issue in acute care hospitals, especially in facilities that provide behavioral health services. Prevention of inpatient falls is a main safety concern in acute inpatient care units, which can lead to restraint use (e.g., applying physical restraint on a patient at high risk for falling). When physical restraint is used improperly, serious injury or death can result.

For clarification, restraints exclude the situations of: (1) applying medical immobilization as a regular part of medical procedures and standard practices to limit mobility or temporary immobilization (e.g., arm restraint during IV administration, body restraint during surgery, and temporary physical restraint before administration of electroconvulsive therapy); (2) using adaptive supports in response to a patient's need (e.g., postural support and orthopedic appliances); (3) applying helmets; and (4) using forensic and correction restrictions for security reasons (Joint Commission, 2007a, 2007b).

The standards for restraint use in acute medical-surgical settings are listed in Table 1. The standards applying to the use of restraints and seclusion in the behavioral health care settings (also called psychiatric facilities or units) are summarized in Table 2.

Table 1. The standards for restraint use and elements of performance for acute medical and surgical inpatient care settings

Standard	Element of performance
Determining a careful approach to restraint use for nonpsychiatric patients	1. The hospital's policies on the use of restraint in the care of nonpsychiatric patients are in place. 2. Clinical justification for the use of restraint is identified and guided by clear criteria present in practice guidelines. 3. When clinical criteria are not available, the qualified staff establishes criteria or guides justification for the relevant patient population and clinical services.

Establishing policies and procedures to guide safe and proper use of restraint	1. The hospital's policies and procedures are developed by appropriate staff and approved by the medical staff, nursing leaders, and others as appropriate.
	2. The policies and procedures for restraint use should include the appropriate details, including:
	  2.1 Protecting the patient and preserving the patient's rights, dignity, and well-being during restraint use
	  2.2 Making a decision based on the patient's assessed needs
	  2.3 Making decisions about applying the least restrictive methods
	  2.4 Ensuring a safe restraint application and removal by qualified staff
	  2.5 Monitoring and reassessing the patient's condition during restraint use by qualified staff
	  2.6 Meeting the patient's physical needs during restraint use
	  2.7 Addressing risks related to vulnerable patient populations (e.g., pediatric, cognitively or physically limited patients)
	  2.8 Making efforts to discuss the issue related to restraint use with the patient and the family around the time of restraint use
	  2.9 Limiting individual restraint orders to physicians
	  2.10 Requiring renewal of restraint orders in accordance with applicable law and regulation
	  2.11 Documenting all restraint episodes in medical records

Standard	Element of performance

Initiating any restraint use according to either an appropriate protocol or an individual order	1. Restraint protocols should include:
	  1.1 Guidelines for assessing the patient
	  1.2 Criteria for applying the restraint
	  1.3 Criteria for monitoring the patient and reassessing the need for restraints
	  1.4 Criteria for removing restraints
	  1.5 Criteria to reflect the hospital's policies and procedures on the appropriate and safe restraint use
	  1.6 Criteria approved by the medical staff, nursing leaders, and others as appropriate
	2. Except for the restraint initiated under a protocol, restraints can be used only on the order of a physician.
	3. An authorized staff maintains and terminates restraint use according to established criteria, the individual patient's needs, and appropriate clinical justification.
	4. An individual order for initiating and renewing restraints must be consistent with the hospital's policies and procedures. Each individual order must identify a rationale for any variation from the hospital's policies and procedures, if any.
	5. If a physician is not available to issue a restraint order, a registered nurse can initiate restraint use based on an appropriate assessment of the patient. In this situation, a physician must be notified within 12 hours of the initiation of restraint. A verbal or written order should be obtained from this physician and included in the corresponding patient's medical record.
	6. If the initiation of restraint is based on a significant change in the patient's condition, the responsible registered nurse must immediately notify a physician. A physician must conduct an examination of the patient, and a written order should be entered into the patient's medical record within 24 hours of the initiation of restraint use.
	7. If the restraint will be continued beyond the first 24 hours, a physician must renew the original order or issue a new order. A renewal or a new order must be based on the result of the examination of the patient conducted by a physician. Such a renewal or new order must be issued no less often than once each calendar day.

Identifying opportunities to reduce the risks related to restraint use by prevention strategies, innovations, and process improvements	1. Hospitals should measure and assess the prevalence of restraint use. 2. Hospitals should identify opportunities to introduce preventive strategies, alternatives to restraint use, and process improvements to reduce the risks related to restraint use.
Monitoring patients while restraints in use	1. An individual patient's needs and the hospital's policies and procedures should be used to establish the frequency, nature, and extent of monitoring of a patient in restraints. 2. A patient in restraints should be monitored at least every 2 hours or sooner. 3. Monitoring should be conducted by qualified staff. Monitoring should be accomplished by direct examination, interaction with the patient, or observation.

Table 1. Continued

Standard	Element of performance

Documenting each episode of restraint use in medical records	1. When restraints are used based on a protocol, the patient's record should reference the protocol or include the protocol.
	2. The hospital's policies and procedures should establish the frequency, format, and content of documentation in the patient's record as related to each episode of restraint use.
	3. Documentation should include:
	    3.1 Relevant orders for restraint use
	    3.2 Findings of patient monitoring
	    3.3 Results of reassessment
	    3.4 Significant changes in the patient's condition

Source: Joint Commission (2007a). *2008 Comprehensive accreditation manual for hospitals: The official handbook* (pp. PC-26 – PC30). Oakbrook Terrace, IL: Joint Commission Resources.

Table 2. The standards for restraint and seclusion use and elements of performance for behavioral health care settings or psychiatric hospitals

Standard	Element of performance

Establish and communicate the hospital's philosophy on the use of restraints and seclusion to all staff members who provide direct care.	1. The hospital's philosophy should address:
	    1.1 Committing to prevent and reduce restraint and seclusion use
	    1.2 Preventing emergency situations that have the potential to lead to restraint or seclusion use
	    1.3 Promoting nonphysical interventions as preferred interventions
	    1.4 Limiting the use of restraints and seclusion to emergency situations
	    1.5 Facilitating the discontinuation of restraint or seclusion use as soon as possible
	    1.6 Raising awareness among staff about the impacts of restraint or seclusion use on patients
	    1.7 Preserving the safety and dignity of the patient when restraint or seclusion is used
	2. The hospital philosophy should be communicated to all staff that provides direct care.

Staffing levels should be set to minimize the use of restraints and seclusion and maximize safety when restraints and seclusion are used.	1. The hospital's staffing levels and assignments should consider:
	    1.1 Acuity levels of the patients
	    1.2 Age and developmental functions of the patients
	    1.3 Frequently seen diagnoses of the patients
	    1.4 Concurrent conditions in the setting
	    1.5 Physical design of the care environment
	    1.6 Staff qualifications

Standard	Element of performance

Staff are competent to minimize the restraint and seclusion use and ensure the patient's safety when restraint use is indicated.	1. Before staff participates in any use of restraints or seclusion, the hospital should ensure they are trained and competent to minimize the use of restraints and seclusion and to apply restraint and seclusion safely.
	2. All staff that provides direct patient care receives ongoing training and demonstrates an understanding of:
	  2.1 The underlying reasons of threatening behaviors revealed by the patient. For example, sometimes a patient may show an aggressive behavior that is related to a patient's medical condition and not related to an emotional condition.
	  2.2 The ways that staff behaviors can affect the patients' behaviors
	  2.3 Using de-escalation, mediation, self-protection, and other techniques (e.g., time-out)
	  2.4 Observation skills to recognize signs of physical distress in patients who are being held, restrained, or secluded
	  2.5 The safe use of restraints, including: physical holding techniques, take-down procedures, and the application and removal of mechanical restraints
	  2.6 How age, developmental functions, gender issues, ethnicity, and history of sexual or physical abuse may affect the way in which a patient reacts to physical contact
	  2.7 Viewpoints of patients who have experienced restraint or seclusion
	3. Observations of the patients in restraints should be conducted at least every 15 minutes. Staff members who are authorized to perform 15-minute assessments should receive ongoing training and be competent in:
	  3.1 Taking vital signs and interpreting their relevance to the physical safety of the patient in restraints or seclusion
	  3.2 Recognizing the nutrition and hydration needs of the patient in restraints or seclusion
	  3.3 Checking the circulation and range of motion in the patient's extremities
	  3.4 Addressing the patient's hygiene and elimination needs
	  3.5 Attending to the patient's physical and psychological status and comfort
	  3.6 Helping the patient in restraints or seclusion meet the behavioral criteria for discontinuing restraints or seclusion
	  3.7 Recognizing the patient's readiness for discontinuing the use of restraints or seclusion
	  3.8 Distinguishing the signs of any incorrect application of restraints
	  3.9 Recognizing the needs and when to contact an appropriate physician to evaluate or treat the patient's physical condition
	4. A sufficient number of staff who provide direct patient care should receive additional training to initiate first aid and cardiopulmonary resuscitation.
	5. The hospital has a plan of providing emergency medical services when needed.

Table 2. Continued

Standard	Element of performance

The initial assessment of each patient at admission should be thorough because the information may help minimize the use of restraint or seclusion.	1. The initial assessment of a patient who is at risk for self-harm should include the following information:
	  1.1 Possible methods, techniques, or tools that may help the patient control behaviors. The patient or family may help in identifying such methods.
	  1.2 Pre-existing medical conditions (e.g., physical disabilities and limitations) that may put the patient at greater risk during restraint or seclusion use
	  1.3 Any history of sexual or physical abuse, which may place the patient at greater psychological risk when restraints or seclusion are used
	  1.4 The patient or family members are educated about the hospital's philosophy and policies on restraint and seclusion use.
	    1.4.1 The family's role (e.g., receiving a notification of a restraint or seclusion use episode) is discussed with the patient.
	    1.4.2 This education is done in concurrence with discussing the patient's right to confidentiality.
	2. The staff members who provides direct patient care should be aware of the patient's behavioral health advance directive, if any.

Nonphysical methods are the preferred interventions in behavior management.	1. Nonphysical methods are always the preferred interventions, including redirecting the patient's focus or using verbal de-escalation.
Restraint or seclusion should be used for emergencies.	1. Restraints or seclusion should be used only when nonphysical interventions are ineffective and when there is an impending risk of a patient who can physically harm self or others. 2. Staff should select an appropriate type of physical intervention based on the information learned from the patient's initial assessment. 3. Hospitals should prohibit restraint or seclusion use for any other purposes, including coercion, intimidation, discipline, convenience, or revenge by staff.

The use of restraints or seclusion should be ordered by a physician.	1. All restraint and seclusion uses are applied and continued according to an order by the physician, who is primarily responsible for the patient's ongoing care, or the physician's designee.
	2. No longer than 1 hour or as soon as possible after the initiation of restraint or seclusion qualified staff must:
	  2.1 Notify and obtain a verbal or written order from the responsible physician.
	  2.2 Consult with the physician about the patient's physical and psychological conditions.
	3. The physician must perform the following tasks on being notified:
	  3.1 Supplying an order
	  3.2 Reviewing with staff about the patient's physical and psychological status
	  3.3 Determining whether restraint or seclusion use should be continued

Standard	Element of performance
	3.4 Providing staff with guidance or ways to help the patient regain control
The patient's family is notified promptly after initiating a restraint or seclusion use.	1. If the patient has consented to have the family informed about care and the family has agreed to be notified, the staff should attempt to contact the family promptly to notify the family of the restraint or seclusion use episode.

A physician must examine the patient in person.	1. The physician, who is primarily responsible for the patient's ongoing care, or the designee, must evaluate the patient in person using the following criteria:
	    1.1 Within 4 hours of the initiation of restraint or seclusion use for patients 18 years old or older
	    1.2 Within 2 hours for pediatric or adolescent patients 17 years old or younger
	    1.3 For Medicare patients, within 1 hour of the initiation of restraint or seclusion
	2. The physician is expected to perform the following tasks:
	    2.1 Working with the patient and staff to identify ways to help the patient regain control
	    2.2 Revising the patient's care plan as needed
	    2.3 Providing a new written order if needed
	3. If the patient is no longer in restraints or seclusion and the original restraint or seclusion order expires, the physician is expected to evaluate the patient in person again within 24 hours of the initiation of restraint or seclusion use.

Written or verbal orders for initiating or continuing restraint or seclusion use should be time limited.	1. Written or verbal orders for restraint or seclusion use should be limited to the following criteria:
	    1.1 Four hours for patients 18 years old or older
	    1.2 Two hours for pediatric or adolescent patients 9-17 years old
	    1.3 One hour for pediatric patients younger than 9 years old
	2. Orders for restraint or seclusion use should not be written as standing orders or on an 'as needed' basis.
	3. If restraint or seclusion use is necessary beyond the expiration of the time-limited order, a new order for restraint or seclusion use must be obtained from the physician (or designee) primarily responsible for the patient's ongoing care.

Patients in restraints or seclusion should be regularly re-evaluated.	1. By the time the restraint or seclusion order expires, the patient must be evaluated in person by the physician, or the designee, who is primarily responsible for the patient's ongoing care.

Source: Joint Commission (2007a). 2008 *Comprehensive accreditation manual for hospitals: The official handbook* (pp. PC-30 – PC41). Oakbrook Terrace, IL: Joint Commission Resources.

Standards to the Use of Restraint and Seclusion

In the process of hospital accreditation, the Joint Commission (2007a) set different standards to medical-surgical (nonpsychiatric) settings and behavioral health care settings for the use of restraints and seclusion. Restraint use in medical-surgical settings differs from that in behavioral health settings. Seclusion only applies to behavioral health care settings, and often occurs in a room set aside for the purpose of seclusion. Seclusion is often used for agitated patients. Restraints may or may not be used when seclusion is applied.

The standards on the use of restraints and seclusion are indicated in the section of provision of care, treatment, and services of the 2008 Comprehensive Accreditation Manual for Hospitals: The Official Handbook (Joint Commission, 2007a). As indicated in this handbook, the standards for the use of restraints in medical-surgical (nonpsychiatric) care areas apply to patients who are:

1. Hospitalized to receive medical or surgical services
2. In the emergency room for assessment, stabilization, or treatment for health care reasons other than behavioral issues
3. In medical observation beds
4. Undergoing same-day or outpatient surgical procedures
5. Receiving rehabilitation as inpatients or outpatients

Risk Factors and Possible Solutions as Suggested by the Joint Commission

According to the data abstracted from the Joint Commission's sentinel event database, restraint- or seclusion-related deaths and injuries represent 3.9% (n = 138) of all 3548 reviewed sentinel events that occurred during 1995-2005. Among the 27 restraint- or seclusion-related sentinel events occurring in 2004 and 2005, 10 events occurred in the behavioral health care units within general hospitals, 10 events in the medical or surgical inpatient care units within general hospitals, and 7 events in psychiatric hospitals.

Among these 27 events, the causes of death were cardiac or respiratory arrest (70%) and suffocation (30%). The five primary factors contributing to these 27 sentinel events were (Joint Commission, 2007b):

1. Therapeutic hold or takedown (26%)
2. Four- or five-point restraint (15%)
3. Wrist restraint (15%)
4. Vest restraint (11%)
5. Seclusion (7%)

The Joint Commission International Center for Patient Safety (1998) also reported five factors that were most likely to contribute to an increased risk of death, including:

1. Restraining a patient in a room that was not under continuous observation by nursing staff
2. Restraining a patient in the supine position, which can predispose the patient to aspiration
3. Restraining a patient in the prone position, which can predispose the patient to suffocation
4. Restraining a patient with deformities that preclude the proper application of the restraint device, especially for applying the vest restraint devices

5.   Restraining of a patient who smokes

Based on the root cause analyses of the reported sentinel events that occurred during 1995-2005, the Joint Commission (2007b) identified four major root causes related to the use of restraints in medical or surgical inpatient care settings, and one root cause associated with the use of restraint and seclusion in behavioral health care settings and psychiatric hospitals. These five root causes and the corresponding prevention strategies are summarized in Table 3. It should be noted that these prevention strategies involve primarily nurses but require the support of the hospital leaders.

Table 3. The major root causes of the reported sentinel events related to restraint or seclusion use and the corresponding prevention strategies for nurses

Root cause	Prevention strategy
Restraint use in medical and surgical inpatient care settings	

Insufficient staff orientation, training, or competence assessment	1. Nursing leaders and managers need to ensure that nurses who provide direct patient care are competent in restraint use and monitoring.
	  1.1 If nurses do not feel well-trained and competent enough in restraint use, they should inform their supervisor for more training and supervision.
	  1.2 Nursing managers or experienced staff can offer guidance to less experienced staff on restraint use.
	2. Nurses must know the alternatives for restraint use, including:
	  2.1 Assessing the patient for hunger, thirst, pain, or discomfort
	  2.2 Discussing with the patient about the unsafe behavior and asking the patient to stop the unsafe behavior and remain calm
	  2.3 Walking with the patient
	  2.4 Adjusting the environment of the patient room to make the patient more comfortable (e.g., furniture arrangement, lighting, and displaying items from home)
	  2.5 Placing a chair or wheelchair at the nurses' station for the patient needing constant observation
	  2.6 Using bed, chair, or door alarms for patients who may wander
	  2.7 Using nondrug alternatives (e.g., massage therapy) to manage pain to avoid symptoms of mental confusion, which may lead to restraint use
	  2.8 Using family visitors or trained sitters to provide constant observation
	3. Hospital and nursing leaders should provide ongoing reinforcing training and education about safe use of restraints and alternatives to restraints.
	4. Nurses can help ensure proper orders for restraint use.
	  4.1 Nursing staff should not implement restraint orders written as 'use physical restraint as needed' or 'prn.'
	  4.2 The restraint orders should be time limited and specific about the type of device to be used and the reason for its use.
	  4.3 Nurses can help ensure that restraint orders meet the hospital's policies in restraint use and are properly documented in the patient records.
	5. Nurses should inform their immediate supervisor about the unsafe staffing levels to provide needed constant observation and to minimize the use of restraints.

Table 3. Continued

Root cause	Prevention strategy

Unsafe care environment, unsafe equipment, and inappropriate device use	1. Nurses must select safe restraint devices according to the needs of the patient populations served.
	2. Nurses must apply restraint devices safely, including, for example:
	   2.1 Tying knots that can be released quickly
	   2.2 Securing bed restraints to the bed springs or frame, or the parts of the bed that move with the patient for an adjustable bed
	   2.3 Applying only soft restraints to older patients and patients with osteoporosis because these patients can be injured by restraint devices
	   2.4 If possible, nurses should avoid high-risk restraint devices, including vest and waist restraint devices and split side rails.
	3. Nurses should ensure a safe care environment for the surrounding area of the patient with restraint use.
	4. Nurses must be aware of the hospital's existing preventive maintenance programs.
	   4.1 When nurses find that restraint devices have not been maintained as required, they should know whom to notify and how.
	   4.2 It is also important to know how to obtain a replacement if needed.

Inadequate initial patient assessment and reassessment	1. Nursing assessment and reassessment on the patient in restraints must be performed in a timely and thorough manner, according to the hospital's policies.
	   1.1 As indicated in the Joint Commission's Sentinel Event Database, all the victims of strangulation were elderly patients who had been placed in a vest restraint. In addition, all victims of death by fire were men who were attempting to smoke or use a cigarette lighter to burn off the restraint.
	2. Nurses must properly assess the patient's nutritional status.
	   2.1 Nursing staff should be aware that a patient's nutritional status can directly affect the cognition level, which may lead to the need for restraint use. When a patient becomes confused or behaves inappropriately or is at risk for fluid and electrolyte imbalance, it is important to assess this patient's nutritional status.
	   2.2 Timely identification of nutritional issues (e.g., dehydration, malnutrition, fluid and electrolyte imbalance, and blood glucose level), especially with elderly patients, is essential.
	3. Nurses should assess the patient's pain management needs.
	   3.1 Agitation or restlessness may indicate an increase in discomfort or pain. Nurses should assess pain on admission and reassess on an ongoing basis to avoid unnecessary restraint use.
	   3.2 Nurses should be aware that patients in restraints may attempt to get out of the restraints to maximize comfort and relieve pain.
	4. Nurses need to assess the patient's toileting needs.
	   4.1 When a patient is in restraints, the responsible nurse should assess the patient's bowel and bladder functions and develop a care plan to meet toileting needs. Scheduled toileting can reduce the anxiety about the needs to eliminate urine or stool by attempting to get out of restraints.
	   4.2 Scheduled toileting can decrease wandering by patients who are unable to express their needs clearly and looking for the bathroom. Without resolving the reasons, wandering may lead to unneeded restraint use.
	5. Nurses should be aware that cognitive issues (e.g., inadequate perception of surroundings and mental disorientation) can lead to restraint use. As a result, nurses must accurately assess the patient's mental cognition in the initial patient assessment.

Root cause	Prevention strategy
	6. Nurses also need to assess the patient's physical strength. Nurses need to know that sometimes confusion seems to increase the patient's physical strength. When interacting with a confused patient, nurses should keep this in mind to be able to protect the patient and themselves from injury. 7. Nurses should identify alternatives for restraint use. If family members are willing to provide one-on-one observation as a restraint alternative, physical restraint would not be necessary. Nurses can teach family members therapeutic holding techniques when they are available to provide one-on-one observation. 8. Nurses must assess each patient for the appropriateness of restraint use. For example, when restraints are used to prevent inpatient falls, the responsible nurse should evaluate the patient's cognitive status, muscle strength and stability while ambulating, agitation, use of medications, and other risks for falls.
Inadequate care provision and plans	1. Nurses should be prepared for any sudden behavioral changes in patients. 1.1 For example, nurses need to aware that patients with head injuries resulting in cognitive or mental impairments may move suddenly and injure themselves or others. Such patients' mental status can limit their understanding or perception of catheters, tubes, IV lines, and other care equipment (e.g., monitor leads). These patients may try to pull a line out or dislodge leads. 2. Nurses must assess patients for risk of dislodging IV lines and other medical equipment. 3. Nurses must use restraints with caution. For example, when a patient needs restraint for safety, the restraint should restrict the patient's movements only to the degree that is needed but could not result in injury or strangulation.
Restraint or seclusion use in behavioral health care settings	
Inadequate observation and monitoring	1. Hospital and nursing leaders and nurses together may develop programs to reduce restraint or seclusion use, including better identification of patients who are more likely to need restraint. 2. Nurses need to have sufficient observation on patients to prevent the need for restraints or seclusion. 3. Nurses can help ensure compliance with requirements related to time limits for restraint or seclusion orders, according to the hospital's policies and processes. 4. Nurses must be knowledgeable about the proper use of physical restraint techniques. 5. According to the hospital's policies, nurses need to observe the patient while in restraints or seclusion and document the observation. 6. The medical needs of the patient in restraints should be assessed by the responsible physicians at admission and addressed as needed. 7. Behavioral health care units and psychiatric hospitals should be equipped to manage medical emergencies (e.g., cardiorespiratory arrest). It is noted that the risk of cardiac events can be increased by psychotropic medications and the physical effects of restraint use.

Source: Joint Commission (2007b). Preventing serious injury or death in physical restraint or seclusion. In R. A. Porché, Jr. (Ed.), *Front line of defense: The role of nurses in preventing sentinel events* (2nd ed., pp. 99-112). Oakbrook Terrace, IL: Joint Commission.

Critical Tips to Prevent Serious Injury or Death in Physical Restraint and Seclusion

Tables 4 and 5 list the critical tips to prevent serious injury or death associated with the use of physical restraints and seclusion. Table 4 was prepared for nurses, who work in acute medical and surgical inpatient care units, and Table 5 was created for families, who are willing to be involved in their hospitalized loved one's inpatient care (e.g., providing one-to-one constant observation).

Table 4. Preventing physical restraint- and seclusion-related serious injuries or deaths: Critical tips for nurses who work in acute, medical, and surgical inpatient care units

Dimension	Tip
Adequate competency for restraint and seclusion use	1. Nurses who provide direct patient care should be competent in restraint use and monitoring. Supervisors and experienced staff can offer guidance to less experience staff on restraint use.
	2. Nurses must ensure proper restraint or seclusion orders. The restraint orders should be time limited and be specific about the type of device to be used and the reason for its use.
	3. When implementing a restraint order, nurses must be sure to apply the ordered restraint devices safely and correctly. For example:
	3.1 Nurses should tie knots that can be released quickly.
	3.2 It is important to secure bed restraints to the bed springs or frame or the parts of the bed that move with the patient for an adjustable bed.
	3.3 Before implementing a restraint order, nurses should also check for the appropriate type of restraint device for the patient served. Nurses should apply only soft restraints to older patients and patients with osteoporosis.
	3.4 When a patient needs restraint for safety, the restraint should restrict the patient's movements only to the degree that is needed but could not result in injury or strangulation.
	4. According to the hospital's policies, nursing assessment and reassessment on the patient's condition and the patient's needs (e.g., toileting, food, and water) while in restraints must be performed in a timely and thorough manner.
	5. Nurses should observe the patient while in restraints or seclusion in a timely manner and document the observation according to the hospital's policies.
	6. Nurses must know the alternatives for restraint or seclusion use. Possible alternatives include:
	6.1 Adjusting the care environment (e.g., the area surrounding the bed) to make the patient more comfortable
	6.2 Assessing the patient for hunger, thirst, pain, or discomfort and providing food, water, and pain management as needed
	6.3 Discussing with the patient about the unsafe behavior and asking him or her to stop the unsafe behavior and remain calm
	6.4 Increasing the frequency of observation to prevent the need for restraint or seclusion use
	6.5 Placing a chair or wheelchair at the nurses' station for the patient who needs constant observation
	6.6 Using bed, chair, and door alarms for patients who may wander
	6.7 Using nondrug alternatives (e.g., massage therapy) to manage pain to avoid symptoms, such as mental confusion, which may lead to restraint use
	6.8 Using family visitors or trained sitters to provide constant observation
	6.9 Walking with the patient

Dimension	Tip
Sufficient staffing to prevent restraint use	1. Nurses must inform their supervisor about the unsafe staffing level to provide needed constant observation and to minimize the use of restraints.
Promoting the safety of the care environment	1. Hospital and nursing leaders must purchase safe restraint devices according to the needs of the patient populations served. 2. Nurses must be aware of the hospital's existing preventive maintenance programs. When nurses find that restraint devices have not been maintained as required, they should know whom to notify and how. It is also important to know how to obtain a replacement if needed. 3. The nurse who observes the patient in restraints must ensure the safety of the patient room and the immediate surrounding area.

Communication to patients and families	1. If the family member is willing to assist in patient care and provide one-on-one constant observation, the responsible nurse must provide educational information to families.
	  1.1 The rationales of providing constant observation should be well communicated between the nurses and the family members. For example, the purposes of providing constant observation can be to prevent falls, wandering, or as an alternative to restraint use.
	  1.2 Nurses must repeat the educational information as often as needed because family visitors may take turns in being with the patient.
	2. When communicating with patients and family members, nurses must communicate and educate patients and their families in an understandable format and using the language preferred. Hospitals should provide interpreters to assist with the education or translate materials.

Table 5. Preventing physical restraint- and seclusion-related serious injuries or deaths: Critical tips for accompanying families

Dimension	Tip

When we, as family members, are used as an alternative to restraint use, we must know the physical and mental conditions of our hospitalized loved one.	1. At admission and anytime during the hospital stay, the patient and family members can help nurses identify alternatives to restraint use.
	2. If family members are willing to provide one-on-one observation as one of the restraint alternatives, physical restraint would not be necessary.
	  2.1 The family member who provides constant observation to the patient must know the current physical and mental conditions of the patient.
	  2.2 The family member also needs to know the patient's risk for falls and endangering himself or herself or others (e.g., wandering, dislodging IV lines and other medical equipment).
	  2.3 The family member should ask for verbal or written (or both) educational instructions from the responsible nurse as related to the hospitalized loved one's needs and care. For example, the responsible nurse can teach family members therapeutic holding techniques when providing one-on-one observation. It is also important for the family member to ask for and know how to use bed rails appropriately to protect the patient.

Table 5. Continued

Dimension	Tip
	3. The accompanying family member should use the call light system to communicate with the responsible nurse when offering one-on-one constant observation.
	4. The family member should ensure that the patient's physical needs are met (e.g., toileting, water, and food).
	4.1 The family member should ask for assistance when transferring the patient as needed, especially for the patient who is on the fall precaution program.
	4.2 The need for assistance should be determined by the responsible nurse and depends on the patient's physical and cognitive conditions.
	5. The family member must report any observed changes in the patient's condition (e.g., becoming more agitated) to the responsible nurse as soon as possible.
	5.1 Any observed changes can be critical and may need to be addressed immediately.
	5.2 The family member must be prepared for any sudden behavioral changes in the patient. For example, the patient with a head injury may have cognitive or mental impairments. Such a patient may move suddenly and injure himself or herself or others. Such patient's mental status can limit the understanding or perception of catheters, tubes, IV lines, and other care equipment (e.g., monitor leads). Such patient may try to pull a line out or dislodge leads.
	6. The family member must get help from the nurse, if needed, to assist the patient use toilet or if the family member must step out of the patient room for a while.
	6.1 Family member should let the nurse know when they will be back as well.
	6.2 The family member is there to assist in nursing care. Despite everything, it is the nurse's responsibility to ensure the patient's safety at all times.
When our hospitalized loved one is in restraints, we also need to understand the physical and mental conditions of our hospitalized loved one.	1. The responsible nurse or the physician must make an effort to discuss the issue related to restraint use with the patient and family members around the time of restraint use.
	1.1 It is important for the patient and family members to know the reasons a certain type of restraint device was used and potential dangers to the patient.
	2. With or without a family member present, the responsible nurse and physician should conduct observations periodically when the patient is in restraints.
	3. When using a restraint and after removing the restraint, the family members should be notified about the most updated physical and mental status of the patient.
	4. After removing the restraint, it is important for the family member to examine the patient's skin condition thoroughly for bruises or signs of early-stage bed sores due to restraint use. If any skin breakdown is noted, the family member must notify the responsible nurse for further examination.

Dimension	Tip
Asking for a safer care environment	1. When family members are providing one-on-one constant observation, they should work with the responsible nurse to ensure a safe care environment in the patient room. 1.1 The family member should make a request for housekeeping to the responsible nurse. The patient's room and bathroom should be clean and dry. 1.2 The family members should ask the responsible nurse to remove unused equipment, if any, from the patient room.

The Joint Commission (2007a) has been promoting reduction of restraint use in the process of hospital accreditation. Hospitals also have being devoting efforts to reduce the use of restraints. Still, restraint- and seclusion-related serious injuries or deaths continue to be a patient safety concern in the acute care and psychiatric settings.

In acute medical and surgical inpatient care units, providing constant observation within a safe care environment is key to minimize restraint use. Family members can be involved in providing constant observation and additional psychological support and comfort to their hospitalized loved one who needs constant observation. Having a family member accompanying the patient, who may require restraint use, is often an alternative to decrease restraint or seclusion use. If so, the design and layout of a patient room should include a comfortable space and seating area for family members.

The facility design should also increase the visibility of patients. This way, nursing staff can provide increased and continuous observation of the patients (with or without restraint use) and minimize the need for restraints. Installing cameras in all patient rooms or designated private rooms for monitoring patients with restraint use from the nurses' station should be considered. Adding windows in alcove doors is another possible facility design consideration for increasing observation and monitoring for the patients with restraints (Reiling & Chernos, 2007).

References

Joint Commission (2007a). *2008 Comprehensive accreditation manual for hospitals: The official handbook*. Oakbrook Terrace, IL: Joint Commission Resources.

Joint Commission (2007b). Preventing serious injury or death in physical restraint or seclusion. In R. A. Porché, Jr. (Ed.), *Front line of defense: The role of nurses in preventing sentinel events* (2nd ed., pp. 99-112). Oakbrook Terrace, IL: Joint Commission.

Joint Commission International Center for Patient Safety (1998). Issue 8-Preventing restraint deaths (November 8, 1998). Available at: http://www.jcipatientsafety.org/147989 (accessed December 8, 2007).

Reiling, J., & Chernos, S. (2007). Human factors in hospital safety design. In P. Carayon (Ed.), *Handbook of human factors and ergonomics in health care and patient safety* (pp. 275-286). Mahwah, NJ: Lawrence Erlbaum Associates.

Inpatient Suicide

Learning from a Patient Case

A male patient, Mr. F, was admitted to a surgical unit for evaluation and observation the afternoon before his planned surgery to remove a lung cancer mass. He was placed in a private room. Prior to his admission, he had a biopsy. The diagnosis and the treatment plan were clear.

The responsible nurse, Nurse A, conducted the admission physical assessment and instructed Mr. F in the usual preoperative care to expect. Nurse A discussed the upcoming surgery with Mr. F and asked whether he had any questions. Mr. F said he was fine and had no questions.

Early that evening, Mr. F kissed his wife good night and told her that he would see her in the morning. Then, his wife left the hospital. Later that evening, Mr. F got himself ready for bed and turned off his light.

About 10:30 P.M., Nurse A heard a loud crash from Mr. F's room and hurried into the room. Nurse A noted that Mr. F was no longer in the room and that the window had been shattered. She ran to the window and saw Mr. F six stories below lying face down. Mr. F was immediately transported to the emergency room, where he was pronounced dead (Joint Commission, 2007a).

Learning from a Patient Case

A 28-year-old male patient, Mr. G, was combative and aggressive on a psychiatric inpatient care unit. Mr. G required restraint and a restraint order was implemented. After Mr. G became more subdued, he was placed in seclusion because there was insufficient staff to provide constant monitoring of his behavior.

In seclusion, Mr. G was alone for a long enough time to remove the drawstring from his gym shorts and tie a slip noose around his neck. Mr. G strangled himself to death (Joint Commission, 2007a).

Knowledge about Inpatient Suicide

The suicide rates in the United States are mostly stable over time, ranging from 12.4 to 10.7/100,000 population. In 2004, the annual suicide rate was 11.5 per 100,000 population, which translated into 89 suicides per day or a suicide every 16 minutes. As a matter of fact, suicide is the eleventh leading cause of death. It is generally estimated that there are 25 attempts for each death by suicide (American Association of Suicidology, 2007).

Suicide distresses families, friends, as well as health care providers. Suicide often prompts guilt in people who think they missed a clue or may have been able to prevent the suicide, if only they had done something differently (Joint Commission, 2007a).

Hospital Standards to Prevent Inpatient Suicides

In the 2008 National Patient Safety Goals for Hospitals, Goal 15, Requirement 15A was meant to identify patients at risk for suicide (Joint Commission, 2007b). This requirement applies to the patients being treated in psychiatric hospitals and for emotional or behavioral disorders in general hospitals. Identification of individual patients at risk for suicide while receiving care in a staffed, round-the-clock care setting is an important first step in protecting and planning the care of these at-risk patients. Recognition of individual patients at risk for suicide following discharge from a hospital is also essential.

As for the compliance solutions, hospitals are expected to implement a risk assessment on all admitted inpatients to identify specific risk factors that may increase or decrease risk for suicide. Each high-risk suicidal patient's immediate safety needs and treatment should be addressed without delay. For these high-risk suicidal patients, hospitals must also provide information, such as a crisis hotline, to patients and their families for crisis situations after the patients are discharged from a hospital (Joint Commission, 2007b).

The purpose of suicide risk assessment is to identify patients at increased risk for suicide. Periodic reassessment is needed to continuously monitor suicide risk over time. However, suicide risk commonly is not considered in patients being admitted to acute inpatient care units for medical or surgical reasons. Suicide risk must be considered in all patients admitted to psychiatric hospitals and to general hospitals for emotional or behavioral disorders and medical or surgical conditions (Joint Commission, 2007a).

Risk Factors and Possible Solutions as Suggested by the Joint Commission

As noted, suicide risk should be considered in all patients being admitted for emotional or behavioral disorders and medical or surgical reasons. Nurses should consider each individual patient's perception of his or her disease and the treatment plan.

For example, patients with cancer may feel hopeless or be depressed because they may view their cancer diagnosis as a death sentence. They are fearful that the cancer treatment will eventually deplete their financial resources. Consequently, in addition to the physical assessment portion, nurses working in medical or surgical inpatient care units should also conduct a thorough psychosocial assessment, including the patient's religious and cultural needs (Joint Commission, 2007a).

Regarding suicide prevention, it is particularly important to note that physicians and nurses tend to make assessment errors at two time points (Joint Commission, 2007a):

1. Soon after the patient is admitted to the hospital
2. When the patient is starting to feel, look, and act better and showing sudden signs of improvement

The commonly mentioned suicide risk factors are summarized in Table 1. In addition, suicide risk is often categorized into four levels (Joint Commission, 2007a):

1. High risk: In this suicidal risk level, a patient would articulate suicidal thoughts and has determined a specific plan.
2. Moderate risk: A patient would express suicidal thoughts without having considered a specific method.
3. Low risk: A patient would verbalize thoughts of death, but not by suicide.
4. Lowest risk: A patient states no thoughts of death.

As for the signs and symptoms of inpatient suicide, nurses also need to watch for patients who have a kind of agitation when they are depressed. Nurses should also watch for a patient's degree of hopelessness by asking one or more of the following questions:

1. Are you feeling hopeless?
2. How long have you been feeling hopeless?
3. What do you think is going to happen to you?
4. What do you think about the future?

For adolescent patient populations, the highest safety risk is that of suicide or self-harm. In most of the instances, adolescents try to harm themselves by, for example, cutting their arms, instead of committing to a completed or attempted suicide. These teen patients also require constant observation and a safe care environment (e.g., free of non-breakaway hardware and sharp objects; Joint Commission, 2006).

According to the Joint Commission's sentinel event database, during 1995-2005, a total of 3548 sentinel events were reviewed and 464 (13.1%) were inpatient suicides (Joint Commission, 2007a). A previous report concluded that about 75% of the suicide events used the methods of hanging in a bathroom, bedroom, or closet. Some other suicide events resulted from patients jumping from a roof or window (Joint Commission International Center for Patient Safety, 1998).

Table 1. The commonly mentioned suicide risk factors

Risk factor	Description
Anger	A person shows rage and uncontrolled temper and seeks revenge.
Anxiety	A person has anxiety or agitation or is unable to sleep.
Behavior or attitude change	A person shows a sudden change in behavior or attitude.
Hopelessness	A person indicates hopelessness.
Ideation	A person expresses or communicates ideation, including: 1. Presence of a suicide plan and final arrangements 2. Threatening to hurt or kill self 3. Talking of wanting to hurt or kill self 4. Looking for ways to kill self by seeking access to firearms, available pills, or other means 5. Talking or writing about death, dying, or suicide
Medical condition	A person suffers from chronic or terminal illness or uncontrollable pain.
Mood change	A person shows a dramatic mood change.
Previous emotional disorders	A person has a history of attempting suicide, depression, or other mood disorders (e.g., schizophrenia and bipolar disorder).
Purposelessness	A person expresses having no reason for living or no sense of purpose in life.
Recent loss	A person experienced a recent loss of, for example, family members or job.
Recklessness	A person acts reckless or engages in risk-taking or self-destructive behaviors or activities.
Substance abuse	A person increases alcohol or drug use.
Trapped	A person is feeling trapped and expresses that there no way out of the current situation.
Victim of assault	A person is a victim of sexual abuse, including incest and domestic violence.
Withdrawal	A person isolates self from friends, family members, and the familiar community.
Witness to a suicide	A person witnessed a suicide.

Sources: American Association of Suicidology (2007). Suicide in the U.S.A. based on current (2004) statistics. Available at: http://www.suicidology.org/associations/1045/files/SuicideInTheUS.pdf (accessed December 8, 2007). Joint Commission (2007a). Preventing suicide. In R. A. Porché, Jr. (Ed.), *Front line of defense: The role of nurses in preventing sentinel events* (2nd ed., pp. 113-128). Oakbrook Terrace, IL: Joint Commission.

Inpatient suicide has been the number one type of sentinel event reviewed by the Joint Commission. Based on the sentinel suicide events occurring from 1995 to 2004, the most frequently reported root cause for suicide events was environmental safety and security (about 90%), followed by patient assessment (about 80%), orientation and training (about 60%), and communication (almost 50%). The suicide events that occurred in 2005 had a similar pattern in the root causes, but there was less emphasis on staff orientation and training (Joint Commission, 2007a).

Based on the root cause analyses of the reported sentinel suicide events occurring in 1995-2005, the Joint Commission (2007a) identified five major root causes related to inpatient suicide. These five root causes and the corresponding prevention strategies are summarized in Table 2. During hospitalization, nurses have most frequent interaction with patients. Consequently, nurses have a key role in the care of potentially suicidal patients in inpatient care settings. It is noted that these prevention strategies involve primarily nurses but also require the support of hospital leaders.

Table 2. The major root causes of the reported sentinel events related to inpatient suicides and the corresponding prevention strategies for nurses

Root cause	Prevention strategy

Unsafe care environment	1. Hospital leaders are required to ensure the design of a safe, accessible, effective, and efficient care environment that meets the needs of the patient served.
	    1.1 Hospitals must meet the challenge of providing a safe care environment while maintaining individual patient's rights (e.g., the rights to privacy and dignity).
	 2. Nurses must assess the care environment to which the patient is assigned (patient room), adjust the patient's location (location of the patient room) if possible, or modify the level of observation accordingly.
	 3. Before moving a high-risk suicidal patient into a patient room, the responsible nurse must be knowledgeable about and aware of the environmental hazards in the patient room. Nurses should advocate for removing these hazards.
	    3.1 Areas and elements in the patient room, that represent an opportunity for a patient intent on committing suicide, include:
	       3.1.1 Door hinges, doorknobs, and door closers
	       3.1.2 Lighting fixtures, closet poles, metal hangers, and non-breakaway curtain rods
	       3.1.3 Non-breakaway bathroom fixtures and disability grab bars
	    3.2 Environmental hazards should be removed whenever possible.
	    3.3 When substantive changes to the environment are not possible, providing close observation, frequent evaluation, or offering one-on-one constant observation should be implemented.

Insufficient staff competence	1. Nurses must know suicide risk factors and should be comfortable with their level of skill and knowledge related to suicide prevention, including:
	    1.1 Assessment skills to determine from the patient's level of agitation, hopelessness, and behavior that a patient is in crisis
	    1.2 An understanding of the importance of the care environment and ensuring that the patient rooms are made as free of hazards as possible
	    1.3 Being aware of the patient's medication and treatment plans and knowing when the patient should receive medications
	 2. Nurses need to ensure their own personal comfort level in caring for suicidal patients.
	    2.1 Many people are fearful of suicide. As part of the orientation and initial training, nursing leaders should help new staff explore their feelings about caring for suicidal patients.
	    2.2 All nurses who care for potentially suicidal patients must be trained in the following subjects:
	       2.2.1 Philosophy of suicide prevention
	       2.2.2 Hospital's approach to suicide risk reduction
	       2.2.3 Suicide warning signs
	       2.2.4 Referral procedures
	       2.2.5 Communication procedures within the hospital
	    2.3 Training programs may include role play to help staff nurses practice their intervening and assessment skills.

Table 2. Continued

Root cause	Prevention strategy
	2.4 Crisis intervention training is also needed, where patients may be aggressive and need restraint or seclusion.
	3. Nurses in the psychiatric unit should be familiar with and consider issues related to a patient's rights, age, and disability-specific needs for safety.
	3.1 Nurses should be well trained about appropriate interaction with psychiatric patients and be aware of the fine line between patient self-determination, patient rights, and restriction of activity and freedom for safety reasons.
	3.2 Nurses must assess possessions for a patient's potential use in self-injury.
	4. Nurses in the psychiatric units must be knowledgeable about detecting and removing contraband.
	4.1 Nurses should be well trained in implementing the hospital's policies and procedures for detecting and removing contraband.
	1. On admission to a psychiatric unit or on return whenever the patient leaves the unit with a pass, patients should be searched for dangerous items, including weapons, sharp items, drugs, lighters, matches, belts, and shoelaces.
Inadequate suicide assessment or reassessment	2. Hospital and nursing leaders and nurses must advocate for a uniform approach to conduct suicide assessment and documentation.
	2.1 A standardized approach can increase the likelihood that the right clinical questions will be asked and relevant information obtained.
	2.2 Hospital and nursing leaders and nurses together need to develop and implement a standard suicidal risk assessment tool to effectively screen patients for suicidal thoughts, gestures, and attempts.
	2.3 Some interventions should be put in place on the basis of specific screening and assessment data (e.g., including in related clinical guidelines or protocols). Actions among nurses must be taken consistent with patient needs.
	3. Nurses should screen all admitted patients for suicidal ideation.
	3.1 Questions about suicide should be asked as sensitively as possible. Nurses should avoid the use of any words or statements that can seem judgmental.
	3.2 Having patients talk about their suicidal thoughts may provide relief for them.
	4. Nurses must be good listeners to ensure the complete answers or responses from patients.
	5. Nurses need to reassess suicidal patients at high-risk times of transition in a 24-hour psychiatric care unit. High-risk times include:
	5.1 The period shortly after a patient is admitted
	5.2 At the time of discharge or at the transition from inpatient care to outpatient services
	5.3 Before granting a high-risk suicidal patient a pass, authorized visits or increased privileges
	6. Before the high-risk suicidal patient is transferred outside the 24-hour psychiatric care unit, the family member(s) must be educated about suicidal warning signs.
Inadequate staffing level	1. Nurses must inform their supervisor of unsafe staffing levels that may prevent providing needed assessment, reassessment, observation, and monitoring.

Root cause	Prevention strategy

Incomplete communication among staff members and inadequate patient information	1. In the psychiatric unit, the physician, nurse, mental health technician, psychiatric aide, social worker, counselor, and psychologist are all part of the team that will have constant or daily contact with patients.
	  1.1 All involved staff should be well-informed about the conditions of their high-risk suicidal patients.
	  1.2 Nurses can help ensure that all the members in the care team are informed about their high-risk suicidal patients.
	2. Nurses can help ensure a complete information transfer of a potentially suicidal patient on admission, including physical and psychiatric histories.
	3. It is essential for nurses to document and communicate key assessment findings to appropriate colleagues.
	  3.1 If assessment findings show that a patient is at high risk for suicide, nurses must inform the responsible physician immediately to be able to implement, for example, one-on-one observation.
	4. Nurses can help ensure complete information transfer during care provision of a potentially suicidal patient.
	  4.1 Information about changes in a patient's behavior may signal a trend and must be communicated to the colleagues on the current and next shift (also called hand-off communication).
	  4.2 All suicidal thoughts, feelings, and behaviors exhibited or expressed by a patient must be clearly communicated to other health care providers, including physicians. Documentation via written notes in the patient chart or oral report is required.
	5. Nurses should help ensure complete information transfer before discharge.
	  5.1 The patient and family member(s) must be informed about what may increase the risk of the return of suicidal ideation (e.g., discontinuation of medications and noncompliance with the treatment plan).
	  5.2 The patient and family member(s) also should be informed about ongoing treatment needs, community resources, and how to access emergency care services after discharge.

Inadequate care planning or care provision	1. Nurses can help ensure completion of all assessments before initiation of a patient's care plan.
	2. Nurses should actively participate in the care planning process and communicate each patient's care plan in detail to the involved members of the care team.
	  2.1 Nurses can help ensure adequate documentation of the care plan and its dissemination to all involved members of the care team.
	  2.2 A patient also needs to accept the care plan if the intended results are to be achieved.
	3. Nurses can help ensure implementation of suicide precautions at the appropriate observation level, as ordered by the responsible physicians.
	4. Nurses should communicate the need to change a patient's observation or monitoring level to the responsible physician.
	5. Nurses can help ensure thorough implementation of the hospital's observation policies and procedures. Nurses can also help identify the occurrence of incomplete observations and take necessary steps to address the situation.
	6. As part of the care provision, nurses must ensure that supervision is adequate to the high-risk suicidal patients during high-risk activities (e.g., when the patient is in the bathroom alone).

Source: Joint Commission (2007a). Preventing suicide. In R. A. Porché, Jr. (Ed.), *Front line of defense: The role of nurses in preventing sentinel events* (2nd ed., pp. 113–128). Oakbrook Terrace, IL: Joint Commission.

Critical Tips to Prevent Inpatient Suicide

For the hospital leaders, facility design considerations are the most basic and important component in preventing inpatient suicides. As suggested by Reiling and Chernos (2007), patient rooms must be designed for maximum visibility for better observation and monitoring. Visibility can be maximized by installing cameras or glass in alcove doors. If family members are willing to provide one-to-one constant observation as an alternative to prevent inpatient suicide, the facility considerations should include a comfortable space and seating area for the accompanying families to remain with their hospitalized loved one at the bedside for a longer period of time.

Patient rooms, especially in psychiatric hospitals and the psychiatric units in general hospitals, should be equipped with, for example, break-away curtain rods and suicide-proof shower heads. Nurses need to pay special attention to ensure that sharp objects or potentially harmful items are not stored in patient rooms. We suggest that patient rooms in acute, medical, or surgical inpatient care units should also have suicide-proof interior designs and equipment because inpatient suicide can occur in these nonpsychiatric units as well. Providing a safe care environment is, indeed, the key to prevent inpatient suicides.

Table 3. Preventing inpatient suicides:
Critical tips for nurses who work in acute inpatient care units

Dimension	Tip
Providing a safe care environment	1. When assigning or reassigning a patient room to a high-risk suicidal patient, it is important for the responsible nurse to assess the care environment to which the patient is assigned. The patient should be placed in a room that is close to the nurses' station to increase monitoring. 2. Before moving a high-risk suicidal patient into a patient room, the responsible nurse must be knowledgeable and aware of the environmental hazards in the patient room and advocate for removing these hazards. 2.1 Environmental hazards should be removed whenever possible. When substantive changes to the environment are not possible, providing close observation, frequent evaluation, or one-on-one constant observation should be implemented.
Adequate staff competency in preventing inpatient suicides	1. Nurses who provide direct patient care should be competent and comfortable in caring for high-risk suicidal patients. In addition, nurses need to ensure their own personal comfort level in caring for suicidal patients. 2. Nurses must be trained and familiar with the hospital's policies and guideline related to suicide prevention. 3. Nurses should screen all admitted patients for suicidal ideation. 4. Nurses must reassess suicidal patients at high-risk times of transition, including the period shortly after a patient is admitted and at the time of discharge. 5. Nurses must ensure that supervision is adequate to the high-risk suicidal patients during high-risk activities (e.g., when the patient is in the bathroom alone).

Dimension	Tip
	6. When caring for a high-risk suicidal patient, the responsible nurse must be knowledgeable about how to detect and remove contraband. Nurses should be trained in implementing the hospital's policies and procedures for detecting and removing contraband.
Adequate staffing level to effectively prevent inpatient suicides	1. Nurses must inform their supervisor about the unsafe staffing level to provide needed constant observation and monitoring.

Sufficient communication to the involved members of the health care team	1. Nurses can help ensure complete information transfer of a potentially suicidal patient on admission, including physical and psychiatric histories.
	2. Nurses can help ensure complete information transfer during care provision of a potentially suicidal patient.
	    2.1 It is essential for nurses to document and communicate key assessment findings to appropriate colleagues. If assessment findings show that a patient is at high risk for suicide, nurses must inform the responsible physician immediately.
	3. Nurses can help ensure thorough implementation of the hospital's observation policies and procedures and implementation of suicide precautions.
	4. Nurses should help ensure complete information transfer before discharge.
	    4.1 The patient and family member(s) must be informed about what may increase the risk of the return of suicidal ideation (e.g., discontinuation of medications and noncompliance with the treatment plan).
	    4.2 The patient and family member(s) also should be informed about ongoing treatment needs, community resources, and methods to access emergency care services after discharge.

Adequate communication to patients and families	1. If a family member is willing to assist in inpatient care and provide one-on-one constant observation, the responsible nurse must provide educational information to the family member.
	    1.1 The rationales of providing constant observation should be well communicated between the family member and the responsible nurse.
	    1.2 The responsible nurse must repeat the educational information as often as needed because the accompanying family member may take turns doing the observation.
	2. When communicating with patients and family members, nurses must communicate with them in an understandable format and using the language preferred. Hospitals should provide interpreters to assist with the education or translate materials.
	3. Before the high-risk suicidal patient is transferred outside the 24-hour inpatient care unit, the family member(s) must be educated about suicide warning signs and be informed about what may increase the risk of the return of suicidal ideation (e.g., discontinuation of medications and noncompliance with the treatment plan).
	    3.1 The patient and family member(s) also should be informed about ongoing treatment needs, community resources, and methods to access emergency care services after discharge.

The risk signs for committing suicide can be subtle. Consequently, nurses must assess suicide risk levels in all patients admitted for emotional or behavioral disorders and medical or surgical conditions. In Tables 3 and 4, we list the critical tips to prevent inpatient suicide. Table 3 is for nurses who work in acute inpatient care units and Table 4 is for patients and families.

Table 4. Preventing inpatient suicides: Critical tips for patients and families

Dimension	Tip

Demanding a safe care environment for our hospitalized loved one	1. We should expect our nurse to remove environmental hazards whenever possible. If we see any hazardous elements in the patient room, we should make a request to our nurse or the unit nurse manager to remove them as soon as possible.
	  1.1 Areas and elements in the patient room that represent an opportunity for a patient intent on committing suicide, include door hinges, doorknobs, door closers, lighting fixtures, closet poles, metal hangers, non-breakaway curtain rods, and non-breakaway bathroom fixtures and disability grab bars.
	2. When family members are visiting or providing one-on-one constant observation, they should work with the responsible nurse to ensure a safe care environment in the patient room.
	3. When visiting the high-risk suicidal patient, visitors should avoid bringing hazardous items with them or for the patient.
	  3.1 It may be safer to ask the responsible nurse to check for us to avoid any hazardous items left with the patient, which may be used for suicide.

Knowing the physical and mental conditions of our hospitalized love one	1. As the family members, we need to be aware of the high-risk times of transition for committing suicide. High-risk times include:
	  1.1 The period shortly after a patient is admitted
	  1.2 At the time of discharge or at the transition from inpatient to outpatient care
	  1.3 Before granting a high-risk suicidal patient a pass, authorized visits, or increased privileges
	2. If family members are willing to provide one-on-one observation for their hospitalized loved one, they would need to be aware of and well-informed about the level of the patient's risk for suicide and endangering himself or herself.
	  2.1 The one-on-one constant observation can be for a short period of time or an extended longer period of time, according to the patient's needs.
	  2.2 The family member should use the call light system as an important way to communicate with the responsible nurse.
	  2.3 The family member must report any observed changes in the patient's mood, attitude, behavior, or physical condition (e.g., becoming more agitated) to the responsible nurse as soon as possible.
	  2.4 Family members must get help from the nurse if they need to use toilet or step out of the patient room for a while. It is the nurse's responsibility to ensure the patient's safety at all times.
	3. The accompanying family should be aware that supervision of a high-risk suicidal patient during high-risk activities is necessary (e.g., when the patient is in the bathroom alone).
	4. With or without a family member present, the responsible physician and nurse should conduct observation and assessment periodically.

Dimension	Tip

Promoting effective communicatio n with our doctor and nurse	1. If family members are willing to participate in inpatient care (e.g., providing one-to-one constant observation), they should ask for verbal or written (or both) educational instructions related to suicide precaution from the responsible nurse. An accompanying family member should know or request the information about:
	  1.1 The rationales of providing constant observation
	  1.2 An update on the patient's condition (e.g., the findings of the routine suicidal risk assessment)
	  1.3 An update on the patient's care plan at least once a day
	2. Before the high-risk suicidal patient is transferred outside a 24-hour inpatient care unit, we must be educated about suicide warning signs and be informed about what may increase the risk of the return of suicidal ideation (e.g., discontinuation of medications and noncompliance with the treatment plan). The patient and family member(s) also should be informed about ongoing treatment needs, community resources, and methods to access emergency care services after discharge.

References

American Association of Suicidology (2007). Suicide in the U.S.A. based on current (2004) statistics. Available at: http://www.suicidology.org/associations/1045/files/SuicideInThe US.pdf (accessed December 8, 2007).

Joint Commission (2006). Goal 15: The organization identifies safety risks inherent in its patient population. In A. Grayson. (Ed.), *Meeting the Joint Commission's 2007 National Patient Safety Goals* (pp. 127-138). Oakbrook Terrace, IL: Joint Commission.

Joint Commission (2007a). Preventing suicide. In R. A. Porché, Jr. (Ed.), *Front line of defense: The role of nurses in preventing sentinel events* (2nd ed., pp. 113-128). Oakbrook Terrace, IL: Joint Commission.

Joint Commission (2007b). 2008 *Comprehensive accreditation manual for hospitals: The official handbook.* Oakbrook Terrace, IL: Joint Commission Resources.

Joint Commission International Center for Patient Safety (1998). Issue 7-Inpateint suicides: Recommendations for prevention (November 6, 1998). Available at: http://www.jcipatientsafety.org/14790 (accessed December 8, 2007).

Reiling, J., & Chernos, S. (2007). Human factors in hospital safety design. In P. Carayon (Ed.), *Handbook of human factors and ergonomics in health care and patient safety* (pp. 275-286). Mahwah, NJ: Lawrence Erlbaum Associates.

Medication Errors

Learning from a Patient Case

On a busy medical inpatient care unit, Nurse A started to administer medications shortly after the beginning of the shift. Nurse A worked in this unit temporarily as a floating nurse, was not familiar with the setting of this unit, and usually worked in pediatrics.

Two elderly male patients shared a semiprivate room: Mr. William Thomas (Tommy was his nickname), who was hospitalized for evaluation of hypotension and was assigned to bed 1, and Mr. Thomas Williams (Tommy was his nickname as well), who had diabetes and cardiovascular disease and was assigned to bed 2. Bed 1 is located by the door of the patient room and bed 2 is further from the door.

As Nurse A entered the patient room, she reminded herself that 'this medication goes to 342, bed 2.' After Nurse A entered room 342, Mr. William Thomas (bed 1) greeted Nurse A and said "You can call me Tommy." Nurse A recalled that the oral hypoglycemic medication was for Mr. Thomas Williams, because Tommy is the nickname of Thomas.

Before Mr. William Thomas took the medication, Nurse A asked to see his identification wristband. Mr. William Thomas told Nurse A that his wristband came off last night, and he had not had a new one yet. Nurse A then asked him to tell her his full name and he said "William Thomas."

Immediately, Nurse A realized that she almost made a medication error by using a room and bed number to identify a patient, making an assumption on the basis of a patient's nickname, and having insufficient patient identification information. This near-miss medication error could have had severe consequences for both patients (Joint Commission, 2007a).

Learning from a Patient Case

A 10-year-old boy with leukemia was to receive intrathecal medications of methotrexate, cytarabine, and hydrocortisone and one IV medication of vincristine. These treatments would usually have been given on the oncology/cancer care unit, but because the oncology unit was full, this boy was admitted to a general medical unit for treatments.

Nurse B prepared the syringes for Physician C and placed all four syringes on a tray on top of a card indicating what was in each syringe. Nurse B and Physician C verbally confirmed each of the intrathecal medications on the tray, but left out the IV medication of vincristine. Physician C started the intrathecal treatment. Nurse B left the patient room momentarily.

After giving methotrexate and cytarabine intrathecally, Physician C picked up the vincristine syringe by mistake and administered this syringe intrathecally. After Physician C finished injecting the vincristine intrathecally, Nurse B returned and found that the hydrocortisone syringe was still on the tray and the IV medication of vincristine was gone.

Immediately, this boy underwent emergency neurosurgery and received intensive care. This 10-year-old boy died a week after the intrathecal injection of vincristine (Joint Commission, 2007a).

Learning from a Legal Case Summary

Mr. P was admitted to Hospital K following an initial emergency room visit to be treated for burns to his back. After having been hospitalized for 3 days, Mr. P claimed that Nurse A forced him to take three large cups of pills. Each cup contained from 6 to 10 different pills. Nurse A said to him that that's what his doctor had prescribed for him to take. Mr. P complained and told Nurse A that he did not believe he was supposed to take all those pills and that he wanted to see his doctor. Nurse A replied back to him that she was in charge right now. So, she was telling him that he was going to take his medications. Mr. P then took all the pills in front of Nurse A. After that, Nurse A left his room.

Short afterward, Nurse A returned back to Mr. P's room and was upset and crying. Nurse A said to Mr. P, "Please tell me you didn't take all the pills." Mr. P replied back to Nurse A that "You made me take them already." Not long after this conversation, Mr. P started feeling woozy and went into cardiac arrest. Mr. P was rushed to the intensive care unit for treatment.

Before Mr. P lost his consciousness, he observed that Nurse A's head nurse immediately fired Nurse A. He also heard that the head nurse blamed Nurse A and said "How you could have made such a mistake as this?" Hospital K admitted that Mr. P received the wrong medications and did not charge him for any hospital expenses associated with correcting what was considered a medication error.

When an action is charged, whether it is considered professional negligence/malpractice or simple negligence depends on whether a health care professional's alleged negligence required the exercise of professional judgment and skills. Medical questions that arose in this case included: (1) whether Nurse A should have known that the amount and type of medications prescribed were unusual for someone with Mr. P's condition; (2) whether Nurse

A should have checked a chart to make sure that these medications were prescribed for Mr. P; and (3) given Mr. P's protestations, whether Nurse A should have consulted with another staff member to confirm that the medications were correct.

Nurse A was not simply affecting a judgment made by another (e.g., the care plan ordered by the responsible physician), but also exercising an independent medical judgment that required Nurse A to evaluate whether the medications were correct. As a result, the court of appeals determined that Mr. P's complaint was professional negligence not ordinary negligence.

Source: NexisLexis®Academic: Federal & State Cases (Case number: A07A1358; November 29, 2007, decided) (accessed on January 1, 2008).

Knowing about Medication Errors

A medication error is defined as any preventable event that may cause or lead to inappropriate medication use or patient harm. The medication may be in the control of the health care providers or patients. Such an event may be associated with a prescribing order communication, medication labeling, packaging, compounding, medication dispensing, distribution, administration, monitoring, medication use, and patient education. Medication errors can lead to adverse medication events (involving some degree of harm from receiving or not receiving a medication) or reactions (concerning an unintended, possibly harmful response). An adverse medication reaction can occur, even when medications are prescribed, dispensed, and administered correctly (Joint Commission, 2007a; National Coordinating Council for Medication Error Reporting and Prevention, 2008a).

Prevalence of Medication Errors

A study conducted in the United States (Burroughs et al., 2007) found that 17% of the surveyed patients encountered medical errors. Among these medical errors, about 44% of the errors patients encountered were related to medications. Indeed, medication errors are concerns to not only patients but also hospitals. Experts estimate that as many as 98,000 people die in any given year from medical errors in US hospitals. A significant number of those deaths would be associated with medication errors (National Coordinating Council for Medication Error Reporting and Prevention, 2008b).

In April 2007, the international steering committee of the Joint Commission International Center for Patient Safety approved a total of nine patient safety solutions for dissemination. Four of these nine patient safety solutions were associated with medication use (Joint Commission International, 2007):

1. Differentiating look-alike and sound-alike medication name
2. Effective control of different concentrated electrolyte solutions
3. Ensuring medication accuracy at transitions of care
4. Avoiding catheter and tubing misconnections

**Table 1. The six processes in a commonly seen medication use system
for inpatient care services**

Process	Responsible party	Action
Process 1: Medication selection and procurement	1. Administrators 2. Clinicians, including physicians, pharmacists, and nurses	1. Establishing formulary 2. Identifying the needed medications and equipment 3. Obtaining and providing needed medications and equipment
Process 2: Safe and secure storage	1. Pharmacists 2. Receiving, security, maintenance, and administrative staff	1. Ensuring proper storage in the receiving area 2. Ensuring proper storage in the pharmacy and on inpatient care units 3. Maintaining the safety and effectiveness of medications
Process 3: Medication prescription and medication order transcription	1. Physicians for medication prescription 2. Nurses for medication order transcription *Note:* Medication order transcription will not be needed only if physicians' orders are transmitted directly to the pharmacy through an electronic order entry system.	1. Medication prescription 1.1 Assessing patients and determining their needs for medications 1.2 Selecting and ordering medications 2. Medication order transcription 2.1 Accurately communicating physician orders to the pharmacy 2.2 Verifying orders that seem inconsistent with the hospital's established safe medication practice
Process 4: Medication preparation and dispensing	1. Pharmacists	1. Purchasing and storing medications 2. Reviewing and confirming medication orders 3. Preparing medications 4. Distributing medications to inpatient care units
Process 5: Medication administration	2. Nurses	1. Reviewing medications dispensed from the pharmacy 2. Assessing patients 3. Administering medications according to hospital policy
Process 6: Medication therapy monitoring	1. Physicians 2. Nurses 3. Pharmacists 4. Patients and families	1. Physicians, nurses and pharmacists: Assessing, reporting, and recording therapeutic, unintended, or adverse effects of medications 2. Patients and families: Observing and reporting therapeutic, unintended, or adverse effects of medications

Source: Joint Commission (2007a). Preventing medication errors. In R. A. Porché, Jr. (Ed.), *Front line of defense: The role of nurses in preventing sentinel events* (2nd ed., pp. 35-58). Oakbrook Terrace, IL: Joint Commission.

In other words, medication errors and associated patient harms can easily occur when mistakes or confusion arise in one or more of these four safety areas.

The Processes in a Medication Use System

As indicated in Table 1, a medication use system includes six processes: (1) medication selection and procurement, (2) safe and secure storage, (3) medication prescription, (4) medication preparation and dispensing, (5) medication administration, and (6) medication therapy monitoring (Joint Commission, 2007a).

These six processes were meant to achieve the common goal of safe, appropriate, effective, and efficient provision of medication therapy to patients who receive the care. These six processes intended to ensure the 'six rights,' which refer to (Joint Commission, 2007a):

1. The right patient
2. The right medication
3. The right dose
4. By the right route
5. At the right time
6. With the right results

Risk Factors and Possible Solutions

Based on the sentinel events reported from 1995 through December 2004, the Joint Commission (2007a) concluded that communication and orientation/training were the two most frequently reported root causes of medication errors at more than 60% each. In 2005, communication and procedural compliance were the two most cited root causes; each accounted for about 80% of the sentinel events related to medication errors. Competency and credentialing was the third most frequently reported cause at more than 50%.

The Joint Commission (2007a) claimed that the roles and responsibilities of nurses as team members were critical to develop a system approach to preventing medication errors and targeting improvement opportunities. Consequently, the Joint Commission (2007a) identified seven root causes and corresponding prevention strategies that focused on the roles of the nurses in preventing medication errors (Table 2).

Table 2. The major root causes of the reported sentinel events related to medication errors and the corresponding prevention strategies for nurses

Root cause	Prevention strategy
Inadequate orientation and training	1. Nurses must comply with hospital medication administration policies and procedures and safe medication policies. 1.1 Nurses' competence in medication administration must be validated before independent medication administration. 1.1.1 Nurses should request training about medications and medication administration devices, if a need arises. 1.1.2 Monitoring the effects of medications is essential and monitoring must include observation for therapeutic, side, and adverse effects.

Table 2. Continued

Root cause	Prevention strategy
	1.2 Nurses need to have a thorough understanding of important pharmacologic and procedural issues surrounding medication administration through training.
	1.2.1 Appropriate training would enable nurses to correlate medications with disease and clinical status.
	1.2.2 Nurses need such knowledge to detect errors and contraindications and anticipate and detect adverse effects.
	1.3 Nurses should understand important pharmacologic and procedural issues related to medication administration, including:
	1.3.1 Common errors surrounding high-risk medications
	1.3.2 Usual doses of frequently administered medications
	1.3.3 Normal infusion rates for frequently prescribed medications
	1.3.4 Potential unintended and adverse effects of the medications administered
	1.3.5 The often increased influence of medications on geriatric and pediatric patients
	2. Nurses must know and use time-honored techniques to reduce medication errors.
	2.1 Nurses must verify each patient's medication dose against the patient's medication administration records (abbreviated as MAR) and available clinical record.
	2.2 Nurses need to pay special attention to the patients, who were transferred from the other care settings, because medication errors frequently occurred in transcription for these patients.
	3. Nurses must reconcile an individual patient's medications.
	4. Hospital, pharmacy, and nursing leaders should adopt the unit-dose systems to reduce medication errors.
	4.1 The unit-dose systems would eliminate the need for multidose concentrates and the need to reconstitute medications and to calculate doses in the inpatient care units by nurses.
	4.2 Medications should be stored in and administered from labeled packages of a single dose, to be ready to be administered when dispensed.
	5. Physicians and nurses should not use potentially confusing abbreviations, acronyms, and symbols.
	6. Physicians and nurses need to monitor medication therapy on the basis of knowledge of therapeutic effects, mechanism of action, side and adverse effects, and the intended effect for each individual patient.
	6.1 The factors that nurses should consider when monitoring the effects of medications on each individual patient should include but are not limited to:
	6.1.1 A patient's demographic characteristics (e.g., age, gender, and cultural or ethnic factors)
	6.1.2 Information about this patient's disease and health condition (e.g., laboratory and radiology results and health history)
	6.1.3 This patient's perceived effects of the medication

Root cause	Prevention strategy

Communication failure
 	
1. Illegible physician handwriting, verbal orders, and incorrect order transcription accounted for a large percentage of medication errors.
2. Insufficient direct communication between the physician who prescribed the medication, the pharmacist who filled the medication, and the nurse who administered the medication, for clarification or verification purposes.
	1. To resolve medication-related concerns before medication administration, a nurse should question the physician who prescribed the medication or the pharmacist who filled the medication order about the choice of medications, administration routes, dosages, interactions, and reactions.
	2. Before medication administration, a nurse should ensure that all orders are clarified and complete.
	3. A nurse should take extra precaution with error-prone medications through increased communication with the physician who prescribed the medication or the pharmacist who filled the medication order.
	4. A nurse must communicate with and educate the patient who receives the medication.
	   4.1 A nurse should identify for the patient or family, each medication the patient is receiving at the time of administration.
	   4.2 The patient or family should be encouraged to ask questions and express concerns.
	   4.3 When a new medication is being given, the responsible nurse should take time to educate the patient or family about the medication, its purpose, and side effects.
	   4.4 Communication with the patient or family about medications may help reduce the likelihood that a patient will receive incorrect medications at a later date.
	   4.5 A patient with adequate information about the medications that he or she is allergic to may be better able to help prevent future allergic reactions.

Failure to ensure safe medication storage and access	1. Nurses should help ensure proper implementation of the hospital's medication storage policies and procedures.
	   1.1 Pharmacists should establish medication storage-related policies and procedures and enforce these policies and procedures through out the hospital.
	   1.2 In inpatient care units, nurses must secure a medication cart whenever it is unattended and make sure that medications are not left unsecured in open areas.
	2. Nurses have a responsibility to guard against medication theft in inpatient care units.
	   2.1 Nurses on each shift must determine whether proper security is in place for emergency medications and the medications kept at the bedside (for the convenience in medication administration by nurses and for training patients on self-administration).
	3. To avoid potential medication errors, nurses should minimize after-hour access to the pharmacy.
	   3.1 When 24-hour on-site pharmacy services are not available, hospitals may adopt safeguards for after-hour access to the pharmacy.
	      3.1.1 The hospital should approve and make a limited set of medications available for inpatient care.
	      3.1.2 These approved medications must be stored in a locked storage space outside the pharmacy.
	      3.1.3 These medications should be accessed only by physicians, physicians' designated personnel, and nurses.

Table 2. Continued

Root cause	Prevention strategy
	3.1.4 Hospitals must develop built-in quality control procedures to ensure accurate medications obtained (e.g., a double-check system).
	3.1.5 Hospitals should have an on-call pharmacist to answer questions and provide medications not available through the system/process described above.
	4. In inpatient care units, floor stock needs should be evaluated on an ongoing basis by the representatives of nursing and pharmacy.
	4.1 Floor stock medications generally should be limited to those for routinely used safe items (e.g., antiseptic and mouthwash solutions) and emergency use.
Insufficient information availability	1. Nurses should have access to reliable and current medication information.
	1.1 Pharmacists, as the medication experts, should be consulted to answer nurses' questions, if any.
	1.2 If a medication is too new to be described in published reference sources that are available in the nurses' station, nurses must receive or obtain appropriate information before medication administration.
	2. Nurses must have timely access to their responsible patients' clinical information and records to assess the appropriateness of medications. Nurses should identify patients properly before medication administration.
Inadequate competence assessment on nurses	1. Hospital and nursing leaders must ensure clinical nurses' ability to meet their performance expectations as stated in the job descriptions as related to medication safety.
	2. Nurses need to assume their personal responsibility for competence, including:
	2.1 Knowing the therapeutic and potential adverse and unintended effects of frequently used medications
	2.2 Obtaining such information when an unfamiliar medication is ordered
	3. Nurses should increase their knowledge and understanding of the types of medication errors occurring, risk factors, root causes, and prevention strategies. Nurses may use such information to identify the potential for sentinel events.
Labeling errors	1. Nurses should administer only properly labeled medications. During the administration process, nurses must check and read the label three times to ensure accuracy, including:
	1.1 When reaching for or preparing the medication
	1.2 Immediately before administering the medication
	1.3 When discarding the container or returning the container to the storage location
	2. Nurses must label all medications that they prepare, even if only one medication was prepared.
	2.1 When a unit-dose system is in place, most of the medications would be labeled. Still, in some situations, medications must be drawn into syringes or poured into medicine cups or basins.

Root cause	Prevention strategy
Unsafe practice environment 1. The working environment was lacking appropriate space and equipment for preparing medication dosages (e.g., poor lighting and unclean work space). 2. During the medication preparation process, nurses encountered interruptions and distractions. 3. Insufficient nursing staff 4. Nurse fatigue may also result in medication errors.	1. Hospital and nursing leaders should support a safe practice environment that allows nurses to take the time and find the space to stop and think to prevent errors in the process of medication preparation. 2. Nurses need to communicate with their supervisors about inappropriate environmental conditions that may compromise safe and accurate preparation of medications (e.g., insufficient nurse staffing).

Source: Joint Commission (2007a). Preventing medication errors. In R. A. Porché, Jr. (Ed.), *Front line of defense: The role of nurses in preventing sentinel events* (2nd ed., pp. 35-58). Oakbrook Terrace, IL: Joint Commission.

Medication Safety: Six Focused Areas

To prevent medication errors, the Joint Commission (2007c) also listed six focused areas that may help clinicians (e.g., physicians, nurses, and pharmacists) improve medication safety at the point of care. These six focused areas were:

1. High-alert medications
2. Look-alike and sound-alike medications
3. Medication labeling
4. Medication reconciliation
5. Patient-controlled analgesia (abbreviated as PCA)
6. Vincristine administration errors (vincristine should be administered only by the IV route not intrathetically).

The top five high-alert medications and common risk factors are listed below (Joint Commission, 2007c):

1. Insulin: Common risk factors included:
    a. When the physician used "U" as an abbreviation for "units" in orders, "U" can be confused with "0" (zero) and result in a 10-fold overdose.
    b. No dose check system was in place.

    c.   Incorrect rates were programmed into an infusion pump.

    d.   Insulin vials in different preparations (concentrations) were often kept in close proximity to each other, and this situation may lead to mix-ups.

    e.   When insulin and heparin vials were kept in close proximity to each other in the same working area on a patient care unit, this situation can lead to mix-ups.

2.   Opiates and narcotics: Common risk factors were:

    a.   Medication errors occurred due to confusion between hydromorphone and morphine.

    b.   Parenteral narcotics were stored on the nurses' station as floor stock and, as a result, were easy to be use inappropriately.

    c.   Incorrect concentration and rates as a result of errors when programming the PCA infusion pump.

    d.   When a patient was receiving PCA, the responsible nurse failed to detect the signs and symptoms of opiate toxicity (e.g., nocturnal hypoxia) and to withdraw and distinguish between oversedation and other complications.

3.   Injectable potassium chloride or phosphate concentrate: Common risk factors included:

    a.   A prescribing order requested for unusual concentrations

    b.   A mix-up between potassium chloride and potassium phosphate occurred.

    c.   Storage of concentrated potassium chloride or potassium phosphate was placed outside the pharmacy (usually on the nurses' station as floor stock).

4.   IV anticoagulants (heparin): Common risk factors can be:

    a.   A multidose container for heparin was provided by the pharmacy.

    b.   The package label was unclear regarding concentration and total volume.

    c.   Nurses were confused between heparin and insulin because both medications had similar measurement units and were often placed in close proximity to each other in the same working area.

5.   Sodium chloride solutions above 0.9%: Common risk factors include:

    a.   Several concentrations or formulations of sodium chloride solutions were available in the pharmacy or on the nurses' station as floor stock.

    b.   Storage of sodium chloride solutions (above 0.9%) was placed outside the pharmacy (usually on the nurses' station as floor stock).

    c.   There was no double-checking system in place.

Medication reconciliation is an important process to ensure patients' medication safety. Patients and their families must participate in the process of reconciling their medications (Joint Commission, 2007c). For a hospitalized patient, medications may be prescribed by multiple physicians (e.g., the primary care physician, physicians at the emergency room, the in-charge physician for inpatient care, and the specialist who comes for consultation) and not filled by a single local pharmacy. Reconciling a patient's medications must be done when a patient is hospitalized. However, medication reconciliation is rarely fully implemented as a medication safety procedure across the care continuum.

A pharmacist, who is a medication expert, may be more suitable to reconcile a patient's medications. However, in the current practice, a nurse who works in an inpatient care unit and admits the patient to the inpatient unit is often obligated to gather the medication information as part of the patient's clinical records.

For each hospitalized patient, the medication information only needs to be gathered once. The same medication information can be passed along to the other professionals in the same health care team and to the nurses who work on different shifts and care for the patient. However, a patient's medication information may need to be updated when medications have been changed during hospital stays.

The Joint Commission (2007c) suggested four steps to effectively reconcile a hospitalized patient's medications. These four steps are:

Step 1: A complete and accurate list of the patient's medications used before being admitted into the hospital should be developed. This list should include the name, dose, route and frequency of each medication, and the time when the last dose is taken. This list may be called a home medication list.

Step 2: A clinician should compare the list of medications developed in step 1 with any new orders for medications after being admitted into an inpatient care unit. It is important to check for duplication, omission of medications, possible medication interaction, and any confusion related to the medication name, dose, or route.

Step 3: A new list of medications should be created that includes the medications a patient is currently taking. It is essential to update this list because orders may change throughout the entire length of stay. This updated list should be consistent with the Medication Administration Record (MAR) of this patient. This list may be called a current medication list.

Step 4: On being discharged home or transferred to another institution, the responsible clinician should use the home medication list (as developed in step 1) and the current medication list (as developed in step 3) to reconcile with the discharge medications. A complete and accurate list of all the medications, which a patient is supposed to take following discharge, should be created. This list should be given to the patient or family (or both), as needed, and should be forwarded to the next health care provider.

National Patient Safety Goals for Promoting the Safety of Medications

In the 2008 National Patient Safety Goals for hospitals, Goal 3 was meant to improve the safety of using medications (Joint Commission, 2007b). As indicated in Requirement 3C, hospitals were required to identify a list of look-alike or sound-alike medications used within the hospital and to take needed actions to prevent errors involving the confusion of these medications. This list should be reviewed at least annually.

As part of Goal 3, Requirement 3D obligated hospitals to label all medications, medication containers, or other solutions (including syringes, medicine cups, and basins) on and off the sterile area to ensure the safe administration of medications. For example, all medication labels must be verified both verbally and visually by two qualified staff members when the person preparing the medication is not the one who will administer the medication. All original containers from medications or solutions should be kept available for reference until the conclusion of the procedure or treatment. Another important factor is that at shift changes or break relief, all medications and solutions (not in the original containers) both on and off the sterile field and their labels must be reviewed by entering and exiting staff (Joint Commission, 2007b).

For Requirement 3E, hospitals also must reduce the likelihood of harm to patients who are undergoing anticoagulation therapy (Joint Commission, 2007b). Anticoagulation, as a high-risk treatment, often leads to adverse medication events because of the complexity of dosing these medications and monitoring the effects. With appropriate staff education, the use of standardized practices for the initiation, maintenance, and monitoring of anticoagulation therapy can reduce the risk of adverse medication events related to the use of heparin, low-molecular-weight heparin, warfarin, and other anticoagulants (Joint Commission, 2007b).

Hospitals were expected to have a policy that addresses baseline and ongoing laboratory tests that are required for heparin and low-molecular-weight heparin therapies. When a hospital provides dietary services, the dietary services should be notified of all patients who are receiving warfarin. The dietary services should respond properly, according to the established food and medication interaction guidelines. Patients and their families also need to be educated about the importance of dietary restrictions and potential for adverse medication reactions and interactions associated with anticoagulation therapy (Joint Commission, 2007b).

Goal 8 was designed to accurately and completely reconcile medications across the continuum of care (Joint Commission, 2007b). As indicated in Requirement 8A, each hospital should have a process for comparing each individual patient's current medications with those ordered for this patient while being hospitalized. It is essential to have the involvement of the patient or family members to create a complete list of the patient's current medications at admission. This complete list of medications should be provided to the patient or family at the time of discharge and be used to communicate to the next health care provider whether within or outside the hospital (Joint Commission, 2007b).

The Joint Commission (2006) also summarized helpful solutions to meet Goal 8, including:

1. Creating a medication reconciliation template/form for gathering information about current medications to help staff see what medications have been reconciled. It is crucial to use open charts, the charts of patients who have been admitted to an inpatient unit for 24 hours, to prevent errors.
2. When conducting a patient interview about the medications taken at admission, it is important to include over-the-counter medications, herbals, dietary supplements, eyedrops, inhalers, patches, and contraceptives.

3. Medication safety can be maximized by putting physicians or their designated personnel in charge of the process of medication reconciliation. If this is done, physicians will not order medications until they receive the patient's current list of medications. It would be helpful to have nurses and pharmacists contribute significantly to this process.

4. It will be helpful to involve a pharmacist in compiling a patient's medication list when a patient is taking more than 10 different medications.

5. Each hospital should develop a time frame for reconciling different types of medications after a patient is admitted into the hospital (e.g., within 4 hours, within 24 hours, or before the next prescribed dose).

6. Including the reasons for changing medications within the medication reconciliation information would help communication among health care providers as to why the patient was shifted to a new type of medication.

7. Including medication reconciliation information in the change-of-shift procedures and the physician's progress notes is essential to promote effective communication among health care providers.

8. It is important to educate patients to bring their medication list with them when being admitted to a hospital or seeing a physician.

Patient Safety Concerns and Initiatives in Inpatient Settings

Hospitals are making efforts to promote safer hospital stays and to prevent medication errors through system-level solutions. For example, some hospitals devote efforts to reconciling medications for the purpose of decreasing medication errors at patient transitions (Leape et al., 2006). According to the 2005 national survey of pharmacy practice in hospital settings in the United States (Pedersen et al., 2007), safe medication systems continue to be in place in most hospitals. For example, 30% of hospitals provided around-the-clock pharmacy services. MARs have become increasingly computerized over the past 6 years. Bar-code technology has been implemented by 9.4% of hospitals, and 32.3% of hospitals have smart infusion pumps.

As for the safe practices for administering medications at the bedside, 96.8% of hospitals regularly verified patient name by oral questioning or examination of the patient's wristband before administering medications, 86% had nurses remove the unit-dose medication from its package immediately before administration at the bedside, and 85.1% had nurses watch the patient take the dose before documenting the administration in the records. Ninety-one percent of hospitals conducted premedication administration order checks (Pedersen et al., 2007). These practices were all intended to prevent medication errors.

Available Technology to Prevent Medication Errors

The Joint Commission (2007a) also illustrated five key systems that are widely available in the current hospital environment:

1. Computerized physician order entry (CPOE) systems: Adopting the CPOE system can reduce medication errors occurring at the ordering and prescribing stages. Such a system allows a physician to use a computer or handheld electronic device to generate a prescription and electronically transfer the order to the pharmacy. Some CPOE systems can be implemented with a proper interface with the pharmacy's computerized systems (e.g., computerized MARs) to reduce medication errors related to transcription from one system to the other system. Available systems have automatic functions or interfaces that allow physicians to look up patients' health records, such as:

   a. Checking a medication's indication against a diagnosis
   b. Warning of possible allergies and medication interactions
   c. Reviewing laboratory test results
   d. Flagging potential medication problems
   e. Displaying a menu of acceptable dosages
   f. Suggesting optimal dosages
   g. Refusing to accept an order until the physician or designated personnel chooses the dose, route, and dosing schedule
   h. Eliminating reliance on handwritten and verbal orders
   i. Suggesting less expensive but equally effective medications

2. Computerized MARs: Adopting the computerized MARs can greatly reduce medication errors as related to transcription (e.g., errors involving legibility of orders). Such a system allows a single document to be shared between pharmacists at the point of dispensing and nurses at the point of administration. This function improves the efficiency and speed delivery of medications and information.

3. Automated dispensing units (ADUs): ADUs are often used in acute care settings to control and improve accountability for: (1) emergency or first-dose medications after pharmacy hours, (2) control of floor stock, and (3) control of and improvement in accountability for narcotic use. With ADUs, nurses may spend less time searching for missing doses and waiting for doses to arrive from the pharmacy. Some more details follow:

   a. ADUs may use an automated unit-dose dispensing machine at each patient bedside or allow medications to be placed on the nurses' stations in a controlled environment in advance of physician orders. Some ADUs use electronic passwords or other means to ensure security, which identify the nurse removing the medication and the patient for whom the dose is intended. With additional user identifications, some systems allow the nurse to open only the drawer in which the correct medication is stored.
   b. Reliance on ADUs can result in problems, such as less checking when obtaining and giving medications and when retrieving a medication from an automated dispenser before a pharmacist screens the order.
   c. Nevertheless, a proper medication control system must be in place so that pharmacists must review all prescriptions to prevent medication errors. This element must not be bypassed after adopting ADUs.

4. Bar-coding technology: Bar-coding technology combined with the ADUs or robotics can be the most sophisticated technology used for medication administration control. More details are described below:

   a. For most of the systems, the patient receiving care will be assigned a bar code on admission. All medication would have a specific bar code. Each nurse who administers medications would have a bar-code reader (also called scanner). Nurses may use a wireless laptop computer (often attached to a medication cart) and a bar-code reader to enable medication administration and immediate online documentation.

   b. After the nurse logs in, the computer would show the patients' MARs this nurse is responsible for. The MAR of the patient receiving care (a paper document) will be scanned first, the medication bar code will be scanned next, and the patient identification wristband will be scanned last. The scanner would sound an alarm if the patient, medication, or order does not match.

   c. All medications must be prepared at the bedside. In addition, documentation must be done shortly after a medication has been administered. For the medications that require a two-nurse check, nurses may perceive this system as an obstacle. It is also essential for nurses to ensure that their patients' wristbands are intact and readable. If not, a new band should be printed before medications are administered.

   d. Most of the Veterans Administration medical centers have been using this technology since 1999. Adopting such bar-coding technology can avert administration errors and near misses related to wrong patient, wrong medication, wrong dose, wrong route, or wrong time. Despite the benefits of bar-coding technology, such systems are not used widely due to the cost. Also, not all the medication manufacturers have bar codes readily printed on the package labels of medications.

5. Automated infusion pumps: Automated, computerized infusion devices can assist nurses in the administration of medications that must be given IV. Dosing limits, standardized concentrations, and other medication administration parameters can be incorporated into the automated infusion devices. The programming function can help prevent errors by staff in programming. Data on programming errors can be recorded automatically. More details follow.

   a. The program on an automated infusion pump can be set up in two ways: (1) a pharmacist first programs and then a nurse validates the program and (2) two nurses together validate the accurate administration information that has been programmed into the device. This validation process is particularly essential when high-risk medications are being delivered (e.g., chemotherapy agents and pain management medications). In the acute care setting, PCA often involves an automated infusion device for pain control.

   b. Regardless of the convenience of using automated infusion pumps, nursing managers must insist on the use of limited types of infusion devices. This is to ensure that all nursing staff have opportunities to receive needed education and training and are knowledgeable about the safety features of the devices being used. Nurses should always make sure that the automated infusion pump is being used as the manufacturer intended with all the safety features engaged (Joint Commission, 2007a).

Technology can help reduce medication errors or problems, but it should not be viewed as a cure-all for medication errors. Most importantly, computerized or automated devices do not eliminate staff's poor performance issues, such as failing to recognize adverse effects of a medication (Joint Commission, 2007a).

Who Is Responsible for Ensuring Medication Safety during Hospital Stays?

A medication error can originate in any stage of the medication use system, including when the physician wrote the order, the pharmacist filled the order, and the nurse administered the medication to the patient. Unfortunately, when a serious medication error occurs that leads to death or serious injury, the nurse who administered the medication is often blamed for giving the medication without questioning the physician who prescribed the medication and the pharmacist who filled the order.

A previous study (Bates et al., 1995) found that medication errors, which resulted in preventable adverse medication events, occurred most often at the stages of ordering (56%) and administration (34%), followed by transcription (6%) and dispensing errors (4%). Errors were much more likely to be intercepted if the error occurred earlier in the process.

For example, 48% of the medication errors were stopped at the ordering stage and, in comparison, 0% at the administration stage. Most adverse medication events resulting from errors happened at the ordering stage, but many also occurred at the administration stage. As a result, prevention strategies should target both ordering and administration stages of the medication delivery process (Bates et al., 1995).

Attributing Medication Errors to the Ones who Administer Medications

The Joint Commission (2007a) suggested that nurses should be trained to correlate medications, disease, and clinical status to correctly detect errors and contraindications and to anticipate and detect adverse effects. However, we argued the appropriateness and logic to require nurses to have a thorough knowledge of all important pharmacologic and procedural issues surrounding medication administration through training.

During the course of medication administration, nurses must adhere to the practice standard of the "five rights" (right medication, right dose, right route, right patient, and right time). Nurses are often expected to identify errors made by physicians who prescribed the medications or pharmacists who dispensed the medications. In reality, licensed nurses (e.g., registered nurses and licensed practical nurses) have limited training and professional knowledge of pharmacology. If hospital and nursing leaders obligated nurses to identify medication errors occurring before they administer medications, it would force nurses to do an impossible task beyond their professional training.

It is important to understand the required pharmacology training that professional nurses must receive during their formal nursing training. Here, we use the traditional 4-year bachelor nursing program offered at the University of Michigan, School of Nursing, Ann Arbor, Michigan, as an example. In this accredited nursing program, a student nurse is only required to take a 4-credit-hour course of "Pharmacology and therapeutics" (about 60 hours total) to be qualified to take the registered nurse licensure examination (the board examination). This one-term course is designed to introduce the fundamental principles of medication action and the essentials of how major medications are used therapeutically in various disease states. Identification and assessment of adverse medication responses and medication-to-medication interactions are also included. The minimum number of credit hours required for graduation is 128 (University of Michigan School of Nursing, 2008a, 2008b). It is obvious that a nurse's training in pharmacology is limited and definitely not sufficient to question the physician who prescribes the medication or the pharmacist who fills the order.

If a nurse is capable of identifying errors made by physicians when prescribing or pharmacists when dispensing medication, this nurse should be licensed to be a physician or pharmacist. It is simply illogical to attribute most of the causes of medication errors to nurses just because they are the ones who administered the medications. It is even more ridiculous to blame nurses for giving the medication without questioning the physician who prescribed the medication and the pharmacist who filled the order.

In practice, nurses are responsible to properly administer the medications as dispensed by the pharmacists. At the same time, hospital leaders must ensure the abilities of physicians and pharmacists to meet their performance expectations as stated in their job descriptions as related to the safety of prescribing and dispensing medications.

Contributors to Medication Errors Performed by Hospital Nursing: Still a Myth

To prevent medication errors, bar coding and advanced decentralized dispensing technology have been introduced to the US health care system. Despite the adoption of new technologies and the implementation of various safety practices for administering medications, medication errors have become an increasingly targeted, crucial safety issue in hospital settings. Medication errors have been linked to nursing care quality, clinical outcomes, characteristics of the work environment, system designs in hospital settings, and nurses' professional knowledge, ethics, and conduct. For example, interruptions have been described as a contributor to medication errors in acute inpatient care settings (Tang et al., 2007).

Collins and associates (2006) observed medical resident rounds in a medical intensive care unit in a US hospital for interruption analysis. This study involved 2-hour observational data. The study findings showed that a distraction or interruption occurred every 5 minutes 10 seconds and preceded a total of two errors on the CPOE system. Collins and associates further classified interruptions into three types:

1. Distraction (9 of 22 observed interruptions; one error): Distraction was defined as an acknowledged stimulus from an external source that was not followed by termination of activity.
2. Distraction with multitasking (3 of 22 observed interruptions): Distraction with multitasking referred to a time period when a distraction caused a clinician to interact in two or more concurrent communication events.
3. Interruption (9 of 22 observed interruptions; one error): Interruption was defined as a cessation of a productive activity for an externally imposed reason before the current task was completed.

In acute care settings, clinical nurses may encounter all three types of interruptions, but what is being interrupted may vary across different types of inpatient care services. As we have observed, due to the nature of the inpatient care services, nurses may encounter more distractions with multitasking than physicians or the nurses who work in the intensive care units.

According to the study by Tang and associates (2007) involving Taiwanese nurses who worked in acute inpatient units, personal negligence and lack of sufficient professional knowledge in pharmacy were the prevailing contributors to medication errors. In practice, nurses who work in acute inpatient units and care for more than one patient in a shift are seldom undisturbed. In the findings of Tang and associates, interruptions were not recognized by clinical nurses as a primary contributor to medication errors. In addition, heavy workload, which has often been linked to nursing shortages and nurse-to-patient ratios as related to case mix and acuity levels, was not identified as the most common contributor. Here, the myths on the links between workload, interruptions, and errors are being challenged.

Tucker and Spear (2006) described the work environment with a special focus on nurses' performance associated with their work systems in six US hospitals. The frequency of work system-related operational failures and their impact on nurse productivity were documented. Operational failures were defined as the inability of a work system to reliably provide supplies, services, or information when, where, and to whom needed.

This study found that nurses experienced an average of 8.4 operational failures per 8-hour shift, involving medications, orders, supplies, staffing, and equipment. The most frequent categories of failure were medication problems, followed by medical orders, supply items, insufficient staffing, and equipment. Nurses also faced frequent interruptions. About 95% of all interruptions were due to patient care issues, such as family members' inquiries about their loved one's medical status. The other interruptions (5%) stemmed from system malfunctions, such as redundant phone messages and pages.

Nurses often understandably provide care for several patients during one shift. Consequently, these nurses may have to juggle multiple operational failures and interruptions related to different patients at the same time. For example, clinical conditions, which were inherent to meeting the needs of patients and their families, made 95% of the interweaving and prioritization of nursing tasks unavoidable (e.g., families' inquiries about their loved one's status and care; Tucker & Spear 2006). Hospital nurses are obligated to respond to such inquiries, nevertheless.

Interruptions in inpatient care units do reflect the nature of nursing practice and are expected. Interruptions, such as answering call lights, are not distractions that should be eliminated. For example, if answering call lights were considered to be less important than completing medical procedures (e.g., preparing medications), patients might try to get out of bed by themselves for toileting. Patients with such urgent physical needs may fall and injure themselves if their nurses neglect them. In the ideal world, both interrupting medication administration and letting a patient fall should not occur.

Challenges for Clinicians in Preventing Medication Errors

We would like to share a story of our observation of a female patient's experience on medication use. The situation occurred at her home the third day after she was discharged from an acute hospital. Understanding the difficulties that a patient may encounter after being discharged is essential to develop a proper medication use system for a hospital. Our observation is summarized below.

> This nursing teacher, who is in her early sixties, has good vision, and is alert and independent, was discharged from an acute hospital after being hospitalized for 7 days for her acute medical problems. She was so glad to be home. When we paid her a visit at her home on the third afternoon after being discharged from the hospital, she was managing to take her medications. She showed us the list of medications she was supposed to take. There were a total of 8 medications in tablets or capsules to be taken by mouth; 3 of them should be taken daily and the other 5 medications twice a day. She complained to us that the names of the medications on the list did not match with the ones on the labels of the medication bottles or packages (7 of them were filled at a pharmacy and the other was an over-the-counter medication).
>
> She was exhausted because she had to figure out which medications and their amounts and frequencies she should take. She said to us that she can only go with the dosage (e.g., the number of milligrams for each tablet). With her permission, we sorted out her medications and prepared a total of 5-day medications in 10 separate zip bags, which were marked to be taken in the morning (A.M.) or afternoon (P.M.).
>
> We were concerned about her health condition and how other recently discharged patients handle their medication administration at home. Medication compliance was a major concern and we wondered what we missed related to this nursing teacher's medication education during her hospital stay and before being discharged. We left in 45 minutes to let her rest per her request.

Despite the fact that this lovely lady had formal nursing training and advanced nursing education, she was still struggling to follow her physician's medical orders. She had less energy and was lethargic and tired. Her major challenge was to match the medication list she was given before being discharged and the medications filled by a pharmacist in a local pharmacy.

It is obvious that our hospital's medication use system is broken. Involving patients and families in preventing medication errors during hospital stays seems to be a mission impossible, even at home. Medication compliance after being discharged is another challenge, though it is not the focus of this book.

During hospital stays, physicians, pharmacists, and nurses are fully responsible for preventing medication errors. We claim that administering and dispensing medications demand professional pharmaceutical knowledge to minimize errors and near misses. To prevent medication errors, we should take a systems approach to determine who is best qualified to dispense and administer medications.

Using Pharmacists or Pharm-techs in Medication Administration

Shifting the responsibility of medication administration in acute inpatient care units from nurses to pharmacists or pharm-techs can be one possible solution to decrease medication errors. Nurses should focus on what they are good at (e.g., patient education, assessment of patients' condition changes and needs); these tasks are also critical to care quality and demand many bedside nursing hours. Nurses are professionally trained to be excellent at caring for patients across the care continuum. Their unique expertise in patient education and assessment should be acknowledged.

In addition, to promote safe practices during medication administration and therapy monitoring, a differentiated job description and responsibilities for physicians, pharmacists, and clinical nurses should be discussed and clarified at the hospital executive level. An error-free, adverse event-free, medication dispensing, administration, and monitoring system demands a well-integrated hospital system.

Should nurses administer medications to patients at the bedside? Or should pharmacists assume this role of administering medication? Should pharmacists be actively involved in providing medication-related patient education and observing for medication-related adverse events? Someone could claim that nurses have been administering medications to inpatients as long as we can remember. However, medication administration does require sufficient knowledge of pharmacology to detect medication errors.

To promote a safe medication use system, we suggest that hospitals should make pharmacists or pharm-techs responsible for medication administration because of pharmacists' expertise in pharmacology. This way, patients can be sure that the health care providers who have expertise in pharmacology are in charge of medication preparation, dispensing, and administration during their entire hospital stay. Pharmacists and pharm-techs should also work with nurses on medication therapy monitoring and medication-related patient education (including discharge plans).

Properly Allocating job Responsibilities among Physicians, Pharmacists, and Nurses in a Medication Use System

By professional training, physicians are meant to diagnose problems, prescribe medications and treatments, and monitor patients' responses to medications. Pharmacists are professionally trained to safely dispense and administer medications and to provide medication-related education and consultation to patients and their families. We do not intend to disregard nurses' value and their contributions to caring for and attending to inpatients' medical needs. It is simply illogical that physicians and pharmacists are willing to spend more time with outpatients and patients, who are ready for discharge, but are less willing to care for inpatients who desperately need intense, professional, lifesaving medical care and services.

Safe hospital stays are critical. We need a medication care system by which pharmacists are stationed in each inpatient care unit around the clock. In current practice, pharmacists have the responsibility to provide medication education and consultation to outpatients and patients who are ready to be discharged. There is no doubt that inpatients deserve professional pharmaceutical knowledge to ensure their medication safety. Pharmacists and physicians must collaborate with clinical nurses, who have most contact with inpatients, to guarantee medication safety at the bedside. Promoting medication safety may demand a systems approach and operational redesign.

If clinical nurses still have to administer medications to their patients, unit-dose systems must be in place to prevent errors during medication administration. Each medication should be stored in and administered from a properly labeled package of a single dose (including medication name, dosage, route, and time to take) when dispensed from the pharmacy. Each medication (including oral or IV solutions) should be ready to be administered by the responsible nurse.

Advancement in Labeling the Package of Each Medication

We suggest that the labeled packages of medications for each patient should come with a list of medications (a paper document for patients to keep), which includes: (1) the patient's name, (2) one additional identifier (e.g., birth date), (3) each medication's scientific and brand names, (4) purpose, (5) dosage, (6) route, (7) time to take, (8) possible adverse medication actions, (9) special instructions, and (10) a picture of the medication printed in color and shown in the real size (if it is a capsule or tablet). This list of medications should also include the name of the physician who prescribed the medications and the name of the pharmacist who filled the medication orders. A telephone number that patients can call for medication consultation should also be included.

This list should be consistent with the corresponding patient's MAR. If a hospital has adopted a computerized MAR system, a program should be written to generate each patient's medications once a day and this list can be printed out at the pharmacy and the nurses' stations.

After administering medications, the labeled packages and the list of medications should be saved for patients to keep. Patients or families should read the medication list and help in making sure that the list includes everything the patient is taking. The labeled packages for each given medication and the list of medications can be used for medication education later on or when the medications are being administered. This medication list and the labeled packages for each given medication can also help patients recognize and visualize the medications that they are taking.

Table 3. Symbols and Braille for instructing patients about medication use

Symbol*	Braille: **A system of writing for the blind that uses characters made up of raised dots***	Description
		Medication to be taken in the morning
		Medication to be taken at noon
		Medication to be taken in the evening
		Medication to be taken before sleep
		Medication to be taken before meal
		Medication to be taken after meal

Symbol*	Braille: **A system of writing for the blind that uses characters made up of raised dots***	Description
		Take one tablet
		Take one-half tablet
		Take two tablets
		For eyes only
		For ears only
		For nose only

* Reprinted with permission from Changhua Christian Hospital, Erlin Branch, Department of Pharmacy, Erlin Township, Changhua County, Taiwan.

It is important to use lay terms and symbols (Table 3 has examples) to help patients with low literacy understand. If needed, the list of medications may be printed in the other languages (e.g., Spanish, Japanese, and Chinese). Most of all, the list of medications should also accommodate the needs of the patients with poor eyesight and the blind (e.g., using Braille, a system of writing for the blind that uses characters made up of raised dots).

Adopting Technologies to Smooth out the Medication Use System

A medication use system involves all six processes of medication selection and procurement, safe and secure storage, prescription, preparation and dispensing, administration, and medication therapy monitoring (Joint Commission, 2007a). For hospital leaders, it is important to adopt both the computerized MAR system and the CPOE system. The CPOE system should also have an appropriate interface to be incorporated with the computerized MAR system.

These two computerized systems together can reduce medication errors associated with transcribing medication orders. Bar-coding technology or similar systems are recommended. The bar-coding technology can act as a gatekeeper to improve the accuracy in patient identification and prevent administering wrong medications and wrong doses to patients.

The ADUs and automated infusion pumps may further reduce medication errors occurring in the process of medication administration, in addition to the advantages of adopting the bar-coding technology.

Table 4 summarizes critical tips for nurses who work in acute inpatient care units to help prevent medication errors.

Table 4. Preventing medication errors:
Critical tips for nurses who work in acute inpatient care units

Dimension	Tip

Obtaining sufficient orientation and training and complying with standards of care related to medication safety	1. Nurses must comply with the hospital's medication safety-related policies and procedures.
	2. Nurses should request training about medications and medication administration devices, if a need arises. Appropriate training would enable nurses to correlate medications with disease and clinical status.
	3. Nurses should understand important pharmacologic and procedural issues related to medication administration, including:
	  3.1 Common errors surrounding high-risk medications
	  3.2 Normal infusion rates for frequently prescribed medications
	  3.3 Potential unintended and adverse effects of the medications administered
	  3.4 The often increased influence of medications on geriatric and pediatric patients
	  3.5 Usual doses of frequently administered medications
	4. Nurses must verify each patient's medication dose against his of her medication administration records and available clinical record.
	5. Nurses need to ensure that medication reconciliation has been completed for individual patient's medications within the time frame, as specified in the hospital's policy.
	  5.1 Nurses need to pay special attention to the patients who were transferred from the other care settings because medication errors frequently occur in transcription for these patients.
	6. Nurses need to monitor medication therapy on the basis of knowledge of therapeutic effects, mechanism of action, side and adverse effects, and the intended effect for each individual patient.
	7. Nurses should not use potentially confusing abbreviations, acronyms, and symbols.

Dimension	Tip

Promoting sufficient communication for clarification and verification purposes	1. Before medication administration, a nurse should ensure that all orders are clarified and complete.
	2. Nurses must resolve medication-related concerns before medication administration. A nurse should take extra precaution with error-prone medications.
	3. Nurses should have access to reliable and current medication information. Pharmacists, as the medication experts, should be consulted to answer nurses' questions if any.
	4. Nurses must have timely access to their responsible patients' clinical information and records to assess the appropriateness of medications.
	5. Nurses must communicate with and educate patients who receive the medications.
	   5.1 A nurse should identify for the patient and family, each medication the patient is receiving at the time of administration.
	   5.2 The patient and family should be encouraged to ask questions and express concerns.
	   5.3 When a new medication is being given, the responsible nurse should take time to educate the patient and family about the medication, its purpose, and side effects.
	   5.4 Communication with the patient and family about medications may help reduce the likelihood that a patient at a later date will receive incorrect medications.

Proper labeling for medications	1. Nurses should administer only properly labeled medications. During the administration process, nurses must check and read the label three times to ensure accuracy, including:
	   1.1 When reaching for or preparing the medication
	   1.2 Immediately before administering the medication
	   1.3 When discarding the container or returning the container to the storage location
	2. Nurses must label all medications that they prepare, even if only one medication was prepared. In some situations, medications must be drawn into syringes or poured into medicine cups or basins.

Ensuring safe medication storage and access	1. Nurses should help ensure proper implementation of the hospital's medication storage policies and procedures. Nurses must secure a medication cart whenever it is unattended and make sure that medications are not left unsecured in open areas. 2. Nurses have a responsibility to guard against medication theft in their working units. Nurses on each shift must determine whether proper security has been provided for emergency medications and the medications kept at the bedside.

Critical Tips for Patients and Families to Prevent Medication Errors during Hospital Stays

During hospitalization, patients and families can only observe the course of medication administration, often performed by nurses (Figures 1 and 2). The huge gap in pharmacology knowledge between our health care providers (physicians, pharmacists, and nurses) and patients and families leads us to a very vulnerable position during hospital stays.

We should ask our doctor or nurse to give us a copy of our most updated medication list or our medication administration record. Each patient has his or her own MAR. This medication list should present the details about the medications we are supposed to take, at least as of that moment.

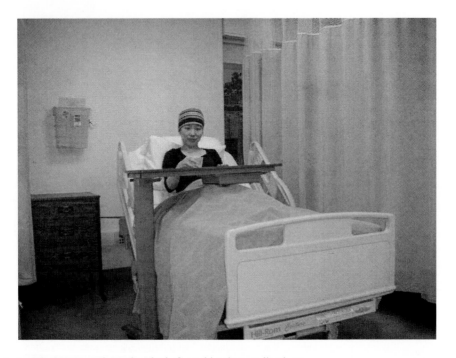

Figure 1. A patient rests on the patient bed after taking her medications.

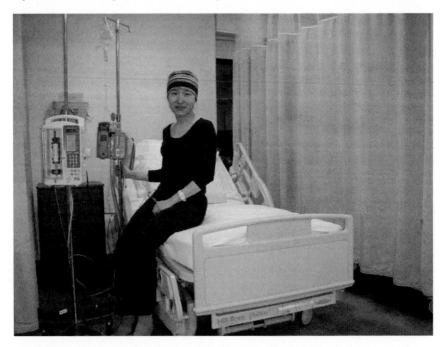

Figure 2. A patient sits on the edge of the bed with her two IV infusion pumps.

We should review this list with our doctor or nurse to find out why we need each medication and what kind of effects we may expect after taking it. With a complete list of our medications and medication education from our doctor or nurse, we may be able to verify the "five rights" (right medication, right dose, right route, right patient, and right time) whenever someone gives us medication of any sort. We should check the medications against our medication list before taking any agents (Roizen & Oz, 2006).

Table 5. Critical information to know to help avoid mistakes with medications:
For hospitalized patients and their families

Question	Issue
	If I am not well enough to do any of the actions indicated below, I should ask a family or friend to help. *Notes:* I should clarify the purposes of my medications with my doctor. I should not take the medications, which I have questions about, until I have my questions answered. If my doctor is not available, my nurse or a hospital pharmacist can help answer some of my questions as well.
Who is responsible for my medications during my hospitalization?	3. My doctor or designated personnel will prescribe the medications needed for my health problem. 4. My doctor must check all of my medications to make sure that they are fine to take together, including my vitamins, herbs, diet supplements, natural remedies, and over-the-counter medications. 5. A pharmacist will check my new medication prescribed by my doctor. This pharmacist should identify whether there are other medications, foods, or drinks that I should not take with my new medication. This action is to help avoid a bad interaction or reaction. 6. A pharmacist will dispense the medications at the pharmacy, according to the orders prescribed by my doctor and forward my medications to the inpatient care unit where I am admitted. 7. Often, a nurse who works in my inpatient care unit will prepare and give the medications to me. 8. Before leaving for the hospital, I need to prepare a list of my home medications I am using and give this list to my doctor and nurse. Another option is bringing all the medication bottles or labels with me to the hospital. This action is very important for my doctor and nurse to reconcile my medications. This list should include but is not limited to: 8.1 Prescription medications 8.2 Over-the-counter medications (e.g., aspirin) 8.3 Vitamins 8.4 Herbs 8.5 Diet supplements 8.6 Natural remedies

Table 5. Continued

Question	Issue
What can I do at the hospital to help avoid mistakes with my medications?	1. I need to make sure that my doctor, nurse, and other health care providers (abbreviated as clinicians) check my wristband and ask my name before giving me medications of any sort (e.g., oral and IV medications); 2. I should not be afraid to tell my clinician if I think I am about to get the wrong medication or therapy. 3. I should know what time I should get my medications. If I do not get them, then I should ask for (e.g., using the call light to call my nurse). 4. I must tell my clinician if I do not feel well after taking a medication. I should ask for help immediately if I think I am experiencing a side effect or reaction. 5. I should get a list of my medications, including the newly prescribed ones. I should read the list carefully and make sure it lists everything I am taking. 6. If I am given IV fluids, I also need to read the bag to find out what is in it. I should ask my clinician how long it should take for the liquid to run out. I must let my clinician know if the liquid is dripping too quickly or slowly.
Questions to ask my doctor	1. How will my new medication help me? 2. Are there other names for this new medication? Does it have a brand or generic name? I must ask my doctor to write the brand name down. 3. Is there any written information about this new medication? I should ask for a copy of written medication information. 4. Can I take this medication with my allergy? I should remind my doctor about my allergies and reactions that I have had to the other medications. 5. Is it safe to take this new medication with my nonprescription ones (e.g., vitamins, herbs, and supplements)? 6. Is there any side effect of this new medication? If I experience side effects or a bad reaction, what should I do? 7. Are there any specific instructions for my new medication (e.g., avoiding certain foods or drinks when taking this new medication)? 8. Can I stop taking this medication as soon as the symptom is relieved? 9. Do I need to swallow or chew the medications? Can I cut or crush it if I need to?

Source: Joint Commission (2008). Speak up: Help avoid mistakes with your medicines. Available at: http://www.jointcommission.org/PatientSafety/SpeakUp/speak_up_med_mistakes.htm (accessed January 1, 2008).

A patient wants a safe hospital stay. Medication errors occur relatively often due to professional or nonprofessional negligence committed by the physician who prescribed the drug, the pharmacist who filled the medication order, or the nurse who administered the medication. We really need to count on our health care providers to provide error-free medication therapy. However, during hospital stays, what a patient or the family can do in preventing medication errors is limited. Asking our hospitals to have a safe medication use system is what we and our communities must do to promote the safety of our medication use. Table 5 lists the critical information essential for hospitalized patients or families as related to safe medication use.

References

Bates, D. W., Cullen, D. J., Laird, N., Petersen, L. A., Small, S. D., Servi, D., Laffel, G., Sweitzer, B. J., Shea, B. F., Hallisey, R., Vander Vleit, M., Nemeskal, R., & Leape, L. (1995). Incidence of adverse medication events and potential adverse medication events: Implications for prevention (ADE Prevention Study Group). *JAMA, 274*(1), 29-34.

Burroughs, T. E., Waterman, A. D., Gallagher, T. H., Waterman, B., Jeffe, D. B., Dunagan, W. C., Garbutt, J., Cohen, M. M., Cira, J., & Fraser, V. J. (2007). Patients' concerns about medical errors during hospitalization. *Joint Commission Journal on Quality and Patient Safety/Joint Commission Resources, 33*(1), 5-14.

Collins, S., Currie, L., Bakken, S., & Cimino, J. J. (2006). Interruptions during the use of a CPOE system for MICU rounds. AMIA Annual Symposium Proceedings/AMIA Symposium, p. 895.

Joint Commission (2006). Goal 3: Improve the safety of using medications. In A. Grayson. (Ed.), *Meeting the Joint Commission's 2007 National Patient Safety Goals* (pp. 37-52). Oakbrook Terrace, IL: Joint Commission.

Joint Commission (2007a). Preventing medication errors. In R. A. Porché, Jr. (Ed.), *Front line of defense: The role of nurses in preventing sentinel events* (2nd ed., pp. 35-58). Oakbrook Terrace, IL: Joint Commission.

Joint Commission (2007b). 2008 *Comprehensive accreditation manual for hospitals: The official handbook*. Oakbrook Terrace, IL: Joint Commission Resources.

Joint Commission (2007c). *Patient safety pocket guide* (2nd ed., pp. 23-68). Oakbrook Terrace, IL: Joint Commission.

Joint Commission (2008). Speak up: Help avoid mistakes with your medicines. Available at: http://www.jointcommission.org/PatientSafety/SpeakUp/speak_up_med_mistakes.htm (accessed January 1, 2008).

Joint Commission International (2007). WHO collaborating center for patient safety solutions: Nine patient safety solutions. Available at: http://www.jcipatientsafety. org/24725 (accessed January 1, 2008).

Leape, L. L., Rogers, G., Hanna, D., Griswold, P., Federico, F., Fenn, C. A., Bates, D. W., Kirle, L., & Clarridge, B. R. (2006). Developing and implementing new safe practices: voluntary adoption through statewide collaboratives. *Quality & Safety in Health Care, 15*(4), 289-95.

National Coordinating Council for Medication Error Reporting and Prevention (2008a). About medication errors: What is a medication error? Available at: http://www. nccmerp.org/aboutMedErrors.html (accessed January 1, 2008).

National Coordinating Council for Medication Error Reporting and Prevention (2008b). Consumer information for safe medication use. Available at: http://www.nccmerp.org/ consumerInfo.html (accessed January 1, 2008).

Pedersen, C. A., Schneider, P. J., & Scheckelhoff, D. J. (2007). ASHP national survey of pharmacy practice in hospital settings: Monitoring and patient education--2006. *American Journal of Health-System Pharmacy, 64*(5), 507-520.

Roizen, M. F., & Oz, W. (2006). *You the smart patient: An insider's handbook for getting the best treatment* (pp. 193-222). New York, NY: Free Press.

Tang, F. I., Sheu, S. J., Yu, S., Wei, I. L., & Chen, C. H. (2007). Nurses relate the contributing factors involved in medication errors. *Journal of Clinical Nursing, 16*(3), 447-457.

Tucker, A. L., & Spear, S. J. (2006). Operational failures and interruptions in hospital nursing. *Health Services Research, 41*(3-Part I), 643-662.

University of Michigan School of Nursing (2008a). Academic programs: B.S.N. curriculum. Available at: http://www.nursing.umich.edu/academics/bsn/curriculum.html and http://www.nursing.umich.edu/academics/bsn/undergrad-courses.html (accessed January 1, 2008).

University of Michigan School of Nursing (2008b). Undergraduate courses. Available at: http://www.nursing.umich.edu/academics/bsn/undergrad-courses.html (accessed January 1, 2008).

Transfusion Errors

Learning from a Patient Case A

In hospital M, Patient A was taken from his inpatient room to the radiology department after a transfusion had been started. Shortly, Patient A developed urticaria and an increased temperature while in the radiology waiting area. He was able to ask for assistance and was transferred back to his inpatient room right away.

Hospital M's transfusion policy did not address the monitoring requirements for the patients when they are removed from their rooms. Consequently, Hospital M reviewed its policy and made revisions. This change in Hospital M's monitoring requirements helped ensure that the patients receiving blood transfusions would be adequately monitored, regardless of their physical locations. In other words, after the blood is administered, ongoing monitoring will be performed to ensure that any adverse events are identified and treated promptly and appropriately (Joint Commission, 2007a).

Learning from a Patient Case B

Patient B just underwent major abdominal surgery and was recovering in the postanesthesia care unit. He became hypotensive. His postoperative hemoglobin level was reported to be quite low. Consequently, his surgeon ordered an immediate transfusion in the postanesthesia care unit, using the blood remaining in the operating room refrigerator from Patient B's earlier surgery.

A unit clerk brought 2 units of blood to the postanesthesia care unit. A nurse administered these 2 blood units to Patient B, without following the patient and blood unit identification and verification procedures. Both blood units were administered to Patient B.

One of the blood units stored in the operating room refrigerator was intended for another patient, not for Patient B. Shortly after finishing the blood transfusion, Patient B developed a hemolytic transfusion reaction and died in the postanesthesia care unit.

Following this sentinel event, this hospital developed a new blood storage policy that prohibited refrigerators in the operating room suites. All blood units should be transported to the operating room only in the patient-specific individual coolers (Joint Commission, 2007a).

Learning from a Legal Case Summary

Mrs. P had difficulties with the birth of her third child. After delivering her child, Mrs. P continued to hemorrhage. The drug and various massaging methods were ineffective. Dr. K, Mrs. P's doctor, decided to perform an emergency hysterectomy and removed Mrs. P's uterus.

While Mrs. P was still in the delivery room, she started to receive two 500-cc units of blood and this was continued after she was moved to the operating room for the hysterectomy surgery. Mrs. P had O+ blood and both blood units were properly matched to be used for her transfusion.

Shortly after moving to the operating room, Dr. K ordered an additional 2 units of blood to be obtained from the hospital blood laboratory. Nurse Aide S, carried the blood to the room adjoining the operating room, where Nurse Aide S was met by Circulating Nurse A. Nurse Aide S and Circulating Nurse A checked the numbers on the blood containers against the numbers indicated on the laboratory slips. Together, they found these numbers to correspond and concluded that these 2 blood units were the correct blood for Mrs. P.

However, they failed to notice that Mrs. Q's name and room number (another inpatient) were on the slips, and Mrs. P's name was not. Both blood units brought to the operation room by Nurse Aide S were A+, which was incompatible with Mrs. P's O+ blood type.

Mrs. P received one full 500-cc unit of the A+ blood and about 100 cc of the second unit before the transfusion error was discovered. The error was discovered by the hospital blood laboratory technician, who handed 2 units of blood to Nurse Aide S. This technician received an inquiry about the blood from personnel in Mrs. Q's room and realized that the blood intended for Mrs. Q had gone to the operating room.

The transfusion was immediately stopped. Dr. K ordered more of the proper O+ blood for Mrs. P and began to give Mrs. P other necessary liquids to dilute the incompatible blood in Mrs. P's system. Fortunately, up to now, Mrs. P exhibited no transfusion reactions.

The hysterectomy proceeded and was completed without any further complications. Mrs. P received a total of 12 units of blood during the surgery. Laboratory tests were done and no kidney damage was noted. The next morning, Dr. K told Mr. and Mrs. P for the first time about the transfusion error episode. Mrs. P was discharged 13 days after her delivery and surgery.

About 11 months later, a lawsuit was filed in trial court. The court of appeals concluded in 1976 that Mrs. P was entitled to the award of $10,000. The court noted that Mrs. P suffered a significant traumatic experience, physically and mentally, because of the blood transfusion error. The amount of the award was justified because that she suffered for only a very short period of time and had no permanent damage.

Source: NexisLexis®Academic: Federal & State Cases (Case number: 12,947; July 7, 1976, decided) (accessed on January 2, 2008).

Learning from a Legal Case Summary

In 1985, Dr. G, a plastic surgeon who practiced in Hospital J, recommended that Ms. C have breast reduction surgery to help alleviate her long-standing back pain and problems. Ms. C elected to have the surgery. Dr. G asked Ms. C to have her own blood stored prior to the surgery. She had a unit of her own blood drawn by the Red Cross in anticipation of her surgery.

During the surgery, Ms. C had a little more than normal blood loss. She received the unit of her own blood.

The next morning (March 26, 1985), a nurse informed Dr. G that Ms. C's hemoglobin level had fallen to 8.2. As a result of this clinical information, Dr. G ordered 2 units of blood. These 2 units of blood were typed and cross-matched before they were administered to Ms. C. As for the sources of the blood, Hospital J received the blood from the Red Cross. The typing and cross-matching were confirmed in Hospital J. However, the blood was not tested for hepatitis, venereal disease, or the AIDS virus because Hospital J did not have the facilities to do so.

Later on March 26, 1985, Ms. C was given a transfusion of a unit of packed red cells, which was collected by the Red Cross on March 7, 1985 from an unidentified person. This blood unit had been tested by the Red Cross for hepatitis and venereal disease, but not for HIV/AIDS virus, because the chapter of the Red Cross did not have the test kits to test blood for the AIDS virus. Shortly after this very unit of blood was donated, the Red Cross received the test kits to test for the AIDS virus and started testing their inventory blood for HIV/AIDS virus.

In August 1986, Ms. C was told that she had been exposed to HIV/AIDS virus when she received the blood transfusion after her breast reduction surgery on March 26, 1985. Ms. C's blood was tested for HIV exposure and the test was positive.

She filed a malpractice and negligence action against Hospital J. The trial court rendered a verdict in favor of Ms. C in the amount of $8,150,000 for her future medical costs. The court of appeals affirmed the trial court's order.

Source: NexisLexis®Academic: Federal & State Cases (Case number: 90AP-599; May 23, 1991, decided) (accessed on January 2, 2008).

A Success Story

The Mayo Clinic is an internationally renowned medical practice based in Rochester, Minnesota, and is affiliated with hospital facilities and a medical school. The Mayo Clinic made an effort to deal with the accountability issues related to transfusion safety. It consolidated all personnel involved in blood transfusion phlebotomy and blood administration activities to become direct employees of the transfusion medicine services. The Mayo Clinic now has a blood transfusion team responsible for phlebotomizing the potential recipient and administering the transfusion to the recipient.

This change gives direct oversight to all transfusion activities to the department of transfusion medicine services. In this system, the phlebotomists, who work for the transfusion medicine services, will be attuned to the importance of proper patient identification. The employees, who are responsible for administering the blood products, will similarly attend to the importance of the proper blood administration (Brooks, 2005).

Knowing about Transfusion Errors

During hospitalization, the use of blood and blood products can be a necessary and potentially lifesaving treatment for many clinical situations (Hussain & Kao, 2005). Recent efforts to make blood transfusion as safe as possible have focused on making the blood in the bag as disease-free as possible. Many of these endeavors have been directed toward infectious complications of blood transfusions (e.g., AIDS, hepatitis B and C, and bacterial contamination). Transfusion safety has improved dramatically although the costs have been equally high. However, blood services will have to continue to deal with emerging pathogens (Brooks, 2005; Joint Commission, 2007a).

The other aspect of safe blood transfusion is related to preventing noninfectious serious hazards of transfusion. These types of transfusion errors include incorrect transfusion (e.g., ABO/Rh incompatibility), under-transfusion, transfusion-related acute lung injury, cardiopulmonary toxicity, and metabolic derangements for massive transfusion. Linden and associates (2000) found that in New York, the transfusion risk of ABO-mismatched blood was 1 in 38,000. These prevalence statistics even exceeded the aggregate risk of all transfusion-associated viral infections at 1 in 50,000 transfusions.

The actual transfusion process is performed primarily in hospitals, but the transfusion process has not been well examined and has held considerably less interest. In fact, most of the blood transfusion errors have occurred in the transfusion process, outside of the blood bank or the department of transfusion medicine services. For example, a patient can receive incorrect blood due to clerical or communication errors (Hussain & Kao, 2005). Consequently, we must turn our attention to enhancing overall blood safety by focusing more on improving the process of blood transfusion.

Errors involving patients, blood specimens, and blood product identification put the patients who receive transfusions at risk. Such errors can result in death for some. A hemolytic transfusion reaction (HTR) often poses a great risk and results in transfusion-related sentinel events. An HTR refers to the hemolysis of a patient's red blood cells due to immunologic incompatibility between the donor and the recipient or due to nonimmune mechanisms. The severity of an HTR depends on the following three factors (Brooks, 2005; Joint Commission, 2007a):

1. The type of incompatibility
2. The quantity of incompatible blood received
3. The elapsed time before initiating treatment for the reaction

Risk Factors and Possible Solutions as Suggested by the Joint Commission

According to the data from the Joint Commission's Sentinel Event Database from 1995 to 2005, transfusion errors accounted for 2.6% (94) of 3548 reported sentinel events. In fact, transfusion administration involves multiple personnel and departments within a hospital. For example, a transfusion administration can involve (Joint Commission, 2007a):

1. A physician who assesses the need of a patient and prescribes a blood transfusion order
2. Laboratory or nursing staff who obtain the blood specimen for typing and cross-matching
3. Laboratory personnel who prepare and label the blood product for transfusion
4. A nurse who administers the blood product

Errors can be made by (Joint Commission, 2007a):

1. A physician writing a transfusion order on the wrong patient chart
2. A blood sample for typing and cross-matching being obtained from the wrong patient
3. Blood product being mislabeled
4. Blood product being labeled correctly but given to the wrong patient

In 2005, for the frequencies of root causes of reported sentinel events, patient assessment was the most often identified root cause for transfusion errors at about 90%, followed by competency and credentialing at about 60%, communication (about 45%), and leadership (about 45%). The Joint Commission (2007a) further identified five major root causes for transfusion errors and the corresponding prevention strategies were developed (Table 1).

Challenges for Clinicians in Preventing Transfusion Errors

Blood transfusion, which is similar to administration of medications, is considered as a kind of medical treatment. The principles for patient identification and monitoring after administration are comparable for medication and transfusion administration. Each hospital may have specific policies or clinical guidelines for medication administration and for transfusion administration.

For example, the verification step in the transfusion procedure requires two staff members to conduct this task together. Except for intrathetical medications, such a requirement is not required for administering most of the medications. In an acute hospital, the medication use system will involve pharmacists who fill the prescriptions. In comparison, the blood transfusion system may involve laboratory staff for typing and cross-matching the blood and the staff in the transfusion medicine services, but not pharmacists.

Table 1. The major root causes of the reported sentinel events on transfusion errors and the corresponding prevention strategies for nurses

Root cause	Prevention strategy

Wrong patient and wrong identification and verification processes
1. Failure to properly identify a patient
2. Inadequate or inaccurate patient identification procedures
3. The hospital's policies and procedures related to transfusion safety insufficient
	1. Hospital leaders should ensure that the identification process is consistent throughout the hospital to avoid transfusion errors.
	  1.1 Nurses must know the hospital's procedure for properly identifying the patient.
	2. Nurses should know how identification information is documented hospital wide.
	  2.1 Nurses must know the specific data and information used to identify patients in the clinical record and on a wristband as appropriate.
	  2.2 Nurses should know how to identify a patient for a transfusion procedure.
	3. Nurses should clarify any confusing patient identification procedures with their supervisors.
	  3.1 Nurses may participate in redesigning the patient identification procedures, if needed.
	4. Nurses or laboratory staff or both must conduct each and every step correctly in the labeling process.
	  4.1 Hospitals should adopt a prepackaged system that includes all the needed equipment for proper specimen and blood unit labeling. This package should include, but is not limited to, wristband sleeve, wristband label, specimen container, labels, and needles.
	5. Before administering blood, nurses must confirm the patient's name with the patient and check the unique patient identifier on the wristband, the blood unit's unique identification number, ABO and Rh type, and the expiration date of the blood.
	  5.1 The administering nurse and the other health care providers should read aloud the information identifying the patient and the unit of blood.
	  5.2 This verification procedure should be conducted at the bedside, if possible.
	  5.3 Confirmation on the transfusion process should be documented by both staff.
	6. Nurses or laboratory staff or both should avoid the use of problematic patient identifiers, such as the room number and bed assignment.

Root cause	Prevention strategy
Insufficient communication and deficient available information	1. Nurses must know how to access their patients' vital information in clinical records, including the prior transfusion history and information concerning a patient's identification. 2. Hospitals may use a standardized transfusion documentation form that details the steps required before giving a patient a unit of blood. Such transfusion documentation can be used as a communication tool. 3. Hospitals need to ensure proper hand-off communication on the recipients among staff (e.g., a physician, nurse, or a radiology or special procedure technician). 3.1 An adequate and accurate hand-off communication would provide needed information to the next staff responsible for the patient's care.

Inadequate patient assessment and monitoring	1. Nurses should check the laboratory values to see whether the transfusion orders for the blood meets the hospital's established criteria. Nurses must confirm the need for the transfusion.
	    1.1 For example, if a patients' hemoglobin or hematocrit value or the platelet count is above the hospital's established level, the responsible nurse may need to check the physicians' notes to learn the rationale for giving the transfusion.
	2. Nurses need to aware of and determine what information is required from the physician's assessment to safely administer the transfusion. Nurses should ensure the availability of key assessment findings and communicate such information to the other members in the health care team.
	3. Nurses must appropriately monitor and observe the patient during and following a transfusion for any transfusion reactions.
	    3.1 Nurses must be able to recognize the signs and symptoms of a transfusion reaction.
	    3.2 If appropriate training is not provided, nurses must request it from their supervisor to ensure that they are properly trained before administering any blood. Transfusion training topics may include but are not limited to:
	        3.2.1 Advantages and disadvantages of different blood component therapy
	        3.2.2 Autologous transfusion
	        3.2.3 Early recognition of transfusion reactions
	        3.2.4 Emergency transfusion before availability of cross-matched blood
	        3.2.5 Equipment used in the transfusion procedure
	        3.2.6 Massive transfusion problems
	        3.2.7 Transfusion criteria
	        3.2.8 Use of platelets, plasma, cryoprecipitate, or plasma derivatives
	        3.2.9 Use of volume expanders other than blood products

Table 1. Continued

Root cause	Prevention strategy

Inadequate staffing levels, orientation, training, or competence assessment	1. Nurses must follow the hospital's established procedures throughout the transfusion process, including the steps for:
	  1.1 Identifying the patient
	  1.2 Labeling the specimen
	  1.3 Sending the specimen to the laboratory for processing
	2. Nurses should learn and be familiar with blood unit types being administered, including autologous, homologous, and directed donor units.
	3. Nurses must know and be competent in appropriate techniques for withdrawing blood from different types of invasive lines. This procedure requires high-quality phlebotomy skills.

Unsafe equipment or care environment
  1. Failure to follow the hospital's patient and blood unit identification and verification process
  2. Failure to follow the hospital's established blood storage policies
	1. Nurses must know the hospital's blood storage and handling policies and procedures.
	2. Hospitals should design transfusion training sessions that involve real-life pressures.
	  2.1 Nurses must be trained in a real-life setting before administering transfusion.
	  2.2 Such training may allow staff to learn from their mistakes, and see how the mistakes are made.
	3. Hospitals and nurses should together determine the barriers that fail to prevent mistransfusion in the transfusion process.
	4. Nurses should know how to use appropriate and available transfusion-related equipment (e.g., infusion pumps). It is also essential to be knowledgeable about the alarm systems on the transfusion equipment, preventive maintenance schedules, and electric safety precautions of related equipment.
	5. Nurses must also act to prevent contamination of blood products and transfusion equipment during storage and handling.

Source: Joint Commission (2007a). Preventing transfusion errors. In R. A. Porché, Jr. (Ed.), *Front line of defense: The role of nurses in preventing sentinel events* (2nd ed., pp. 59-71). Oakbrook Terrace, IL: Joint Commission.

Demand a Blood Transfusion Team: A System Approach

To prevent transfusion errors, a system approach is needed. If possible, a hospital should have its own blood transfusion team that is responsible for phlebotomizing the potential recipient and administering the transfusion to the recipient. For example, the Mayo Clinic has a blood transfusion team responsible for phlebotomizing the potential recipient and administering the transfusion to the recipient (Brooks, 2005; see *A success story* at the beginning of this chapter). Depending on the size of the hospital and resources available, each hospital may create a new position within the hospital to coordinate all transfusion activities. This general type of position may be labeled a "transfusion safety officer" (Books, 2005).

Adopting Technologies to Improve Safety of Blood Transfusions

For hospital executives, it is important to adopt both the bar-coding technology and the computerized medication administration records to improve accuracy in patient identification and prevent wrong-patient and incorrect blood unit errors. Other technologies, which have similar functions as the bar-coding technology, are smart chip and biometrics technologies. However, the bar-coding technology is relatively more acceptable than the other two technologies in the US hospital environment. Adopting the bar-coding technology or similar technologies is indeed the hospital's judgment call (Brooks, 2005).

As for the bar-coding technology, for most of the systems, the patient receiving care will be assigned a bar code on admission. All blood units would have a specific bar code. Each nurse who administers blood units would have a bar-code reader (also called scanner). Nurses may use a wireless laptop computer attached to a medication cart and a bar-code reader to initiate the verification and identification process. When adopting the bar-coding technology, all verification steps must be prepared at the bedside (Joint Commission, 2007b). This technology can effectively prevent transfusion errors due to staff's inappropriate or incomplete patient identification and verification tasks.

Advancement in Labeling Blood Units Ready to be Administered

We suggest that each labeled blood unit should come with a list of information, including, but not limited to, the recipient/patient's name, the unique patient identifier (being matched with the information on the wristband), the ABO and Rh blood type of the recipient, ABO and Rh type of the blood, the expiration date of the blood, and the physician's name who orders the transfusion on the label. The information on the label of a blood unit should be consistent with the corresponding patient's MAR and the slip from the blood bank or the department of transfusion medicine services.

To enhance the likelihood of ABO-matched transfusions, Brooks (2005) suggested that retyping all patients who do not have a historical ABO type on their clinical records is important and essential. This additional step would not require a great expenditure of resources. Until a patient has had two separate determinations of blood type, this patient should be issued only type O blood.

Training on Transfusion Safety

Regularly providing on-the-job training related to transfusion safety to hospital personnel at all levels and including related materials in the new staff orientation are essential. Transfusion administration involves multiple personnel and departments within a hospital—from ordering the blood transfusion, to collecting the specimen, to administering the blood components. Staff members who perform any tasks in the blood transfusion preparation and administration procedures need to be constantly reminded of the proper way to perform their tasks.

Errors can be made by a physician who wrote an order on the wrong patient chart, a blood sample that was obtained from the wrong patient, the blood product that was mislabeled, or the blood product that was labeled correctly but given to the wrong patient (Joint Commission, 2007a). Consequently, training on blood transfusion-related procedures and tasks should have a special emphasis on proper patient and blood product identification.

Table 2 summarizes a list of critical tips for nurses who work in acute inpatient care units to help prevent transfusion errors.

Critical Tips for Patients and Families to Prevent Transfusion Errors

The entire transfusion administration procedures often involve: (1) a physician, who assesses the need of a patient and prescribes a blood transfusion order; (2) a laboratory or nursing staff, who obtains the blood specimen for typing and cross-matching; (3) a laboratory technician, who prepares and labels the blood product for transfusion; and (4) a nurse, who administers the blood product (Joint Commission, 2007a). Regardless, if our doctor has prescribed a blood transfusion for us, we can only observe the processes of obtaining the blood specimen from us (for typing and cross-matching) and administering the blood product to us (including the patient identification procedure if this procedure is performed at bedside). These two tasks are often performed by nurses who work in inpatient care units.

Table 2. Preventing transfusion errors:
Critical tips for nurses who work in acute inpatient care units

Dimension	Tip
Performing accurate patient identification procedures	1. Nurses must know the hospital's policies and procedures and the specific data and information for properly identifying the patient (e.g., in the clinical record and on a wristband). 2. Nurses must follow the hospital's established procedures throughout the entire transfusion process, including the steps for: 2.1 Identifying the patient 2.2 Labeling the specimen 2.3 Sending the specimen to the laboratory for processing 3. Before administering blood, nurses must confirm the patient's name with the patient and check the unique patient identifier on the wristband, the blood unit's unique identification number, ABO and Rh type, and the expiration date of the blood. 3.1 The administering nurse and the other health care provider (a total of two staff members) should read aloud the information identifying the patient and the unit of blood. This verification procedure should be conducted at the bedside, if possible. 3.2 Confirmation on the transfusion process should be documented by both staff. 3.3 Nurses should avoid the use of problematic patient identifiers, such as the room number and bed assignment.

Dimension	Tip
Sufficient hand-off communications among staff members	1. Nurses must know how to access their patients' vital information in clinical records, including the prior transfusion history and information concerning a patient's identification. 2. Nurses must ensure proper hand-off communication on the blood recipient (patient) among staff to provide needed information to the next staff responsible for the recipient's care.

Adequate patient assessment and monitoring	1. Before administering blood, nurses should check the laboratory values to see whether the transfusion order for the blood meets the hospital's established criteria and confirm the need for the transfusion.
	2. Nurses must appropriately monitor and observe the patient during and following a transfusion for any transfusion reactions.
	  2.1 Nurses must be able to recognize the signs and symptoms of a transfusion reaction.
	  2.2 Nurses should learn and be familiar with blood unit types being administered, including autologous, homologous, and directed donor units.
	  2.3 Nurses must know and be competent in appropriate techniques for withdrawing blood from different types of invasive lines, according to the hospital's established policies and procedures.
	  2.4 Nurses must ensure that they have been properly trained before administering any blood. If appropriate transfusion training was not provided, nurses must request transfusion training from their supervisor. Nurses must be trained in a real-life setting before administering transfusion.

Promoting a safe care environment	1. Nurses must know the hospital's blood storage and handling policies and procedures. 2. Nurses should know how to use appropriate and available transfusion-related equipment (e.g., infusion pumps), including the alarm systems on the transfusion equipment, preventive maintenance schedules, and electric safety precautions of related equipment. 3. Nurses must also act to prevent contamination of blood products and transfusion equipment during storage and handling.

We really need to rely on our nurses to deliver an error-free blood transfusion, however. As a result, Table 3 lists the critical information and tips that are essential for hospitalized patients and their families to know in their efforts to avoid transfusion errors. These tips may help us prevent wrong-patient and wrong-product errors due to insufficient patient identification procedures and avoid any treatment delays related to possible transfusion reactions.

Table 3. Critical information to know to help avoid transfusion errors:
Tips for patients and families

Question	Issue
	If I am not well enough to do any of the actions indicated below, I should ask a family or friend to help.

What can I do to help avoid transfusion errors?	1. If a blood transfusion is ordered by my doctor, I should ask my doctor:
	    1.1 The purpose for receiving the blood transfusion
	    1.2 The blood unit type to be administered
	    1.3 Possible transfusion reactions that I may experience and should report to my nurse
	        1.3.1 A transfusion reaction refers to any adverse event that occurs due to a blood transfusion. Doctors who prescribe transfusion orders must always balance the risk of a transfusion reaction against the anticipated benefit of a blood transfusion.
	        1.3.2 Transfusion-related adverse events can take the form of (Wikipedia, 2008):
	            1.3.2.1 An allergic reaction
	            1.3.2.2 A transfusion-related infection
	            1.3.2.3 Hemolysis related to an incompatible blood type
	            1.3.2.4 An alteration of the immune system related to the transfusion
	2. Before receiving blood transfusion, I need to make sure that my nurse checks my wristband and asks my name. This is important to ensure no wrong-patient error.
	3. Before receiving the blood, I should tell my nurse my blood type (ABO and Rh type). If the blood I am receiving is different from my blood type, I should question for possible blood incompatibility.
	4. I should not be afraid to tell my nurse if I think I am about to get a transfusion of the wrong-type blood.
	5. I must tell my nurse if I do not feel well while receiving or after the blood transfusion. I should ask for help immediately if I think I am experiencing a transfusion reaction.
	6. I should ask my nurse how long the transfusion should take for the blood to run out. I must let my nurse know if the blood is dripping too quickly or slowly.

What kind of transfusion reactions should I pay attention to?	1. The types of transfusion reactions that I may experience, include (Wikipedia, 2008):
	    1.1 Acute hemolytic reaction: A medical emergency results from rapid destruction of the donor red blood cells by the recipient's antibodies. The most common cause is clerical error (e.g., a patient receives a wrong unit of blood). Symptoms include fever, chills, back pain, and pink or red urine. This reaction may cause a serious complication of acute renal failure.
	    1.2 Anaphylactic/severe allergic reaction (1 per 30,000-50,000 units transfused): A medical emergency that requires prompt treatment and may be life-threatening. This reaction often occurs in people with selective IgA deficiency. However, these people are often asymptomatic and may not know they have IgA deficiency until an anaphylactic reaction occurs.
	    1.3 Bacterial infection (1 in 50,000 platelet transfusions and 1 in 500,000 red blood cell transfusions)

Question		Issue
	1.4	Febrile nonhemolytic transfusion reaction (1 per 2 million units transfused): The most common adverse reaction but clinically benign and no lasting side effect or problems. Symptoms include fever and shortness of breath 1-6 hours after receiving the transfusion.
	1.5	Iron overload (1 in 12-20 units of red blood cells transfused): Recipients who receive several red blood cell transfusions can develop iron overload, which can damage the liver, heart, kidneys, and pancreas.
	1.6	Transfusion-associated acute lung injury (1 in 2000 units transfused): This reaction is a syndrome of acute respiratory distress and often related to fever, noncardiogenic pulmonary edema, and hypotension. Symptoms can be mild to life-threatening and the mortality rate is less than 10%. The recipients often recover fully within 96 hours.
	1.7	Transfusion-associated graft-versus-host disease: This fatal reaction refers to an immune attack by transfused cells against the recipient (e.g., immunosuppressed patients). It is a common complication of stem cell transplantation but a rare complication of blood transfusion.
	1.8	Volume overload (also called transfusion-associated circulatory overload): Recipients with impaired cardiac function (e.g., congestive heart failure) can experience volume overload following blood transfusion, which may lead to edema, shortness of breath while not lying flat, and shortness of breath while lying flat.
What kind of treatment would I receive if I experienced transfusion reactions?	1.	Stopping the transfusion immediately is the most important medical treatment in dealing with a presumed transfusion reaction.
	2.	Hospital and nurses must save the remaining blood and IV tubing for testing. According to each hospital's policy, tests on the blood product for possible bacterial contamination and tests on the recipient for hemolysis may be required.
	3.	Most hospitals have transfusion reaction protocols in place.

Source: Wikipedia (2008). Transfusion reaction. Available at: http://en.wikipedia.org/wiki/Transfusion_reaction (accessed January 2, 2008).

References

Brooks, J. P. (2005). Reengineering transfusion and cellular therapy processes hospitalwide: ensuring the safe utilization of blood products. *Transfusion, 45*(4 Suppl.), 159S-171S.

Hussain, E., & Kao, E. (2005). Medication safety and transfusion errors in the ICU and beyond. *Critical Care Clinics, 21*(1), 91-110, ix.

Joint Commission (2007a). Preventing transfusion errors. In R. A. Porché, Jr. (Ed.), *Front line of defense: The role of nurses in preventing sentinel events* (2nd ed., pp. 59-71). Oakbrook Terrace, IL: Joint Commission.

Joint Commission (2007b). Preventing medication errors. In R. A. Porché, Jr. (Ed.), *Front line of defense: The role of nurses in preventing sentinel events* (2nd ed., pp. 35-58). Oakbrook Terrace, IL: Joint Commission.

Linden, J. V., Wagner, K., Voytovich, A. E., & Sheehan, J. (2000). Transfusion errors in New York State: An analysis of 10 years' experience. *Transfusion, 40*(10), 1207-1213.

Wikipedia (2008). Transfusion reaction. Available at: http://en.wikipedia.org/wiki/Transfusion_reaction (accessed January 2, 2008).

Wrong-Site Surgery

Learning from a Patient Case A

Nurse A, who worked in the preoperative preparation area and the operating room, reviewed Patient B's medical record and found that Patient B's history and physical examination were completed by an internist. The history and physical examination showed that Patient B has bilateral arthritis of the knees and concluded that Patient B had been scheduled for a total knee replacement. However, there was no indication of which knee. The surgeon also had no preoperative notes included in Patient B's medical record because Patient B was admitted the day of the surgery.

Patient B did not speak English fluently and had limited abilities to read English. Nurse A completed the informed consent solely on the basis of the information noted in the operating room schedule, which called for a right-sided total knee replacement. The total knee replacement surgery was performed on the wrong knee (Joint Commission, 2007a).

Learning from a Patient Case B

As a routine, Surgeon C's office staff mailed informed consents to patients prior to their scheduled surgeries. Patients were instructed to sign the consent form and take it to the hospital on the day of surgery.

An elderly female patient, Mrs. D, received an informed consent form for a cervical laminectomy with fusion. Mrs. D did not recall whether Surgeon C mentioned fusion. Mrs. D called her son, who accompanied her during her doctor visit when the surgery was discussed. Mrs. D's son, a physician, explained to Mrs. D that her scheduled surgery should be a lumbar laminectomy. The fusion part was wrong and the procedure site was also inaccurate. If Mrs. D had not noticed the error on the informed consent, a wrong-site surgery and wrong procedure would have been done (Joint Commission, 2007a).

Learning from a Patient Case

In a busy morning, an elderly Hispanic patient, Mr. E, came to the preoperative preparation and holding area for a carpal tunnel procedure. Nurse F worked in the preoperative preparation and holding area and admitted Mr. E. Mr. E's family was asked to remain in the waiting area.

Mr. E's history and physical examination did not indicate that Mr. E had some memory problems. Consequently, a mental evaluation was not included as part of Nurse F's evaluation. Nurse F was also unaware that in some cultures, including Hispanic cultures, patients tend to agree with whatever authority figures say, even when they disagree with authority figures (e.g., doctors and nurses).

The surgery schedule had the wrong wrist specified for Mr. E's surgery. Nurse F asked Mr. E the question: "We're performing the surgery on your left wrist, is that right?" Mr. E responded "yes" to Nurse F's question. The surgery was done on the wrong wrist (Joint Commission, 2007a).

Learning from a Patient Case

In the preoperative preparation and holding area, Nurse G verified with a male patient, Mr. H, that his arthroscopic surgery was for the right knee as posted on the surgery schedule and the consent form. Before the surgery, Surgeon F talked to Mr. H in the holding area and placed a dot above Mr. H's left knee. The dot was marked on the wrong knee.

Shortly, Mr. H was transferred into the operating room. Surgeon F and Nurse G did not communicate about the procedure site and the procedure site was not verified again. Mr. H was anesthetized and the operation started. Unfortunately, Surgeon F performed the surgery on the wrong knee, that is, the knee Surgeon F placed a dot above (Joint Commission, 2007a).

Learning from a Patient Case

To comply with the Joint Commission's hospital accreditation requirements, Hospital J had adopted the Universal Protocol for Preventing Wrong Site, Wrong Procedure, Wrong Person Surgery™. The nurse manager for the preoperative preparation and holding area and the operating room had indicated to her nursing staff that the time-out must be conducted before surgeons start procedures.

Patient K was admitted to have an arthroscopic procedure on his left knee. In the operating room, according to Hospital J's policies, Nurse L reminded Surgeon M that a time-out should be conducted before starting the procedure on Patient K. Surgeon M was mad and replied back to Nurse L that he knew what he was doing and did not need outsiders telling him how to do his work.

Immediately, Surgeon M removed the drape from Patient K's right knee and picked up the scalpel. Surgeon M made an incision despite Nurse L's protest that the right knee was not marked and the clinical records indicated the procedure was to be performed on the left knee.

After making the incision, Surgeon M moved the drape covering Patient K's left knee and saw that the left knee had been marked. As a matter of fact, the site was not marked by Surgeon M himself.

The incision on the right knee was closed and the operation on the left knee began (Joint Commission, 2007a).

Learning from a Legal Case Summary

Patient M underwent a cerebral vascular ultrasound in July 1999. This preoperative diagnostic test showed 80% stenosis of the right internal carotid artery. Dr. R, who practiced in Hospital D, scheduled Patient M for a carotid endarterectomy on his right carotid artery to be conducted at Hospital D.

In September 1999, Dr. R performed surgery on Patient M, carotid endarterectomy surgery on the left side instead of the stenosed right carotid artery. Shortly after this wrong-site surgery error, Patient M underwent a second carotid endarterectomy surgery at Hospital D and this time the surgery was on the correct site—the right internal carotid artery.

Patient M asserted that he had suffered injuries attributed to the unnecessary surgery on his left carotid artery with accompanying physical and emotional pain, suffering, distress, and scarring. Patient M filed a malpractice action after Dr. R's erroneous operation on his healthy left carotid artery.

Dr. R and Hospital D filed demurrers to Patient M's claims for punitive damages set forth in Patient M's medical malpractice complaint. The court denied the demurrer to Patient M's claim for punitive damages as to Dr. R, but granted the demurrer to Patient M's claim for punitive damages as to Hospital D.

Source: NexisLexis®Academic: Federal & State Cases (Case number: 01-CV-2062; December 7, 1001, decided) (access on January 4, 2008).

Knowing about Patient Harms Related to Wrong-Site Surgery

The Joint Commission has made significant efforts to address wrong-site surgery, performance of the wrong procedure, and surgeries operated on the wrong body part and on the wrong patient (Joint Commission, 2007a). Wrong-site surgery constituted 12.5% of the 3548 sentinel events reported to the Joint Commission from 1995 to 2005. Most of them were orthopedic cases. These sentinel events involved surgery on the wrong side (59%), surgery on another wrong site (19%), surgery on the wrong patient (12%), and the wrong surgical procedure (10%). More than 50% of the events happened in ambulatory surgery units within hospitals and 29% occurred in inpatient operating rooms (Joint Commission, 2007a).

Wrong-site surgery is usually preventable. In practice and traditionally, surgeons have the primary responsibility for ensuring that the surgical procedure will be performed on the correct site. However, prevention of wrong-site surgery does demand the cooperation and interdependence of all health care staff members, including physicians, anesthesia providers, and nurses (Joint Commission, 2007a).

In 2004, the Universal Protocol for Preventing Wrong Site, Wrong Procedure, Wrong Person Surgery™ became one of the Joint Commission requirements for all accredited hospitals (Joint Commission, 2003a). This universal protocol is intended to achieve the goal of preventing wrong-site, wrong-procedure, and wrong-person surgery. In the process of developing this protocol, a consensus was reached among the experts from the relevant clinical specialties and professional disciplines. This consensus included eight key principles (Joint Commission, 2003a):

1. Wrong-site, wrong-procedure, and wrong-person surgery can and must be prevented.
2. It is necessary to use multiple, complementary strategies to achieve the goal of eliminating wrong-site, wrong-procedure, and wrong-person surgery.
3. Effective communication and active involvement among all members of the surgical team are essential.
4. If possible, the patient or a legally designated representative should be involved in the surgical-site verification process.
5. Consistent implementation of a standardized verification process would be most effective.
6. A standardized verification process should be flexible enough to allow for appropriate adaptation when required to meet specific patient needs.
7. A requirement for site marking should concentrate on patients involving right or left distinction, multiple body structures (e.g., both fingers and toes), or levels (e.g., a specific section of the spine).
8. A universal protocol should be applicable or adaptable to all operative and other invasive procedures, including procedures done in settings other than the operating room.

In accord with these principles, the *Universal Protocol for Preventing Wrong Site, Wrong Procedure, Wrong Person Surgery* provided implementation requirements and had three main components: (1) a preoperative verification process, (2) marking the operative site, and (3) conducting a time-out immediately before starting the procedure. The aims and processes of these three main components are described below (Joint Commission, 2003a, 2003b, 2006):

1. A preoperative verification process
   1. Aim: This step was meant to ensure that all of the relevant documents, the history and physical examination, the signed informed consent, relevant images, and any required implants and special equipment are available prior to the start of the procedure.

1.1.1 Reviewed clinical records must be consistent with each other, with the patient's expectations, and with the surgical team's understanding of the intended patient, procedure, and site.

1.1.2 Missing information or discrepancies should be addressed and resolved before starting a procedure. A preoperative verification checklist was suggested to ensure availability.

1.2 Process: This ongoing process of information gathering and verification should occur during the following time points or situations, if applicable:

1.2.1 At the time the surgery or procedure is scheduled

1.2.2 At the time of admission into the hospital

1.2.3 Any time the responsibility for care of the patient is transferred to another health care provider

1.2.4 Conducting this process with the patient's involvement when he or she is awake and alert

1.2.5 Before the patient leaves the preoperative area or enters the procedure or operating room

2. Marking the operative site

2.1. Aim: This step was meant to identify unambiguously the intended site of incision or insertion.

2.2. Process: For procedures involving right or left distinction, multiple structures (such as fingers and toes), or multiple levels (such as the exact vertebral level on spine), the intended site must be marked, such that the mark will be visible after the patient has been prepped and draped. Requirements were also indicated:

2.1.1 Making the mark only at or near the incision site

2.1.2 The mark must be unambiguous. It is suggested to use initials or "YES" or a line representing the proposed incision. An "X" may be ambiguous.

2.1.3 The mark must be visible after the patient is prepped and draped.

2.1.4 The mark should be made using a marker that is sufficiently permanent to remain visible after completion of the skin prep.

2.1.5 The method of marking and type of mark must be consistent throughout the hospital. Adhesive site markers should not be used as the sole means of marking the surgical site.

2.1.6 The surgeon or physician who will perform the procedure should do the site marking.

2.1.7 Marking should take place with the patient involved, awake, and aware, if possible.

2.1.8 The final verification of the site mark should take place during the time-out.

2.1.9 A defined procedure must be in place in the hospital for patients who refuse site marking.

2.3. Exemptions: The action of marking the operative site should be exempted in the following situations:

2.3.1. Single-organ surgical cases (e.g., cardiac surgery and cesarean section)

2.3.2. Intervention cases for which the catheter or instrument insertion site may not be predetermined (e.g., cardiac catheterization)

2.3.3. Teeth

2.3.4. Premature infants for whom the mark can cause a permanent tattoo

2.3.5. Cases in which the surgeon or physician performing the procedure is in continuous attendance with the patient, from the time of decision to do the procedure and getting consent from the patient through to the conduct of the procedure

3. Conducting a time-out immediately before starting the procedure

   3.1   Aim: The purpose of this step was meant to conduct a final verification of the correct patient, procedure, site, and implants, if applicable.

   3.2   Process: This step involves active communication among all members of the surgical team and should be consistently initiated by a designated member of the team.

      3.2.1 This procedure should be conducted in a "fail-safe" mode that the procedure will not start until any questions or concerns are resolved.

      3.2.2 This procedure must be conducted in the location where the operation or procedure will be performed and performed immediately before starting the operation or procedure.

      3.2.3 This procedure should be briefly documented and may include a checklist. A checklist should include, at least, the following information:

         3.2.3.1 Agreement on the surgery or procedure to be done

         3.2.3.2 Accurate patient identity

         3.2.3.3 Correct surgical or procedure side and site

         3.2.3.4 Accurate patient position on the operating table

         3.2.3.5 Availability of correct implants and any special equipment or special requirements, as applicable

      3.2.4 The hospital must have processes and systems in place for resolving differences in staff responses during the time-out.

Risk Factors and Possible Solutions as Suggested by the Joint Commission

The Joint Commission (2001) identified several situational factors that may increase the risk of performing wrong-site surgery:

1. Emergency surgical cases
2. Multiple procedures scheduled to be conducted on the same patient during one trip to the operating room
3. Patients with unusual physical characteristics (e.g., morbid obesity or physical deformity)

4. Surgical procedures involving unusual equipment or set up in the operating room

5. Surgical procedures conducted under unusual time pressures (e.g., an unusual start time and staff-perceived time pressure to speed up the preoperative procedures)

6. Change from the scheduled operating room

7. More than one surgeon involved in the surgical case

According to the data from the Joint Commission's Sentinel Event Database, communication was the most often identified root cause for wrong-site surgery at about 80%, followed by orientation and training at about 50%, and procedural compliance at about 30%. For most of the errors related to wrong-site surgery, multiple causes were identified. The Joint Commission (2007a) analyzed four major root causes for wrong-site surgery in depth and developed the corresponding prevention strategies for each of these root causes for nurses (Table 1).

**Table 1. The major root causes of the reported sentinel events
related to wrong-site surgery**

Root cause	Prevention strategy

Communication failure
 	
1. Inaccurate or incomplete communication among staff members
2. Team members hesitant to point out possible errors owing to the intensely hierarchical culture of the operating room
3. Failure to involve the patient, family, or advocate in the identification and verification processes, including the informed consent process and the site-marking process
	1. During transitions of care, nurses who work in the inpatient unit or the preoperative holding area must communicate to the next health care provider the information about the site of surgery.
	   1.1 The method used for communicating patient information should be part of a formal, structured process and should be described in the hospital's policies.
	   1.2 Documentation in clinical records and verbal communication together help enhance information transfer.
	   1.3 Nurses who work in the preoperative holding area must:
	      1.3.1 Receive a report from the nurse caring for the patient previously
	      1.3.2 Review relevant clinical records
	      1.3.3 Verify the information with the patient
	      1.3.4 Document the findings properly
	   1.4 In the operating room, the entire surgical team (including the surgeon) must be informed of the surgical site and be involved in the verification process.
	2. Hospitals must identify and correct the source of communication problems to the extent possible.
	3. Hospital and nursing leaders and nurses should continuously identify processes that can be improved.
	   3.1 Nurses should communicate with their immediate supervisor about a flawed informed consent process, if any.
	   3.2 Nurses who work in inpatient care units or the preoperative holding area must ensure that the signed informed consent form is obtained from the patient before they administer medications that alter the level of consciousness or state of alertness of the patient.
	4. Nurses and the surgical team should avoid using abbreviations when communicating about surgical sites and procedures.

Table 1. Continued

Root cause	Prevention strategy
Incomplete preoperative patient assessment	1. In each preoperative assessment, nurses can help ensure proper identification of the surgical site and procedure, particularly when multiple specialists are seeing one individual patient for multiple problems. 2. In each preoperative assessment, nurses must ensure availability of critical clinical information for each patient, including: 2.1 Information on the informed consent form 2.2 Medical record 2.3 Imaging studies 2.4 Any other sources for verifying the site 3. Nurses must ensure that the preoperative assessment is complete by knowing the populations served by the hospital (e.g., some patients may have a tendency to agree with authority figures). Nurses should seek other methods of verification when needed.
Incorrect patient verification process, and lacking adequate information	1. Nurses and the surgical team members must know and follow the *Universal Protocol for Preventing Wrong Site, Wrong Procedure, Wrong Person Surgery.* 2. Nurses are often involved in preparing a patient for surgery. Nurses must understand the hospital's verification policies and processes. 2.1 Hospital and nursing leaders must ensure sufficient staff with proper orientation and training to follow the established patient verification policies and procedures. 2.2 Hospital and nursing leaders must also evaluate staff competence in verification policies and procedures on a regular basis. 3. The nurse who prepares the patient for surgery must review all clinical information provided and take an active role in verifying the proper patient and surgical site. 3.1 The site must be verified verbally with the patient, the family, or the advocate. 3.2 Certain patient populations may require special attention, when the proper patient and site are verified, including: 3.2.1 Patients who are unable to communicate due to age (e.g., infants and young toddlers) 3.2.2 Patients who do not speak English 3.2.3 Patients with cognitive impairment (e.g., dementia) 3.2.4 Patients with temporary communication impairment 4. Nurses should be aware of the policy and procedure for marking the site. The surgeon who will perform the procedure should mark the site himself or herself, while the patient is still awake and able to participate in the site-marking process. 5. Nurses in the operating room can help ensure the use and availability of critical information. A checklist may help identify the needed information. 6. Nurses may facilitate the surgical team in the use of a time-out before the procedure begins. The time-out process should include but is not limited to: 6.1 Patient identity 6.2 Accurate surgical side and site 6.3 Agreement with the patient and among all team members on the procedure to be done 6.4 Correct patient position to the operating table 6.5 Availability of correct implants and special equipment, if any

Root cause	Prevention strategy
Traditional, hierarchical hospital culture	1. Hospitals should obtain information about the near misses from staff nurses so that common factors in the near misses can be identified. 2. Hospitals should ask staff nurses and understand what aspects of the *Universal Protocol for Preventing Wrong Site, Wrong Procedure and Wrong Person Surgery* they believe to be difficult to implement. When specific concerns are known, these concerns can be addressed. 3. Hospitals should acknowledge positive behaviors of staff nurses and positive aspects of the current practices in the operating room, as related to preventing wrong-site surgery. 4. Some surgeons and other surgical team members may participate in surgical or other invasive procedures at more than one hospital, surgical center, office, or clinic. If the procedures and tools for identification and verification of the patient and procedure were the same through out the medical community, wrong-site surgery-related errors could be reduced. Consequently, the hospital may need to consider collaboration with surgeons and nurses throughout the community to standardize the implementation of the *Universal Protocol for Preventing Wrong Site, Wrong Procedure and Wrong Person Surgery.*

Source: Joint Commission (2007a). Preventing wrong-site surgery. In R. A. Porché, Jr. (Ed.), *Front line of defense: The role of nurses in preventing sentinel events* (2nd ed., pp. 87-98). Oakbrook Terrace, IL: Joint Commission.

Challenges for Clinicians in Preventing Wrong-Site Surgery

Wrong-site surgery is usually preventable. Surgeons, as the lead in the surgical team in the operating room, have the primary responsibility for ensuring that the surgical procedure is being performed on the correct site. However, prevention of wrong-site surgery does demand the cooperation and interdependence of all involved clinicians, including the surgical team members (surgeons, anesthesia providers, and nurses) and the staff working in the inpatient care units (physicians and nurses) (Joint Commission, 2007a).

For example, a patient can be admitted to an inpatient unit prior to the surgery. On the day of surgery, this patient will be transferred to the preoperative holding area and then to the operating room. After the surgery, this patient may stay in the recovery room for a while and then be transferred back to an inpatient unit before being discharged home.

When a task involves multiple departments and personnel (e.g., the patient identification and verification processes for correct surgical site), error tends to occur during transitions of care. As human nature, most of the clinicians may think that the other clinicians will conduct the same identification and verification processes again later on. Consequently, careless identification and verification processes can be performed.

At the same time, clinicians may assume that the ones who have conducted the same patient identification and verification processes must have done a thorough job on this very patient. Because many personnel have checked for the same thing, there is no need to verify whether the patient, the procedure, and the surgical site are correct again.

Besides, the last patient identification and verification will be done in the operating room. However, if a time-out is not called and the patient identification and verification processes are not done thoroughly just before starting surgery, a wrong-site surgery could easily occur.

It is important that nurses perform the patient identification and verification processes comprehensively according to the hospital polices and the *Universal Protocol for Preventing Wrong Site, Wrong Procedure, Wrong Person Surgery*. Hospital and nurse leaders must evaluate staff competence in verification policies and procedures on a regular basis. Table 2 summarizes critical tips for nurses who work in acute inpatient care units to help prevent wrong-site surgery.

Table 2. Preventing wrong-site surgery:
Critical tips for nurses who work in acute inpatient care units

Dimension	Tip

Ensuring complete preoperative patient assessment	1. In each preoperative assessment, nurses can help ensure proper identification of the surgical site and procedure, particularly when multiple specialists are seeing one individual patient for multiple problems.
	 2. In each preoperative assessment, nurses must ensure availability of critical clinical information for each patient, including:
	   2.1 Information on the informed consent form
	   2.2 Medical record
	   2.3 Imaging studies and any other sources for verifying the site
	 3. Nurses must ensure that the signed informed consent form is obtained from the patient or a designated advocate, before they administer medications that alter the level of consciousness or state of alertness of the patient.

Performance of correct patient verification process	1. Nurses must understand the hospital's verification policies and processes.
	   1.1 Nurses must know and follow the *Universal Protocol for Preventing Wrong Site, Wrong Procedure, Wrong Person Surgery.*
	   1.2 Nursing leaders must ensure sufficient nursing staff with proper orientation and training to follow the established patient verification policies and procedures.
	   1.3 Nursing leaders must also evaluate nursing staff competence in verification policies and procedures on a regular basis.
	 2. The nurse who prepares the patient for surgery must review all clinical information provided and take an active role in verifying the proper patient and surgical site.
	   2.1 The site should be verified verbally with the patient, the family, or an advocate, as appropriate.
	   2.2 Nurses must aware that certain patient populations may require special attention, when performing the patient identification processes, including:
	     2.2.1 Patients who are unable to communicate due to age (e.g., infants and young toddlers)
	     2.2.2 Patients who do not speak English (a translator will be needed to perform the verification processes)
	     2.2.3 Patients with cognitive impairment
	     2.2.4 Patients with temporary communication impairment
	 3. Nurses should be aware of the policy and procedure for marking the site.

Dimension	Tip
	3.1 For example, the surgeon who will perform the procedure should mark the site himself or herself while the patient is still awake and able to participate in the site-marking process. 4. If a procedure is conducted in the acute inpatient care unit, the patient's responsible nurse may facilitate the health care team in using a time-out before the procedure begins. The time-out process should include but is not limited to: 4.1 Patient identity 4.2 Accurate procedure side and site 4.3 Agreement with the patient and among all health care team members on the procedure to be done 4.4 Correct patient position required for the procedure 4.5 Availability of special equipment, if any
Promoting effective communication during transitions of care	1. During transitions of care (from an inpatient care unit to the preoperative holding area), nurses must communicate with the next health care provider the information about the site of surgery, according to the hospital's policies. 1.1 Documentation in clinical records and verbal communication together help enhance information transfer. 2. Nurses should avoid using abbreviations when communicating about surgical sites and procedures with nursing colleagues and the other health care providers. 3. Nursing leaders and nurses should continuously identify processes that can be improved.

Table 3. Ensuring a safe surgery:
Essential information for patients and families to know

Time frame	Concern and question to ask
General principles	1. If I am not well enough to do any of the actions indicated below, I should ask a family or friend to help. 2. Most of the surgical or procedural terms can be difficult to understand and remember. It is important to ask my doctor or surgeon to explain to me in lay terms or plain English and provide me a written information of, for example, the name of the surgery or procedure, the surgical side, and site. 3. It is my body and I have the right to understand exactly what procedure will be performed on my body. I must have my questions answered before I sign the informed consent form for the surgery to be performed on my body. 4. In the current health care environment, many patients are asked to arrive the hospital on the morning of the scheduled surgery. If so, it is important for me to know and completely understand all the details related to the surgery in advance and before leaving for the hospital (e.g., at the doctor office visit).
Preparing for my surgery	1. I should write down the questions and take the question list with me when I see my doctor. Questions to ask my doctor and surgeon include but are not limited to: 1.1 Are there any medications (e.g., prescription or over-the-counter drugs) that I should not take before my surgery? 1.2 Can I eat or drink before my surgery? 1.3 Are there any special instructions I should pay attention to? 2. I should ask my family or a friend to take me to and from the hospital or surgery facility. 3. If possible, I should arrange for someone to be with me for the entire hospital stay to ensure that I get the postoperative care I need. 4. Immediately before I leave home for the hospital, I need to make sure that:

Table 3. Continued

Time frame	Concern and question to ask
	4.1 I have taken a shower, washed my hair, and removed any nail polish from my fingers and toes. 4.2 I should not wear any make-up. 4.3 I must leave my jewelry and other valuables at home. 4.4 I should ask the family or a friend who will accompany me to the hospital to keep my important documents and some emergency money after I am admitted into the hospital, especially during the period when I am in the preoperative and holding area and the operating room.

When I am in the hospital	1. A surgeon or nurse will ask me to sign an informed consent from. I should read this form carefully. If I am not well enough to read, I should ask a family member or friend to help.
	2. Before signing the informed consent form, I must have an opportunity to talk to my surgeon about the surgery. I should make sure that all my questions have been answered before I sign the informed consent form.
	3. I should make sure that the informed consent form has correct information of:
	    3.1 My name
	    3.2 The kind of surgery I will have
	    3.3 The risk of my surgery
	4. To prevent wrong-site surgery, my surgeon, nurse, and the other surgical team members may ask me the following questions many times, including:
	    4.1 Who I am
	    4.2 What kind of surgery I am having
	    4.3 The part of my body to be operated on
	5. My doctor and nurse must verify that the information on the informed consent form and my understanding about the surgery are consistent with the information indicated on my medical record.

Just before the surgery	1. My surgeon who will perform my surgery will make a mark on my body part to be operated on. I or my family should participate in this process to make sure that my surgeon marks only the correct body part and nowhere else. 2. Marking should be done when I am awake. If I cannot be awake for the marking, my family or friend can watch my surgeon conducting the marking process for me. 3. I should ask my surgeon whether he or she will take a time-out just before starting my surgery. I should let my surgeon know that, taking a time-out is important to me to reduce the risks of potential harms and errors related to wrong-site surgery.

After the surgery	1. Depending on the surgery, most of the patients spend a few days at an inpatient care unit after the surgery.
	2. After the surgery, if I experience any pain, I should tell my doctor and nurse about my pain.
	3. I should ask questions about the medications that are given to me, especially any new medications.
	    3.1 I must remind my clinicians about any allergies that I have to medications.
	    3.2 If I have any additional questions or concerns about the medications, I should talk to my doctor or nurse before taking them.
	4. For a new medication, I may ask my doctor, nurse, or pharmacist the following:
	    4.1 What is it?
	    4.2 What is the purpose in taking this new medication?
	    4.3 Are there any side effects?

Time frame	Concern and question to ask
	5. If I am given any IV fluids, I should ask my doctor or nurse how long the liquid should take to run out. It is important to tell my nurse if the liquid seems to be dripping too quickly or slowly.
	6. Before being discharged home, I must ask my doctor: 6.1 Whether I will need therapy or medications after I leave the hospital? 6.2 When can I resume activities, including work, exercise, and traveling?

Source: Joint Commission (2007b). Speak Up™: Help avoid mistakes in your surgery. Available at: http://www.jointcommission.org/NR/rdonlyres/2020EE90-CBD6-482D-8FE3-24593431A313/0/wrong_site_brochure.pdf (accessed on January 4, 2008).

Critical Tips for Patients and Families to Prevent Wrong-Site Surgery

In an inpatient care unit (patient rooms) and the preoperative holding area, a patient, the family, or a patient advocate can observe and be involved in the processes of identification and verification for correct procedure side and site. A patient should also participate in marking the surgical site.

If our physician or surgeon gave us written information about our scheduled surgery, we should make sure that the surgery and procedure site indicated on this written information are exactly the same as printed on the informed consent form for this surgery. In the processes of identification and verification for correct procedure side and site, it is critical for us to ensure that the correct surgery and site are accurately communicated among our health care providers and us. We must communicate directly with our surgeon who will perform the procedure about the surgery to be done or with our physician about the procedure. We should not agree with our surgeon or doctor if the information about our surgery and procedure site is incorrect.

After being transferred into the operating room, the surgical team members, especially the surgeons, are primarily responsible for reidentifying and reverifying the surgical side and site to prevent wrong-site surgery. This final check is called a time-out, which should always be conducted immediately before the surgery starts. In the operating room, patients often are under the influence of medications and may have temporary communication impairment or be unconsciousness. We can only depend on the surgical team members and hope that they will conduct a time-out to prevent wrong-site surgery. As a matter of fact, what a patient and the family can do in preventing wrong-site surgery is limited.

We seek surgery for better health and quality of life, though surgeries do carry certain risks. Before we are transferred into the operating room, we can make our hospital care safer by actively communicating with our doctors and nurses in the processes of identification and verification for correct procedure side and site. Table 3 lists the critical information that is essential for a patient and the family to know in their efforts to ensure safe surgery.

References

Joint Commission (2001). Sentinel event alert (Issue 24-December 5, 2001): A follow-up review of wrong site surgery. Available at: http://www.jointcommission.org/ SentinelEvents/SentinelEventAlert/sea_24htm (accessed on January 2, 2008).

Joint Commission (2003a). Universal Protocol for Preventing Wrong site, Wrong Procedure, Wrong person Surgery™. Available at: http://www.jointcommission.org/NR/ rdonlyres/E3C600EB-043B-4E86-B04E-CA4A89AD5433/0/universal_protocol.pdf (accessed on January 2, 2008).

Joint Commission (2003b). Implementation expectations for the Universal Protocol for Preventing Wrong Site, Wrong Procedure and Wrong Person Surgery™. Available at: http://www.jointcommission.org/NR/rdonlyres/DEC4A816-ED52-4C04-AF8C-FEBA74A732EA/0/up_guidelines.pdf (accessed on January 2, 2008).

Joint Commission (2006). Universal protocol 1: The organization fulfills the expectations set forth in the Universal Protocol for Preventing Wrong site, Wrong Procedure, Wrong Person Surgery™ and associated implementation guidelines. In A. Grayson. (Ed.), *Meeting the Joint Commission's 2007 National Patient Safety Goals* (pp. 139-156). Oakbrook Terrace, IL: Joint Commission.

Joint Commission (2007a). Preventing wrong-site surgery. In R. A. Porché, Jr. (Ed.), *Front line of defense: The role of nurses in preventing sentinel events* (2nd ed., pp. 87-98). Oakbrook Terrace, IL: Joint Commission.

Joint Commission (2007b). Speak Up™: Help avoid mistakes in your surgery. Available at: http://www.jointcommission.org/NR/rdonlyres/2020EE90-CBD6-482D-8FE3-24593431A313/0/wrong_site_brochure.pdf (accessed on January 4, 2008).

Treatment Delays

Learning from a Patient Case

In hospital A, all the telemetry monitors were centralized in a single location and monitored by two monitor watchers at 24 hours a day, 7 days a week. Patient B in Unit H was being monitored by one of the old monitors that had not been operating properly. At 1:30 A.M., Patient B developed a life-threatening arrhythmia. Because of the monitor equipment's inoperative alarm system, the monitor watcher did not notice the arrhythmia for 25 to 30 minutes (estimated by the monitor watcher).

The monitor watcher, Ms. C, thought that something must be wrong within the equipment. She placed a call to the nurses' station of Unit H to notify the responsible nurse to assess Patient B but no one answered the call.

Ms. C sensed a possible prolonged delay and was not aware of how long the patient had had ventricular tachycardia. Ms. C called a code for Patient B's room. The code team arrived at the unit and found that all nursing staff members, including the responsible nurse of Patient B, were trying to respond to a code on another patient within Unit H. The responsible nurse of Patient B was not aware that Patient B had developed a life-threatening arrhythmia.

Resuscitation was initiated by the code team but was not successful. Death was deemed to be the consequence of missed detection of a fatal arrhythmia because of equipment failure (Joint Commission, 2007).

Knowing about Treatment Delays

Treatment delays can occur when desired care, services, or treatments are not provided in the time frame required to meet a patient's care needs. Treatment delays may result in inconvenience to patients and their families (e.g., an extended hospital stay), serious physical or psychological injury, or death in the worst scenario. A hospital's care system that provides effective and safe care, treatments, and services and the ability of the hospital staff to move patients through the health care processes are keys to maintaining timely care deliveries (Joint Commission, 2007).

A hospital care system for inpatient care services includes the phases of: (1) accessing the hospital; (2) admitting to the hospital; (3) receiving care within the hospital; and (4) being discharged from the hospital. In the processes of delivering inpatient care services, nurses are integrally involved in each of these phases. In each phase of care during hospitalization, there are many opportunities where system failures may occur, and these system failures may lead to delays in treatment. Delays in treatment can lead to unexpected and adverse consequences (Joint Commission, 2007).

The process of establishing care priorities should be based on identified needs for each individual patient. This process can collapse at any of the following situations (Joint Commission, 2007):

1. Delays in performing and documenting a patient's medical history, physical assessment, and reassessment
2. Delays in testing and obtaining test results
3. Delays in implementing care guidelines (e.g., a clinical pathway for a certain medical problem)
4. Delays in replacing or repairing broken or inoperative equipment

From the perspective of information management, treatment can be delayed in the following cases (Joint Commission, 2007):

1. The information systems of the ambulatory care and emergency department are not part of the hospital's retrieval system.
2. Information is not tracked.
3. Information is not transmitted in time.
4. Information related to patient care is not stored in a central location.
5. Paper-based clinical records may not be present and their location may be unknown.
6. Physicians do not act on the updated patient information appropriately.

In acute, medical, and surgical inpatient care units, nurses are well positioned to help reduce the likelihood of adverse events resulting from treatment delays. However, physicians are indeed the key members in the health care team to ensure that each individual patient's care plan is properly in place and implemented thoroughly. Each individual patient's care plan should be modified according to changes in a patient's condition on the basis of the findings of monitoring, reassessment, and test results.

Risk Factors and Possible Solutions as Suggested by the Joint Commission

Among the sentinel events reported to the Joint Commission from 1995 to 2005 (a total of 3548 events), delay in treatment accounted for 7.6% (269 events) of reported events. Communication was the most often identified root cause for delay in treatment at about 85%, followed by patient assessment at about 70%, procedural compliance at about 50%, availability of information and continuum of care at about 40 % each (Joint Commission, 2007).

The Joint Commission (2007) further conducted an in-depth analysis on five major root causes for delay in treatment and identified strategies that nurses can adopt to reduce the likelihood of treatment delay-related deaths and injuries. Table 1 lists the prevention strategies related to inpatient care.

Table 1. The major root causes of the reported sentinel events related to treatment delays and the corresponding prevention strategies for nurses

Root cause	Prevention strategy

Inadequate communication among physicians, nurses, and laboratory staff	1. Nurses who work in inpatient care units must ensure effective communication of information related to patients' needs from one shift to the next.
	  1.1 Implementing a standardized approach to hand-off communications (e.g., an opportunity for nurses to ask and respond to questions related to patients) can prevent some adverse events related to inadequate communication.
	  1.2 Using both in-person shift reports and written documentation would promote effective communication.
	  1.3 Nurses should receive and understand all the required information at the beginning of the shift.
	2. According to hospital policies, nurses should respond promptly and appropriately to critical information received from other disciplines.
	  2.1 Hospitals should have a system in place that flags critical test results (e.g., laboratory and radiographic studies) received from the laboratories in an effective manner. For example, a system of panic-value reporting should be implemented.
	  2.2 Nurses should also know the critical values defined for various tests so they can ensure that the responsible physicians receive timely notification of abnormal or other time-sensitive results.

Table 1. Continued

Root cause	Prevention strategy

Insufficient staff orientation, training, and staffing	1. Hospitals should consider standardizing the procedure used to process clinical data (e.g., test results).
	   1.1 Processes should be designed to minimize variation; variation increases the likelihood of error.
	   1.2 A system may include:
	      1.2.1 Presenting all test results to the physician at a scheduled time of day so the physician can review these test results and determine what action needs to be taken
	      1.2.2 Nurses can place the critical tests results, as defined by the hospital policy, needing attention from the physician.
	2. Hospitals must ensure the competence of all staff members to meet patients' needs in a timely manner.
	3. If nurses are not comfortable with their knowledge or skills, they should request additional training to ensure their own competence for the tasks they are assigned to do.
	4. Nursing leaders need to ensure that nurses are able to provide care in a timely and effective manner, including sufficient staffing.
	   4.1 Nurses also need to inform their supervisor of unsafe staffing situations.

Inadequate assessment	1. Nurses should perform initial nursing assessment within the time frame as specified in the hospital policy.
	2. Hospitals must ensure sufficient nurse staffing and training to perform assessments in a timely manner.
	3. Nurses must reassess their patients regularly to monitor care interventions.
	   3.1 Appropriate nursing care must involve regularly assessing each individual patient's response to care.
	   3.2 Delays in reassessing or monitoring the patients' conditions can also lead to undesirable occurrences.
	4. Nurses must evaluate each individual patient's present condition and compare it with the previously reported condition.
	   4.1 Nurses' ability to identify that a patient's condition is getting worse can be crucial to this patient's survival (e.g., alerting the responsible physician for changes in conditions).

Inadequate information management	1. The transmission of data and information must be timely and accurate among physicians, nurses, and the laboratory staff.
	   1.1 Nurses must document the care provided and the patients' response to the care.
	   1.2 Timely completion of clinical records is important to ensure care quality and prevent adverse events related to treatment delays.
	   1.3 Hospital leaders need to ensure that clinical records are designed in a way that information filed in the record can been seen and acted on by the appropriate clinicians (usually the responsible physicians).

Root cause	Prevention strategy
	2. Hospital leaders should ensure availability of the clinical records to all staff requiring the information to provide safe and timely care. 2.1 For example, some hospitals implemented electronic record systems, which make up-to-date clinical records available and permit authorized staff access from multiple locations.

Unsafe care environment	1. Nurses need to help ensure that the equipment and technology being used (e.g., for monitoring, delivering drugs, and ventilating patients) are in optimal functioning order.
	  1.1 The function of equipment is vital to the timely provision of safe care.
	  1.2 Nurses must comply with the hospital policy and procedures related to equipment maintenance and ensure that faulty equipment is repaired.
	2. Nurses may participate on the teams that evaluate the purchase of new equipment and help identify new equipment that may reduce the likelihood of adverse events related to equipment failures.
	  2.1 Nurses can also participate in the development of hospital policies and procedures related to the new equipment.
	3. Hospital and nursing leaders must ensure that nurses receive adequately training on proper and safe equipment use.
	4. Hospital and nursing leaders need to have the design and implementation of redundant or back-up systems to help ensure patient safety, in case equipment failures occur.

Source: Joint Commission (2007). Preventing treatment delays. In R. A. Porché, Jr. (Ed.), *Front line of defense: The role of nurses in preventing sentinel events* (2nd ed., pp. 129-140). Oakbrook Terrace, IL: Joint Commission.

Challenges for Clinicians in Preventing Treatment Delays

In inpatient care settings, physicians determine the diagnosis, prescribe medications and treatments, and order laboratory tests or imaging studies. If a patient's condition changes, the responsible physician must initiate a new care plan, prescribe new medications, or order treatments, tests, or procedures as needed.

However, physicians are usually not available to monitor their patients' conditions at the bedside on a regular basis. Consequently, physicians often count on nurses to initiate communication with them on changes in a patient's condition and critical laboratory test results. Nurses are obligated to ensure that medical treatments are delivered correctly and in a timely manner and that care plans (including assessment, reassessment, and monitoring) are implemented accordingly. Nurses must practice and act on physician orders.

If an error occurred as related to treatment delays, hospital leaders tend to blame nurses for inappropriate training and insufficient communication with the responsible physicians. Rarely are such errors identified as attributable to the physicians' irresponsibility. It is illogical to depend on nurses' experience and make nurses obligated to alert physicians about their patients' critical laboratory results, for example. Hospitals should have policies in place to prevent physicians' negligence on assessing and monitoring their patients' needs.

Where are the responsible physicians? Regardless of being a new or experienced physician, it is a physician's responsibility to actively follow up with the conditions of their patients' and act on any changes. The laboratory results should be read by the responsible physician who ordered the test. If needed, the responsible physician should initiate new treatments, medications, or procedures.

Nurses must follow the hospital's policies on documentation and ensure that the documentation on their responsible patients is thorough and clear. In acute inpatient care units, using verbal communication by telephone calls to enhance communication with physicians is still viable and needed. However, physicians should make sure that they read their patients' clinical records and nurses' notes at least once a day to ensure their orders have been carried out appropriately as intended.

Table 2 lists our suggested prevention strategies for nurses to prevent treatment delays in acute inpatient care settings.

Table 2. Preventing treatment delays:
Critical tips for nurses who work in acute inpatient care units

Dimension	Strategy

Ensuring a safe practice environment and having sufficient training for the assigned tasks	1. If nurses are not comfortable with their knowledge or skills, they should request additional training to ensure their own competence for the tasks they are assigned to do.
	2. Nurses need to inform their supervisor of unsafe staffing situations.
	3. Nurses need to help ensure the equipment and technology being used (e.g., for monitoring, and delivering drugs) are in optimal functioning order.
	  3.1 Equipment function is vital to the timely provision of safe care.
	  3.2 Nurses must comply with the hospital policy and procedures related to equipment maintenance and ensure that faulty equipment is repaired.

Performing initial assessment in a timely manner and conducting reassessment according to the hospital policy	1. Nurses should perform initial nursing assessment within the time frame as specified in the hospital policy. 2. Nurses must observe and reassess their responsible patients regularly and carefully monitor care interventions.
Ensuring adequate documentation and information management	1. Nurses must document the care provided and the patients' response to the care. 2. Timely completion of clinical records is important to ensure care quality and to prevent adverse events related to treatment delays.

Dimension	Strategy
Promoting effective communication with physicians, nurse colleagues, the laboratory staff, and other health care providers	1. Nurses must ensure effective communication of information related to patients' needs from one shift to the next. 1.1 Implementing a standardized approach to hand-off communications can prevent harms and errors related to inadequate communication. 1.2 In-person shift reports and written documentation are both critical to promote effective communication of patient information during shift change. 2. Nurses should respond promptly and appropriately to critical information received from other disciplines. 2.1 Nurses should know the critical values defined for commonly seen tests in their working units. 2.2 Nurses should include abnormal test values in hand-off communications to ensure continuity of care. 2.3 The responsible physician has the assumed responsibility to interpret the test results and act on the test results as needed. As appropriate toward patient safety, nurses should ensure that the responsible physicians receive timely notification of abnormal or other time-sensitive results.
Promoting effective communication with patients and their families	1. Nurses should not interpret laboratory test and imaging study results to patients and their families before the responsible physicians complete interpreting the test results and document their interpretations on the clinical records. 2. If a patient and the family ask for the test results (especially the ones that have not been read by the responsible physician), the responsible nurse should contact the responsible physician and forward the patient's request to the physician. 2.1 Before contacting the responsible physician, it is important for the responsible nurse to understand the main concerns or issues that the patient and the family have (e.g., treatment plans, changes in the patient's condition). 2.2 Following up with the patient's requests and concerns may ease the patient's anxiety and worry about the health condition. 3. Understanding the patient's and family's concerns is one of the ways to offer psychological support to the patient, which is one of the nurse's roles in practice. 4. It is important for nurses to explain to patients and their families about their ongoing treatments, including oral medications and IV fluids.

Table 3. Preventing treatment delays: Tips for patients and families

Dimension	Tip
	If I am not well enough to do any of the actions indicated below, I should ask a family or friend to help.

Letting my doctor and nurse know my feeling and observed changes of my body	1. If I sense any changes in my body, I should tell my nurse right away and let my doctor know.
	  1.1 Changes in my body may link to new medications, treatments, or procedures and may possibly indicate that I need additional treatments.
	  1.2 I must express my pain, discomfort, or change in my body to my doctor and nurse to prevent treatment delays.

Knowing my health condition and care plan from my doctor and nurse	1. I should ask my doctor or nurse what kind of laboratory tests or imaging studies I had or will have during this hospital stay. It will be extremely helpful to ask for written information.
	2. If my doctor has ordered a laboratory test or imaging study for me, I should ask when the test will be performed and when I can get the results. Are there any specific instructions that I should pay attention to before taking the tests?
	  2.1 Tests may include laboratory tests on blood, urine, sputum, or other specimens (e.g., obtained through biopsy) and image studies (e.g., x-ray);
	  2.2 I should make a list of the tests I have undergone and follow up the test results with my doctor and nurse.
	  2.3 I must request the test result and my doctor's interpretation of the test results. I should feel comfortable expressing my desire to know my test results.
	  2.4 If my doctor is not in the unit, I should tell my nurse my desire to know my test results and my doctor's interpretation.
	3. I or my family should request an update about any change in my health condition (improvement or worsening) at least once a day during the entire hospital stays.
	  3.1 It is important to know when my doctor will come to see me so my family can be with me when my doctor is explaining my condition and treatment plan. My family can ask questions and take notes for me, if needed.
	  3.2 I should also feel comfortable asking my nurse about my treatment and care plan. In most of the hospital, there are at least two shifts per day. I should ask my nurse about my treatment and care plan to be given during his or her shift.

Critical Tips for Patients and Families to Prevent Treatment Delays

What patients and their families can do to prevent treatment delays is limited. Before we as patients or families can be involved in preventing treatment delays, we must know our updated care plan and what kind of treatments, laboratory tests, or imaging studies we had and are going to have. Without knowing what is happening to our body and our care plan, we are uninformed, even after we have been harmed due to treatment delays.

To prevent treatment delays, a collaborative relationship among physicians, nurses, patients, and families is needed and this relationship must be based on open communication held on a regular basis, including effective information exchange on the existing and emerging clinical issues and treatments. Only when we are well informed about our care plan, can we assist our caregivers in preventing harms as a consequence of treatment delays.

Hospitalization can be extremely stressful and exhausting to patients and families physically, psychologically, and financially. Anxiety and worries can build up before or immediately after being admitted to the hospital. Understanding our care plan and any changes in our health condition is essential to help manage and decrease our anxiety and worries.

We must communicate with our responsible physician and nurse regularly. For example, we should request an update about any changes in our health condition and care plan (including new treatment and tests) from our doctor at least once a day during the entire hospital stay. We may ask our doctor when to expect a visit, at which time it would be helpful to have a family or friend at the bedside with us. Our family or friend may help us take notes. We should also ask our nurse about our ongoing treatments and medications and any update to our care plan. Table 3 lists the tips for patients and families to be involved in the efforts of preventing treatment delays during hospital stays.

References

Joint Commission (2007). Preventing treatment delays. In R. A. Porch, Jr. (Ed.), *Front line of defense: The role of nurses in preventing sentinel events* (2nd ed., pp. 129-140). Oakbrook Terrace, IL: Joint Commission.

Operative and Postoperative Errors and Complications

Learning from a Patient Case A

Before leaving for the operating room, Patient A had a central venous line inserted by Dr. B (a surgical resident), when Patient A was waiting in his patient room in a surgical inpatient care unit. Dr. B ordered a chest x-ray to determine the position of this recently inserted catheter (the central venous line). Before the result of the x-ray was available, Dr. B had to leave Patient A's room to attend to a seriously ill patient in the emergency room.

After Patient A was sent to the operating room, the clerk of the inpatient care unit, where Patient A was staying, received the radiology report and filed the x-ray report for Dr. B to review later. The report indicated the presence of a dangerous pneumothorax.

Dr. B did not get a chance to review the x-ray report before Patient A's procedure started. In addition, this critical radiology report was not sent to the operating room because the radiology department did not routinely communicate the urgency of the report to the physician who ordered the x-ray study. The clerk in the inpatient care unit also did not know what information should be directed to the operating room. Moreover, the surgical team members in the operating room did not notice that a piece of vital information was missing.

Because of inadequate communication at several points, Patient A experienced cardiopulmonary arrest during the surgical procedure (Joint Commission, 2007).

Learning from a Patient Case B

When Nurse C was conducting the preoperative assessment of Patient D for a scheduled colonoscopy, Patient D told Nurse C that he was also scheduled for a cardiac stress test 3 days later. However, Patient D did not recall why he was having the cardiac stress test. Nurse C failed to bring this information to the gastroenterologist's attention before starting the procedure. Shortly after completing the colonoscopy procedure, Patient D developed chest pain in the recovery room and was diagnosed with a myocardial infarction.

A hospital committee reviewed this adverse event and determined that Patient D's preoperative assessment was incomplete. The colonoscopy procedure should have been rescheduled pending the cardiac stress test results (Joint Commission, 2007).

Learning from a Patient Case

On a surgical inpatient care unit, Nurse E was assigned to care for 5 patients. Patient F was in surgery at the beginning of Nurse E's day shift, and the other 4 patients had surgery performed the day before. Around noon, Patient F was transferred back to the surgical unit. Nurse E accompanied the patient to his room and assisted postanesthesia care staff in getting Patient F into bed. Nurse E took report from the postanesthesia care staff and began postoperative care.

Nurse E checked Patient F's vital signs and dressing and determined that the dressing needed to be changed. Nurse E left Patient F's room to obtain supplies for dressing change. On her way back to Patient F's room, she also attended to the need of one of her other patients; this patient had methicillin-resistant Staphylococcus aureus infection. Nurse E started the procedure of changing Patient F's dressing right way. Unfortunately, Nurse E failed to wash her hands before entering Patient F's room and before changing Patient F's dressing. Although Nurse E wore gloves for the dressing change, she opened the clean dressing package and arranged supplies before putting on the gloves.

Three days later, Patient F developed a fever. The skin around the incision site was red and thick drainage was coming out from the surgical wound. A culture of the wound drainage showed methicillin-resistant S. aureus.

Patient F recovered from this surgical site infection and was discharged eventually. His hospital stay was prolonged by 3 weeks. Patient F needed another 3 months after discharge to recover before returning to the lifestyle he had before undergoing the surgery.

A hospital committee's investigation concluded that this surgical site infection was a result of Nurse E's failure to follow the handwashing procedure. Patient F's surgical site infection led to additional discomfort and risk for Patient F, additional treatment and medications, a longer hospitalization, and a longer recovery period (Joint Commission, 2007).

A Success Story

Jewish Hospital Downtown and St. Mary's Health Care, located in Louisville, Kentucky, were determined to use a multidisciplinary team approach and concentrate their efforts on reducing the incidence of surgical site infections in patients undergoing total joint replacements. This multidisciplinary team immediately adopted several changes to reduce surgical site infections. The success was maintained with ongoing data review. The successful changes that this multidisciplinary team adopted included (Institute for Healthcare Improvement, 2006):

1. Implementing Hibiclens bath or shower in preprocedure skin preparation. Hibiclens baths or showers have been recommended by Centers for Disease Control and Prevention. If a patient is having problems with infections, particularly with gram-positive organisms, Hibiclens should be added to the bath water.

2. Providing education to orthopedic office managers and nurses about the purpose of using chlorhexidine (also called Hibiclens) for body baths or showers

3. Adopting the clipper method for hair removal on the surgical site

4. Monitoring blood glucose for all patients undergoing total joint replacements

5. Providing education to orthopedic surgeons and anesthesia teams regarding the prophylactic antibiotic protocols

6. Staffing preoperative personnel for flexible hours to ensure appropriate delivery and timing of antibiotics for patients scheduled for surgery at 7:30 A.M.

7. Anesthesia being responsible for pushed IV medication of Kefzol (IV antibiotic) to ensure a therapeutic time frame of 30 minutes prior to the incision time

8. Using a stamp to notify inpatient care units and pharmacy of preoperative antibiotic timing, surgery end time, and timing for discontinuation of antibiotics

9. Developing a postoperative order set to include the appropriate prophylactic antibiotic protocol

Knowing about Operative and Postoperative Errors and Complications

Efforts relevant to prevention of sentinel events associated with operative and postoperative errors and complications start before a patient arrives in the operating room and continue in the postanesthesia recovery unit, an intensive care unit, and the inpatient care unit. As operative volume increases, so does the risk for errors, complications, and sentinel events.

Brennan and associates (1991) conducted a study on selected acute care, nonpsychiatric hospitals in New York State in 1984. They found that adverse events occurred in 3.7% of the hospitalizations and 27.6% of the adverse events were due to negligence. Among these adverse events, about 48% were related to surgery (including orthopedic, neurologic, thoracic, cardiac, vascular, and general surgery). Among these surgery-related adverse events, medication complications were the most common type of adverse event (19%), followed by wound infections (14%) and technical complications (13%).

Data from the Joint Commission's Sentinel Event Database from 1995 to 2005 showed that operative and postoperative errors and complications accounted for 12.5% of all sentinel events, and wrong-site surgery errors were involved in 12.8% of all sentinel events. In other words, surgery-related errors and complications accounted for a total of 25.3% of the reported sentinel events, which was almost double the rate of patient suicide-related events (13.1%) and the rate of medication error-related events (10.1%; Joint Commission, 2007). Overall, operative and postoperative errors and complications have been identified as one of the major sentinel event types.

Epidemic of Operative and Postoperative Errors and Complications

As indicated in the document of *Operative and Post-Operative Complications: Lessons for the Future* published by the Joint Commission (2000) on February 4, 2000, 84% of the operative and postoperative complications resulted in patient deaths and 16% resulted in serious injury. As for the time periods when these complications occurred, 58% of the complications happened during the postoperative period, 23% during the operative procedures, 13% during postanesthesia recovery, and 6% during anesthesia induction.

Among these complications, 90% occurred in relation to nonemergent procedures. These reported complications were most frequently associated with the following types of procedures (Joint Commission, 2000):

1. Head and neck surgery
2. Interventional endoscopies
3. Interventional imaging
4. Open abdominal surgery
5. Orthopedic surgery
6. Thoracic surgery
7. Tube or catheter insertion

The most frequent reported operative or postoperative complications by the types of procedures were (Joint Commission, 2000):

1. Acute respiratory failure resulting from open orthopedic procedures (including cardiac arrest in the operating room)
2. Burns resulting from an electric scalpel (also called electrocautery) used with a flammable pre-solution
3. Endoscopic procedures, including gastrointestinal or non-gastrointestinal procedures with perforation of adjacent organs (e.g., liver lacerations were the most frequent complications of abdominal and thoracic endoscopic surgeries)
4. Imaging-directed percutaneous biopsy or tube placement resulting in liver laceration, peritonitis, or respiratory arrest while patients were temporarily off prescribed oxygen during the procedure
5. Inserting a central venous catheter into an artery by mistake
6. Inserting a nasogastric feeding tube into the trachea or a bronchus by mistake
7. Massive fluid overload from absorption of irrigation fluids during genitourinary (also called gynecologic) procedures

The Institute for Healthcare Improvement (2008a) claimed that postoperative infection has been a major cause of patient injury, mortality, and increased health care costs. It is estimated that 2.6% of nearly 30 million operations or procedures are complicated by surgical site infections each year. Based on the data collected in 1992, each infection was estimated to increase a hospital stay by 7 days and add over $3000 in charges. The Institute for Healthcare

Improvement (2008a) suggested appropriate preoperative administration of antibiotics as being effective in preventing surgical site infections.

In the national initiative led by Institute for Healthcare Improvement "Protecting 5 Million Lives Campaign" to reduce surgical complications, four goals and corresponding changes in care have been recommended (Institute for Healthcare Improvement, 2007):

1. Preventing surgical site infection: Possible changes for improvement included:
   a. Appropriate use of antibiotics
   b. Proper hair removal on the surgical site
   c. Tight postoperative glucose control for major cardiac surgery patients
   d. Immediate postoperative normothermia for colorectal surgery patients
2. Prescribing β-blockers for patients who are taking β-blockers prior to admission to the hospital or the operating room: Possible changes were:
   a. Identifying patients who have been taking β-blockers before surgery to ensure that they are continued after surgery
   b. Educating patients and families to inform their surgeon and anesthesiologist that they have been taking β-blocker medications
   c. Developing standard postoperative order sets or protocols that include provision of β-blockers for patients who received β-blockers before surgery
   d. Implementing medication reconciliation to ensure that postoperative orders include necessary preoperative medications, such as β-blockers
   e. Educating patients and their families about the importance of continuing β-blockers after surgery.
3. Using venous thromboembolism prophylaxis: Possible changes for improvement included:
   a. Developing standard order sets for prophylaxis
   b. Depending on the needs for different surgical procedures, developing protocols for providing prophylaxis
   c. Providing education and training for staff about the importance of venous thromboembolism prophylaxis
   d. Educating patients before surgery about the prophylaxis they will receive to reduce risk
4. Preventing ventilator-associated pneumonia: Not all surgical patients will receive postoperative mechanical ventilation. However, patients who will receive postoperative mechanical ventilation can be at risk for ventilator-associated pneumonia as one of the most serious types of pneumonia.
   a. Ventilator-associated pneumonia is an airways infection that must have developed more than 48 hours after the patient has been on mechanical ventilation.
   b. The Institute for Healthcare Improvement (2008a, 2008b) suggested that hospitals consider using the "ventilator bundle" for all surgical patients receiving postoperative mechanical ventilation, particular those ventilated for more than 24 hours. The "ventilator bundle" is a series of interventions related to ventilator care. The key components of the "ventilator bundle" include:

    i.   Elevation of the head of the patient bed

    ii. Implementing daily "sedation vacations" and assessment of readiness to wean from the ventilator

    iii. Ordering peptic ulcer disease prophylaxis

    iv. Applying deep venous thrombosis prophylaxis

Risk Factors and Possible Solutions as Suggested by the Joint Commission

Among the sentinel events reported to the Joint Commission from 1995 to 2005, communication was the most often identified root cause for operative and postoperative errors and complications at about 75%, followed by patient assessment at about 54%, procedural compliance at about 43%, care planning at about 40 %, and availability of patient information at about 33% (Joint Commission, 2007).

A lack of a complete preoperative assessment was one of the causes associated with various operative adverse events. Lacking a complete preoperative assessment involved (Joint Commission, 2007):

1. Failure to capture changes in a patient's health condition
2. Failure to consider the existence of a patient's preexisting disease(s)
3. Failure to plan appropriately for the postoperative care due to insufficient information
4. Inappropriate choice of anesthetic, surgical procedure, and medications due to lack of information
5. Missing laboratory data

Possible adverse events as related to operative and postoperative errors and complications and corresponding causes were (Joint Commission, 2007):

1. Anaphylactic reactions: Failure to identify a patient with a medication allergy
2. Bleeding situations: Failure to identify the use of anticoagulants before invasive procedures
3. Cardiac arrest: Failure to identify the use of dietary supplements containing stimulants
4. Serious respiratory responses with sedation: Failure to identify a patient with sleep apnea

As for postoperative monitoring, hospital policies should address the differences in required monitoring for different surgeries or procedures. After undergoing a surgical procedure, all patients, including outpatients, inpatients, and same-day surgery patients, should have postoperative monitoring. Some patients may come to an operating room's postanesthesia care unit or may be transferred directly from the operating room to an intensive care unit. Other patients may return to their patient rooms in an inpatient care unit right after surgery. Hand-off communications are important in any of these situations (Joint Commission, 2007).

The Joint Commission (2007) conducted an in-depth analysis on major root causes for operative and postoperative errors and complications and identified strategies that nurses can adopt to reduce the likelihood of related deaths and injuries. Table 1 lists the prevention strategies related to inpatient care.

Table 1. The major root causes of the reported sentinel events
related to operative and postoperative errors and complications
and the corresponding prevention strategies for nurses

Root cause	Prevention strategy

Failure to follow established policies and procedures	1. Hospital and nurse leaders should establish policies and procedures to reduce the risk of operative and postoperative errors and adverse events.
	   1.1 Nurse leaders must monitor consistency of compliance with the hospital policies and procedures.
	   1.2 Nurse leaders should collect and analyze compliance data on a regular basis.
	2. Nurse leaders should standardize procedures across care settings within the hospital to help ensure uniform performance of patient care processes.
	   2.1 It is also important to develop and use standardized procedures for high-risk activities (e.g., conscious sedation, emergency care, pain management, and hyperalimentation) to help reduce the likelihood of adverse events.
	3. Nurses must feel comfortable enough about established communication channels to promptly and freely question unclear or inappropriate orders.
	4. Nurses who work in the inpatient care units and staff members who work in the preoperative area and operating room must communicate clearly across units about the proper use of antibiotics so maximum effectiveness of antibiotic use can be achieved.
	   4.1 In most of the situations, the use of prophylactic antibiotics is recommended.
	   4.2 When prophylactic antibiotics are planned to be given before surgery, the timing of administration is crucial.
	5. Nurses must know the prevalent organisms associated with surgical site infections, including methicillin-resistant *Staphylococcus aureus* (abbreviated as MRSA).
	6. Nurses should be aware and use evidence-based practice guidelines to reduce the occurrence of surgical site infections, including:
	   6.1 Proper use of prophylactic antibiotics
	   6.2 Clipping rather than shaving the skin at the surgical site
	   6.3 Cleaning the skin preoperatively (e.g., showering with a solution such as chlorhexidine)
	   6.4 Before surgery, control of blood glucose levels at 100 mg/dL or less for patients with or without diabetes

Table 1. Continued

Root cause	Prevention strategy

Inadequate staff competence and credentialing (physicians)	1. Hospital and nurse leaders should develop a mechanism for identifying the privileges held by the physicians before the physicians perform any invasive procedures in the emergency room or on an inpatient care unit.
	   1.1 This mechanism is important to ensure that physicians performing procedures are qualified to do so.
	   1.2 During the day, nurse managers are usually responsible for checking with the medical staff office. During the evening and night, the hospital should have a mechanism in place for nurses to verify the privileges of physicians, if needed.
	2. Nurse leaders should ensure that the job descriptions and competence requirements for clinical nurses accurately reflect the job being performed (e.g., the performance of actual skills and tasks performed by nurses on the job).

Insufficient communication among health care providers	1. Hospital and nursing leaders should develop clinical practice guidelines to enhance communication.
	   1.1 Clinical practice guidelines offer an excellent opportunity to guarantee that the needed communication and issues are addressed.
	   1.2 When designing clinical practice guidelines, essential communication should be considered at each step.
	2. Nursing leaders and nurses should develop a means to ensure that all required information is present in the patient record or with the patient before the patient is transported to the operating room.
	   2.1 A checklist of items needed for surgery can help nurses decrease reliance on memory and provide consistency.
	   2.2 Involving two nurses in verifying the items indicated on the checklist can help respond to human issues that nurses often encounter, including stress, fatigue, and time pressures.
	3. Nurses should use documentation as a communication tool.
	   3.1 Nurse leaders should provide training for clinical nurses about the information on forms used by other disciplines. For example, by being able to interpret the anesthesia record, nurses would be able to follow specific events, review vital signs, identify medications and fluids used during the surgical procedure, and understand plans for the recovery period.
	4. Nurses can help ensure effective interdepartmental communication.
	   4.1 Nurse leaders and nurses may consider working with radiology staff to develop a system for rapid communication of selected abnormal results (e.g., pneumothorax).
	   4.2 Within each inpatient care unit, nurse managers and nurses can develop a system whereby no result reports will be filed for later review without initial review by a nurse. Unit clerks can be educated to recognize results that demand immediate attention.

Inadequate preoperative assessment and postoperative monitoring	1. Nurses can help ensure that preoperative assessments are available and accurate in the patient records.
	   1.1 Nurses should be familiar with the scope and assessment time frames, as specified in hospital policies.
	   1.2 Nurses should also be familiar with the components required in the history and physical examination, the nursing assessment, and consultant assessments.
	2. Nurses should compare available information in the assessments, laboratory reports, other parts of the medical record, and other patient care documents to ensure the consistency of data.

Root cause	Prevention strategy

	3. Nurses must know and follow the hospital's postoperative monitoring policies through appropriate and sufficient training, orientation, and competence assessment.
	4. Nurse leaders and nurses should use high-quality monitoring documentation forms.
	    4.1 A monitoring documentation form can remind nurses about activities and documentation that must be completed.
	    4.2 A form should clearly identify the elements to be monitored, the time frame involved, and the discharge criteria.
	    4.3 A well-designed form can be handy to the recorder and the reviewer.
	5. Nurses must know what to monitor and understand how to use and interpret the collected data.

Poor procedural compliance associated with insufficient staffing and inefficient operating systems	1. Nurse leaders, managers, and nurses need to work together to determine whether staffing practices (e.g., nurse-to-patient ratios) adversely affect the care provided. If so, it is important to devise a workable staffing plan to reduce or eliminate the adverse effects.
	2. Nurses must obtain information from postanesthesia care staff in time to plan backup coverage for breaks and other times when the assigned nurse may not be immediately available.
	    2.1 Postanesthesia care staff often telephone the inpatient care units before patients are returned to their rooms.
	    2.2 If needed due to insufficient staffing, nurses may consider working with postanesthesia care staff to develop a means for earlier communication.
	3. Nurse leaders, managers, and nurses should evaluate how and where supplies for dressing changes and other frequently performed procedures are stored.
	4. Nursing managers and nurses need to develop a system for easy notification of appropriate personnel (e.g., unit clerks) when equipment needs maintenance or supplies need to be stocked.
	    4.1 Supplies also include alcohol-based waterless hand cleaner.
	    4.2 Nursing managers may request a pocket-sized hand sanitizer for ready availability of hand-cleaning supplies.
	5. Nursing managers and nurses should request that hand lotions or creams be available wherever hands may be washed to reduce irritation to skin.
	6. Nurses should teach patients about proper hand hygiene and what to expect from staff members who care for them.
	    6.1 Nurses should also encourage patients to ask staff whether they have washed their hands before entering their room and touching them for treatments or procedures.

Source: Joint Commission (2007). Preventing operating and postoperative errors and complications. In R. A. Porché, Jr. (Ed.), *Front line of defense: The role of nurses in preventing sentinel events* (2nd ed., pp. 21-34). Oakbrook Terrace, IL: Joint Commission.

Challenges for Clinicians in Preventing Operative and Postoperative Errors and Complications

Based on the findings at the initial assessment, reassessment, and monitoring, physicians determine each individual patient's diagnoses, prescribe medications and treatments, and order laboratory tests or imaging studies, as needed. Nurses who work in an inpatient care unit must practice and act on these orders.

**Table 2. Preventing operative and postoperative errors and complications:
Critical tips for nurses who work in acute inpatient care units**

Dimension	Strategy
Following the hospital's established policies and procedures and the standards of nursing practice	1. Nurses should practice according to the hospital's established clinical practice guidelines, if any, to ensure uniform performance of patient care processes and prevent postoperative complications.
Ensuring adequate preoperative assessment and postoperative monitoring	1. Before transporting patients to the operating room, nurses can help ensure that all the required preoperative assessments are available. 2. Before transporting patients to the operating room, nurses should compare available information in the assessments, laboratory reports, other parts of the medical record, and other patient care documents to ensure the consistency of data. 3. Nurses must know and follow the hospital's postoperative monitoring policies through appropriate and sufficient training, orientation, and competence assessment. 3.1 Nurses must know what to monitor and understand how to use and interpret the collected monitoring data.
Preventing surgical site infections	1. Nurses should be aware of and use the hospital's established practice guidelines to reduce the occurrence of surgical site infections. 2. Nurses must know the prevalent organisms associated with surgical site infections, including methicillin-resistant *Staphylococcus aureus* (abbreviated as MRSA); 3. Nurses should teach patients about proper hand hygiene to protect themselves and what to expect from staff members who care for them. 3.1 Nurses should also encourage patients to ask staff whether they have washed their hands before entering their room and touching them for any treatments or procedures. 4. Nurses in the inpatient care units and staff in the preoperative area and operating room must communicate clearly about the proper use of antibiotics, so maximum effectiveness of antibiotic use can be achieved.

Promoting effective communication	1. Nurses should practice according to the hospital's established clinical practice guidelines to ensure effective patient monitoring and consistent communication.
	2. Nurses should use written documentation as a communication tool within the inpatient care units and with the staff in the other departments to prevent miscommunication and misinterpretation.
	    2.1 Both verbal communication and written documentation are essential for clarification during hand-off communications.
	3. Within each inpatient care unit, nurse managers and nurses can develop a system by which result reports will not be filed for later review by physicians without initial review by a nurse. After being reviewed by a nurse, the unit clerk can file the reports.
	4. Nursing managers and nurses should develop a means to ensure that all required information is present in the patient's record or with the patient.
	    4.1 A checklist of items needed for surgery can help nurses decrease reliance on memory and provide consistency.
	    4.2 To ensure accuracy, the patient identification and verification processes before transporting patients to the operating room should be conducted by two nurses together.

Dimension	Strategy
	5. To ensure patient safety, nurses must feel comfortable enough about established communication channels to promptly and freely question unclear or inappropriate orders before and after surgery.
Ensuring a safe practice environment	1. Nurse leaders, managers, and nurses need to work together to determine whether staffing practices adversely affect the care safety and quality provided (e.g., nurse-to-patient ratios). If so, it is important to devise a workable staffing plan to reduce or eliminate the adverse effects. 2. Nurse leaders, managers, and nurses should evaluate how and where supplies for dressing changes and other frequently performed procedures are stored. 3. Nursing managers and nurses need to develop a system for easy notification of appropriate personnel when equipment requires maintenance or supplies need to be stocked.

Nurses who work in acute inpatient care units must also follow the hospital's established policies, procedures, and standards of nursing practice to prevent operative and postoperative errors and complications, including adequate preoperative assessment and postoperative monitoring procedures. Effective hand-off communications are always critical in preventing errors. To prevent surgical site infections, nurses must practice good handwashing hygiene. Nurses should also teach patients about proper handwashing hygiene for themselves and what to expect from the staff members who care for them. Table 2 lists our suggested strategies for nurses to prevent operative and postoperative errors and complications in acute inpatient care settings.

Critical Tips for Patients and Families to Prevent Operative and Postoperative Errors and Complications

Patients and their families have limited ability to prevent operative and postoperative errors and complications because patients and their families do not usually have sufficient quality and quantity of professional medical knowledge to make a judgment or question their physicians, nurses, or the other health care providers who provide care for them. Most of all, medical practice has become so specialized that even professionally trained nurses may also experience difficulties in understanding all the surgical terms, procedures, and treatment plans in a specialized area in which they do not practice.

One retired nursing professor shared with us her story about her health seeking experience. She is in her mid-eighties and still very alert. She has undergone several major surgeries, including a mastectomy, spinal surgery with fusion, and total hip replacement for both of her hips.

She told us that often she was unable to understand what her internist (a doctor who specializes in internal medicine) was telling her about her diseases during her doctor office visits. She has been seeing this internist for over 20 years. Still, her internist has not been able to successfully communicate with her about her diseases and care needs in lay terms that she can understand without consulting her physician friend. She often must ask her physician friend, who lives in California, to explain to her again what's going on in her body.

She believed that most of the other patients have even more difficulty understanding what their doctors were telling them. We agreed with her and understand how frustrating such situation can be with our doctors.

This huge gap in professional medical knowledge cannot be changed, however. As a matter of fact, as patients we usually have no idea whether the care, treatments, or procedures we are receiving are up to the standards of medical or nursing practices. For example, it is difficult to tell whether we are sufficiently monitored after surgery.

What we can do to prevent operative and postoperative errors and complications is limited, but we may still be able to make a big difference. For example, we can help prevent surgical site infections. After surgery, we can ask our health care providers (e.g., physicians, nurses, and nursing attendants), as a reminder, whether they have washed their hands before entering our room and touching us for performing any treatments or procedures. We should also ask our doctors and nurses to clean their stethoscopes with alcohol before they use their stethoscopes on us (Roizen & Oz, 2006).

We also must tell our physicians and nurses when we experience pain, discomfort, or changes in our health conditions. If we have a wound dressing, a catheter, or a drainage tube, we should tell our nurses when the dressing becomes wet or loose. Until we are told to change our wound dressing ourselves, we should not touch our surgical site, IV site, and any other open wound. If we are able to get up, we should wash our hands with soap and water several times a day, especially after hugging or shaking hands with a visitor. If we are not mobile, we can use an alcohol sanitizing gel (Roizen & Oz, 2006).

As always, we must communicate with our responsible physician and nurse on a regular basis about our health condition and updated care plan. Most of all, we should ask our surgeon what potential postoperative complications of our surgery we should look for and what we should do if complications occur. We must be aware of possible postoperative complications and have our questions answered by our surgeon before the surgery.

Table 3 summarizes the tips for patients and families to be involved in the efforts of preventing operative and postoperative errors and complications.

**Table 3. Preventing operative and postoperative errors and complications:
Tips for patients and families**

Dimension	Tip
	If I am not well enough to do any of the actions indicated below, I should ask a family or friend to help.
Letting my doctor and nurse know my feelings and observed changes in my body before and after surgery	1. I should ask my surgeon what complications I should watch for after surgery and what I should do if complications occur. 2. If I sense any changes in my body, I should tell my nurse right away and let my doctor know. 2.1 I must express any pain, discomfort, or change in my body to my doctor and nurse. Any of these symptoms may indicate that a complication has developed. 3. I must communicate with my responsible physician and nurse on a regular basis about my health condition and updated care plan.

Dimension	Tip
Helping ensure a safe care environment: Preventing surgical site infections	1. I should remind the health care providers who care for me (e.g., physicians, nurses, and nurse aides) to wash their hands before entering my room and touching me for performing any treatments or procedures. 2. I should ask my doctor and nurse to clean their stethoscope with alcohol before they uses the stethoscope on me. 3. If I have a wound dressing, a catheter, or a drainage tube, I should tell my nurse when the dressing becomes wet or loose. 4. Until I am told to manage my wound myself, I should not touch my surgical site, IV site, and any other open wound. 4.1 I should ask my nurse how to take care of my wound shortly after surgery (e.g., the day after the surgery). 5. If I am able to get up, I should wash my hands with soap and water several times a day, especially after hugging or shaking hands with a visitor. If I am not mobile, I can use an alcohol sanitizing gel.

References

Brennan, T. A., Leape, L. L., Laird, N. M., Hebert, L., Localio, A. R., Lawthers, A. G., Newhouse, J. P, Weiler, P. C., & Hiatt, H. H. (1991). Incidence of adverse events and negligence in hospitalized patients. Results of the Harvard Medical Practice Study I. *New England Journal of Medicine*, *324*(6), 370-376.

Institute for Healthcare Improvement (2006). Improvement report: It's hip to get the antibiotic in. Available at: http://www.ihi.org/IHI/Topics/PatientSafety/SurgicalSite Infections/ImprovementStories/It'sHipToGetTheAntibioticIn.htm (accessed January 8, 2008).

Institute for Healthcare Improvement (2007). Getting started kit: Reduce surgical complications how to guide. Available at: http://www.ihi.org/NR/rdonlyres/ AC9AAEED-7516-4371-8810-8BF45B8CE9C2/0/SCIPHowtoGuide.doc (accessed January 8, 2008).

Institute for Healthcare Improvement (2008a). Surgical site infections: Case for improvement. Available at: http://www.ihi.org/IHI/Topics/PatientSafety/SurgicalSite Infections/ (accessed January 8, 2008).

Institute for Healthcare Improvement (2008b). Implement the ventilator bundle. Available at: http://www.ihi.org/IHI/Topics/CriticalCare/IntensiveCare/Changes/ImplementtheVentilat orBundle.htm (accessed January 8, 2008).

Joint Commission (2000). Issue 12-Operative and post-operative complications: Lessons for the future. Available at: http://www.jcipatientsafety.org/14776/ (accessed January 6, 2008).

Joint Commission (2007). Preventing operating and postoperative errors and complications. In R. A. Porché, Jr. (Ed.), *Front line of defense: The role of nurses in preventing sentinel events* (2nd ed., pp. 21-34). Oakbrook Terrace, IL: Joint Commission.

Roizen, M. F., & Oz, M. C. (2006). *You the smart patient: An insider's handbook for getting the best treatment* (pp. 193-222). New York, NY: Free Press.

Health Care-associated Infections

Learning from a Patient Case

In Hospital A, the neurovascular inpatient care unit had many patients who were 65 years or older. These patients were being treated for stroke and other neurovascular conditions. Most of the patient rooms were semiprivate rooms, with each room having two patients.

Several patients in this neurovascular unit had urinary catheters. Most of the patients used bedside commodes or bedpans for toileting because of insufficient mobility to get to the bathroom. Urinary tract infections seemed to occur frequently in this unit.

Ciprofloxacin is the antibiotic used most often to treat the urinary tract infections. However, the use of antimicrobials is the most important risk factor for the development of Clostridium difficile-associated diseases. C. difficile is a bacterium that often causes diarrhea and serious intestinal conditions.

Frequent handwashing was enforced to prevent staff members from transferring pathogens among patients. Unfortunately, an outbreak of C. difficile-associated diarrhea still occurred on this neurovascular unit. About 15% of the patients were infected. Two patients developed complications of intestinal perforation and sepsis and required admission to the intensive care unit. Fortunately, no patients died. Thus, hospitalization was prolonged for all of the patients infected with C. difficile. (Joint Commission, 2007a).

Learning from a Legal Case Summary

Mrs. K underwent cervical disc surgery at Hospital W on August 5, 1997. During Mrs. K's recovery at Hospital W, Mr. and Mrs. K noticed that the nursing staff never wore gloves while inserting IV catheters into Mrs. K's arms and never washed their hands before attempting to insert the needles. On at least nine occasions, when the IV needle came out of Mrs. K's vein (failed IV insertion attempts), nurses, who were not wearing gloves, stuck Mrs. K multiple times with the same needle.

On one occasion, Mrs. K's tubing became disconnected and fell onto her bed sheet. A nurse, who was not wearing gloves, picked up the tube and reconnected it to the IV tubing without changing the needle. One time, Mr. K questioned one nurse regarding Hospital W's handwashing practices, but his question was ignored.

On August 8, 1997, Mrs. K was released. However, she still had tenderness and soreness on her right arm at the sites of the multiple failed IV insertion attempts. She had a temperature of 100°F at the time of her release, indicating the presence of an infection.

Three weeks after being discharged from Hospital W, a small cut on her leg turned into a serious open wound, which ulcerated and deepened. Skin lesions continued to develop on her body, including the IV sites. Mrs. K was diagnosed with pyoderma gangrenosum, which was characterized by continuous infections from open skin wounds. Pyoderma gangrenosum is a permanent, devastating illness that causes tissue to become necrotic, leading to deep ulcers. When deep ulcers occur, they can lead to chronic wounds. This illness often occurs on the legs and is thought to be due to immune system dysfunction.

The evidence showed that the nurses at Hospital W violated the standard of care in the non-aseptic manner in which these nurses handled Mrs. K's IV therapy. There was a reasonable degree of medical certainty that Mrs. K contracted a Staphylococcus aureus infection in Hospital W and that this infection triggered Mrs. K's illness of pyoderma gangrenosum. Mrs. K's S. aureus infection resulted from failure to use aseptic, sterile procedures.

Mrs. K and Mr. K filed a medical malpractice action against Hospital W that Hospital W's nursing staff had breached the applicable standard of care when they administered IV therapy. This violation of the applicable standard of care caused Mrs. K to contract a S. aureus infection, which triggered her current illness of pyoderma gangrenosum.

Source: NexisLexis®Academic: Federal & State Cases (Case number: A03A0780; June 17, 2003, decided) (accessed on January 11, 2008).

Learning from a Legal Case Summary

Dr. B was a family practitioner at Hospital P from 1980 until June 1991. In March 1989, Dr. B developed a series of skin conditions on his face, hands, arms, and head. He started treating these conditions himself. In June 1990, Dr. B developed nodular lesions on his hands and forearms. In September 1990, Dr. B consulted a dermatologist who diagnosed the lesions as exudative dermatitis and ordered an HIV test. Dr. B tested HIV seropositive.

In early October 1990, Dr. B met with the Minnesota Board of Medical Examiners (abbreviated as the Board) regarding his medical practice. The Board advised Dr. B to wear two pairs of gloves when caring for patients and to refrain from performing surgery. Dr. B complied with the Board's requirements and voluntarily stopped delivering babies.

After meeting the Board, Dr. B performed one gynecologic examination on Patient T in late October 1990 and another one in early January 1991, during the time he suffered from dermatitis.

After Dr. B performed the second gynecologic examination on Patient T, Dr. B met with the Board again. As a result of this meeting, Dr. B was prohibited from delivering babies, performing surgery, and conducting invasive procedures using a sharp instrument in a patient's body cavity.

In May 1991, the Board and the Minnesota Department of Health contacted 336 patients on whom Dr. B performed one or more invasive procedures while gloved, during the period that Dr. B suffered from exudative dermatitis. Dr. B also sent letters (dated June 17, 1991 and signed by Dr. B) to these 336 patients to explain his situation. A total of 325 patients obtained HIV tests and none of them tested HIV seropositive; 3 patients refused testing, 7 could not be located and 1 had died of causes unrelated to AIDS.

Dr. B discontinued his medical practice in June 1991. He died of AIDS-related complications in September 1991.

Over 50 former patients filed complaints against Dr. B and Hospital P. Patient T was one of these 50 former patients. She brought this action against Dr. B and Hospital P for emotional damages she allegedly suffered on learning that Dr. B had performed two gynecologic procedures on her while he was infected with HIV and was suffering from open sores on his hands and forearms.

The Supreme Court of Minnesota reinstated summary judgment in favor of Dr. B and Hospital P on Patient T's emotional distress claims. The reasons are summarized below:

1. Patient T, who failed to allege actual exposure to HIV, was not in personal physical danger of contracting HIV and was not within a zone of danger for the purposes of establishing a claim for negligent infliction of emotional distress. In fact, Dr. B did comply with the restrictions imposed by the Board and did not place Patient T at any reasonable risk of contracting HIV.

2. Patient T failed to establish that Dr. B's conduct was either intentional or reckless for the purposes of a claim for intentional infliction of emotional distress.

3. Patient T also did not allege that Dr. B performed a different medical procedure from that to which she consented. In addition, Dr. B's conduct did not significantly increase the risk that Patient T would contract HIV. As a result, Patient T's claim for battery failed.

4. Dr. B's undisclosed risk of HIV exposure did not materialize in harm to Patient T because Patient T tested negative for the HIV antibody. So, Patient T was unable to establish a claim for negligent nondisclosure.

This legal case highlighted the conflict between Dr. B's self-interest in his ability to continue his medical practice and his patient's right to full information when determining whether to consent to procedures and treatments. Patients do have the right to information about actual and substantial risks to their health. At the same time, patients should have the right to information about risks that they consider personally important to their health.

It was common knowledge among medical professionals that the risk of HIV transmission under the circumstances presented in this legal case was low. As of 1995, there had been no known case of HIV transmission from a physician to a patient. The theoretical risk of HIV transmission from an infected health care worker to a patient during invasive procedures is minute. The general public probably did not share this common knowledge.

As a matter of fact, having a low risk for HIV transmission does not mean that there was no risk at all. Also, having a low risk for HIV transmission may have caused a reasonable patient to seek treatment from another physician to avoid a possible severe consequence. These were the rationales the Minnesota Board of Medical Examiners used to restrict Dr. B from delivering babies, performing surgery, and doing invasive procedures using a sharp instrument in a patient's body cavity.

Source: NexisLexis®Academic: Federal & State Cases (Case number: C6-93-1203, C5-93-1306, C4-93-1328; February 10, 1995, filed) (accessed on January 14, 2008).

Learning from a Legal Case Summary

Nurse A was the assistant head nurse in the pediatric unit at Hospital N. On December 8, 1990, during her shift that night and into the next morning, Nurse A was responsible for the care of 9 infants, including Baby C. As indicated in the hospital record, Baby C tested positive for HIV, which causes AIDS. During Nurse A's shift on December 8, Dr. D (a second-year resident) and Dr. T (a first-year resident) were also responsible for the treatment of Baby C.

At about 5:30 A.M. on December 9, when Nurse A was changing Baby C's diaper, a needle left in Baby C's crib penetrated Nurse A's right thumb to the bones. The needle was immediately removed and discarded by Nurse A. The needle was discarded before it could be tested for the presence of HIV. Nurse A was then treated in Hospital N's emergency room with drugs for exposure to hepatitis and was advised to take zidovudine (AZT) tablets as a preventive measure against AIDS. Nurse A was given an HIV antibody test right away, which was negative.

Nurse A recalled that Dr. T told her around 3:00 A.M. on December 9 that she was going to draw blood from Baby C. Although Nurse A did not see Dr. T draw blood from Baby C, Nurse A did see Dr. T holding a vial of blood afterward. Nurse A was stuck by the needle in Baby C's crib less than 3 hours later.

On December 10, 1990, a physician's assistant employed by Hospital N allegedly advised Nurse A to assume that she was HIV positive until the HIV tests showed otherwise. This physician's assistant also advised Nurse A to take AZT tablets, to use condoms when having intercourse with her husband, and to avoid kissing family members or sharing utensils with them. Nurse A did take the AZT tablets for 6 months and then discontinued the medication due to its side effects.

In August 1991, Nurse A began an action to recover her damages from Hospital N for the negligent infliction of emotional distress, which was caused by her fear of contracting AIDS. Nurse A's fear of contracting AIDS was commonly referred to as an "AIDS phobia" claim. Nurse A sought damages for the period from 1990, when the incident occurred, to the year 2005. As claimed by Nurse A, on the theory if Nurse A was free of the HIV-associated diseases by the year 2005, she would have no further risk of developing AIDS. On the other side, according to Hospital N, there was a consensus in the medical community that 95% of all persons who will ultimately test positive for the HIV virus will do so within 6 months of exposure and that current tests for the presence of the virus were 99% reliable.

In November 1993, Nurse A was examined by a physician retained by Hospital N. This physician determined that Nurse A showed no signs of HIV-associated diseases. Regardless of this result, Nurse A refused to take a blood test to determine whether she was HIV positive. In an order dated September 21, 1995, the court determined that Nurse A was not required to submit an HIV antibody test to maintain a cause of action for negligent infliction of emotional distress caused by her fear of contracting AIDS based on her having been stuck with a potentially contaminated needle left in the crib of an infant who was HIV positive.

The Supreme Court ordered Hospital N to pay Nurse A for those damages suffered during the first 6 months following Nurse A's potential exposure to HIV. Nurse A's fear of contracting AIDS should be limited to those damages suffered during the first 6 months following her potential exposure to HIV on December 9, 1999, unless Nurse A presented evidence that she tested positive for HIV.

Source: NexisLexis®Academic: Federal & State Cases (Case number: 95-03066, 95-10151, 96-08460, 96-08461; October 15, 1996, decided) (accessed on January 12, 2008).

Knowing about Health Care-associated Infections

Health care-associated infections are defined as infections that patients acquire during the course of receiving treatment for other conditions within a hospital or other health care facility (Centers for Disease Control and Prevention, 2007a). The effects of health care-associated infections on patients range from relatively minor (e.g., requiring a longer period of treatment with antibiotics) to devastating (e.g., dying of the infection; Joint Commission, 2007a).

Health care-associated infections are among the top 10 leading causes of death in the United States (Centers for Disease Control and Prevention, 2007a). The Centers for Disease Control and Prevention have been striving to understand how health care-associated infections occur and to develop appropriate interventions because health care-associated infections may result in death. Overall, urinary tract infections accounted for 32% of all health care-associated infections, followed by surgical site infections (22%), bloodstream infections (15%), and pneumonia (14%; Centers for Disease Control and Prevention, 2007b).

It was estimated that in 2002, the number of health care-associated infections was approximately 1.7 million in US hospitals. Among these 1.7 million, 417,946 (25%) infections occurred among adults and children in intensive care units, 1,266,851 (74%) infections among adults and children in inpatient care units (other than intensive care units), 33,269 (2%) infections among newborns in high-risk nurseries, and 19,059 (1%) infections among newborns in well-baby nurseries (Klevens et al., 2007). It is noted that most of the infections occurred in inpatient care units other than intensive care units.

Overall, the estimated number of deaths related to health care-associated infections was 98,987 deaths due to pneumonia or lung infections at about 31%, as the most frequently seen infection, followed by bloodstream infections, urinary tract infections, surgical site infections, and infections of other sites. For the infection-related deaths occurring in inpatient care units, urinary tract infections were the most commonly seen type, followed by surgical site infections, bloodstream infections, and pneumonia (Klevens et al., 2007).

Infectious Diseases that Patients May Acquire during Hospital Stays

The Centers for Disease Control and Prevention (2006) identified the following infectious diseases that may be transmitted within hospitals and, for that reason, are possible health care-associated infections:

1. Acinetobacter drug resistance: Acinetobacter are bacteria commonly found in soil and water and also found on the skin of healthy people (e.g., health care providers). Many types of Acinetobacter exist and all can cause human diseases among very ill patients in intensive care units and inpatient care settings, but rarely occur outside of hospitals. *Acinetobacter baumannii* accounted for about 80% of reported infections.

2. Blood-borne pathogens: This type of infection is considered as an occupational infection. Health care providers are at risk for occupational exposure to blood-borne pathogens, including hepatitis B virus, hepatitis C virus, HIV, and viral hemorrhagic fever involving Ebola and Marburg. Exposures often occur through needle sticks or cuts from the other types of sharp instruments that have been contaminated with an infected patient's blood. Exposures can also occur through contact of the eye, nose, mouth, or skin with a patient's blood.

3. *Burkholderia cepacia*: *B. cepacia* refers to a group of bacteria that can be found in soil and water. *B. cepacia* bacteria pose little medical risk to healthy people. However, patients who have weakened immune systems or chronic lung disease (particularly cystic fibrosis) may be susceptible to infections with *B. cepacia*. Unfortunately, *B. cepacia* infections are often resistant to common antibiotics.

4. Chickenpox (also called varicella): Chickenpox is a highly contagious disease in hospitals, which is caused by varicella-zoster virus through airborne transmission. Sources for health care-associated exposure may include patients, visitors, and hospital workers who are infected with varicella.

5. *Clostridium difficile*: *C. difficile* is a bacterium that often causes diarrhea and serious intestinal conditions (e.g., colitis).

6. *Clostridium sordellii*: *C. sordellii* is a rare bacterium that causes pneumonia, endocarditis, arthritis, peritonitis, and myonecrossi. Women are at highest risk of infections from *C. sordellii* following a live birth or spontaneous, medical, or surgical abortion. Severe toxic shock syndrome is most often linked to gynecologic infections in women and infections of the umbilical stump in newborns.

7. Creutzfeldt-Jakob disease (CJD): CJD disease is a rapidly progressive, invariably fatal neurodegenerative disorder that is caused by an abnormal isoform of a cellular glycoprotein know as the prion protein. The estimated

annual incidence of CJD worldwide, including the United States, is about one patient case per one million people.

8. Gastrointestinal infections: Acute gastrointestinal infections may be caused by a variety of agents, including bacteria, viruses, and protozoa. Transmission of agents within hospitals usually results from contact with infected individuals, from consumption of contaminated food, water, or other beverages, or from exposure to contaminated objects or environmental surfaces. Airborne transmission may occur, but rarely.

9. Hepatitis A: Health care-associated hepatitis A, as one of the occupational infections, does not occur frequently. The transmission of health care-associated hepatitis A from patients to health care providers usually involves activities that increase the risk of fecal-oral contamination (e.g., not washing hands after handling an infected infant, and sharing food, beverages, or cigarettes). The transmission usually happens when the source patient has unrecognized hepatitis and has diarrhea or fecal incontinence.

10. Hepatitis B: Health care-associated hepatitis B is considered as one type of occupational infections. Hepatitis B is caused by the hepatitis B virus that attacks the liver and may result in lifelong infection, liver cirrhosis, liver cancer, liver failure, and death. Hepatitis B virus spreads when a small amount of blood from an infected person enters the body of a person who is not infected. Health care providers, who have received hepatitis B vaccine and have developed immunity to the virus, are at no risk for infection. For a susceptible person, who does not have immunity to the hepatitis B virus, the risk from a single needle stick or a cut exposure to hepatitis B virus-infected blood ranges from 6% to 30%.

11. Hepatitis C: Health care-associated hepatitis C is perceived as one type of occupational infection. Hepatitis C is caused by hepatitis C virus, which can be found in the blood of persons who have hepatitis C. The average risk from a single needle stick or a cut exposure to hepatitis C virus-infected blood is approximately 1.8%.

12. HIV/AIDS: Health care providers can be exposed to blood-borne pathogens of HIV. Exposures can occur through needle sticks or cuts from other sharp instruments contaminated with an infected patient's blood or through contact of the eye, nose, mouth, or skin with a patient's blood. Most of the exposures do not result in infection. Transmission of HIV from health care providers to patients in hospitals is rare. Proper sterilization and disinfection procedures are required to prevent transmission of HIV.

13. Influenza (also called flu): Flu symptoms include fever, headache, tiredness, dry cough, sore throat, nasal congestion, and body aches. It is important to use a tissue to cover mouth and nose when coughing and sneezing and to clean hands with soap and water or with alcohol gels or wipes right away. During hospital stays, patients may be asked to wear a mask if they are coughing or sneezing.

14. Methicillin-resistant *Staphylococcus aureus* (MRSA): Methicillin-resistant *S. aureus* is a type of bacteria that is resistant to methicillin and other more

common antibiotics, including oxacillin, penicillin, and amoxicillin. *S. aureus* infections often occur among hospitalized patients who have weakened immune systems.

15. Mumps: Mumps is transmitted by contact with mumps virus-holding respiratory secretions, including saliva. The portals of entry are the nose and mouth. Unilateral or bilateral parotitis occurred in approximately 50% of unvaccinated patients who were infected with mumps. About 30% to 35% of infected patients had nonspecific, flulike symptoms without parotitis and the remainder was asymptomatic. An effective vaccination program for health care providers is the best approach to prevent health care-associated mumps transmission in hospitals.

16. Norovirus: Noroviruses are a group of related, single-stranded RNA, non-enveloped viruses that cause acute gastroenteritis in humans. Noroviruses are highly contagious and are transmitted through primarily the fecal-oral route or through a droplet route from vomitus. Dehydration is the most common complication. Infected patients may require IV replacement fluids.

17. *Parvovirus* B19: *Parvovirus* B19 (also called fifth disease) is a virus that only infects humans. *Parvovirus* B19 is a mild rash illness that occurs most commonly in children; about 50% of all adults have ever been infected during childhood or adolescence. The ill child typically has a slapped-cheek rash on the face and a lacy red rash on the trunk and limbs. Animal parvoviruses exist but they do not infect humans. In addition, humans cannot catch *parvovirus* B19 from a parvovirus-infected dog or cat.

18. Pneumonia: Pneumonia has accounted for about 15% of all infections occurring in hospitals. The primary risk factor for acquiring health care-associated bacterial pneumonia in hospitals is mechanical ventilation with its needed endotracheal intubation. Among health care-associated pneumonia infections, more than 50% are acquired in either medical intensive care units or coronary care units.

19. Rubella: Rubella is a mild febrile rash illness in children and adults. Infected patients may also have symptoms of lymphadenopathy, malaise, or conjunctivitis. Arthralgia and arthritis can occur in about 70% of infected adult and adolescent females.

20. Severe acute respiratory syndrome (SARS): SARS is a viral respiratory illness caused by a coronavirus, called SARS-associated coronavirus (SARS-CoV). SARS was first reported in Asia in February 2003. SARS-CoV is transmitted most readily by respiratory droplets produced when an infected person coughs or sneezes. At the beginning, infected patients may have a high fever, headache, an overall feeling of discomfort, body aches, or mild respiratory symptoms. About 10% to 20% of infected patients have diarrhea. About 2 to 7 days after onset, infected patients may develop a dry cough and most patients develop pneumonia. At present, there is no known SARS transmission anywhere in the world; the most recent human cases were reported in China in April 2004 in an outbreak resulting from laboratory-acquired infections.

21. *Streptococcus pneumoniae* drug resistance: *S. pneumoniae* is a leading cause of morbidity and mortality in the United States. It is estimated that each year *S. pneumoniae* causes 3000 cases of meningitis, 50,000 cases of bacteremia, 500,000 cases of pneumonia, and 7,000,000 cases of otitis media. Penicillin-resistant and multidrug-resistant strains of *S. pneumoniae* have begun to emerge in the United States and have been widespreaded in some communities.

22. Tuberculosis: Transmission of tuberculosis in hospitals has been associated with close contact with patients who have infectious tuberculosis, particularly when health care providers are performing cough-inducing procedures (e.g., bronchoscopy and sputum induction). Transmission of tuberculosis is a recognized risk to both patients and health care providers. Patient cases of multidrug-resistant tuberculosis have been recognized and are more difficult to treat.

23. Vancomycin-intermediate *Staphylococcus aureus* (VISA) and vancomycin-resistant *S. aureus* (VRSA): VISA and VRSA are two specific types of antimicrobial-resistant staphylococcus bacteria; VISA and VRSA cannot be successfully treated with vancomycin because these bacteria are no longer susceptible to the drug. Fortunately, all VISA and VRSA isolates are still susceptible to other antibiotics approved by the US Food and Drug Administration.

24. Vancomycin-resistant enterococci (VRE): Enterococci are bacteria that normally exist in the human intestines and in the female genital tract. Enteroccocci sometimes can cause infections, and in some instances, become resistant to vancomycin, which is the antibiotic most often used to treat infections caused by enterococci. Most of the vancomycin-resistant enterococci infections occur in hospitals.

25. Viral hemorrhagic fever: Viral hemorrhagic fever, which includes Ebola and the Marburg virus, can be transmitted within hospitals. Ebola hemorrhagic fever is a severe, often fatal disease that has appeared sporadically since its initial recognition in 1976.

Possible Conditions Related to Acquiring Health Care-associated Infections

Health care providers as well as contaminated equipment and clothing can transfer health care-associated infections from a patient to another patient and from a patient to a health care worker (Joint Commission, 2007a). An effective infection prevention and control program should be able to protect patients from the transmission of infectious diseases and from the conditions attributable to the care they receive. Preventing the transmission of infectious diseases from patients to health care providers is also an important aspect of infection control (Centers for Disease Control and Prevention, 2005).

In the modern hospital environments, many types of invasive devices and surgical treatments have been used to help patients recover. For various treatment purposes (e.g., IV therapy), medical devices and surgical procedures go around patients' natural defenses against invading microorganisms (e.g., skin). Consequently, use of invasive devices and surgical treatments has been linked to lung, bloodstream, and urinary tract infections. Hospitals are also obligated to protect patients from device-associated and procedure-associated infections (Centers for Disease Control and Prevention, 2007c).

Device-associated and procedure-associated conditions that patients may encounter within a hospital include (Centers for Disease Control and Prevention, 2007c):

1.   Catheter-associated urinary tract infections
2.   Dialysis-associated infections
3.   Foot spa-associated and hot tub-associated infections
4.   Infections occurring during tissue transplantation
5.   Intravascular catheter-associated bloodstream infections
6.   Surgical site infections
7.   Ventilator-associated pneumonia (also abbreviated as VAP)

Reducing Health Care-associated Infections as One of the National Patient Safety Goals

In the 2008 National Patient Safety Goals for hospitals, Goal 7 was established to reduce the risk of health care-associated infections. Hospitals are required to comply with current World Health Organization's hand hygiene guidelines or the hand hygiene guidelines developed by the Centers for Disease Control and Prevention to reduce the transmission of infectious agents by health care providers to patients (Joint Commission, 2008).

Health care-associated infections are indeed preventable. The most effective preventive method is good hand hygiene. Improved adherence to hand hygiene by washing hands with soap and water or using alcohol-based hand rubs is crucial to reduce transmission of antimicrobial-resistant organisms and reduce overall health care-associated infection rates. In addition, the use of gloves should not eliminate the need for hand hygiene and the use of hand hygiene also should not eliminate the need for gloves. In fact, gloves can reduce hand contamination by 70% to 80%, prevent cross-contamination, and protect patients and health care providers from contracting infectious diseases (Joint Commission, 2007b).

At the same time, the Joint Commission (2008) required hospitals to undergo a root cause analysis on the patients who unexpectedly died or suffered major permanent loss of function because of having health care-associated infections. These patient cases should be managed as sentinel events. The root cause analysis should attempt to answer: (1) why the patient acquired an infection and (2) given the fact of the infection, why the patient died or suffered permanent loss of function. In each root cause analysis, hospitals are required to address the management of care on the patient before and after the identification of infection (Joint Commission, 2008).

Despite this, the Joint Commission (2007a) has claimed that hand washing has been used inconsistently and sometimes is done inadequately among health care providers (e.g., physicians and nurses). For example, nurses' compliance with hand washing is often based on the number of opportunities to wash their hands and depends on what they are doing for each of their patients, not just on the number of patients.

Based on previous studies, Lautenbach (2001) summarized possible barriers to individual handwashing, including:

1. Health care providers' belief that their compliance level with hand hygiene guidelines was better than it actually was
2. Not integrating individual handwashing into health care providers' daily practice
3. Skin damage from frequent use of soaps and detergents
4. The time required for proper handwashing (at least 15 seconds)
5. To promote good hand hygiene, the Joint Commission (2007b) suggested seven tips for convincing health care providers to always wash their hands:
6. Respected staff leaders should make an extra effort to be good role models by consistently practicing good hand hygiene.
7. Hospitals should install dispensers of alcohol-based hand rubs inside or just outside each patient room. Alcohol-based hand rub gel dispensers can be placed in egress or exit corridors but not alcohol-based hand rub foam dispensers. It is important for hospitals to follow the advice of state and local fire marshals for the safest placement of alcohol-based hand rub gel or foam dispensers.
8. Hospitals are encouraged to install speakers outside the doors of each patient room in high-risk departments or units. Speakers would replay a recorded reminder every time a staff member leaves the room that says "Please remember to wash your hands before leaving room xxx."
9. Hospital leaders should let health care providers know that they will be monitored from time to time to ensure that handwashing is performed consistently.
10. Hospitals should measure the volume of alcohol-based hand rubs used per 1000 patient-days and keep staff members informed of the results.
11. Encourage staff members to remind one another to wash their hands before and after each patient contact.
12. Educate patients to ask their health care providers whether they have washed their hands. For example, some hospitals have staff members who provide direct care to patients wear buttons that say "Ask me if I washed my hands."

Risk Factors and Possible Solutions as Suggested by the Joint Commission

Of the infection-associated sentinel events reported to the Joint Commission in 2005, communication was the most often identified root cause for health care-associated infections and complications at about 75%, followed by environmental safety and security (50%), procedural compliance (38%), competency and credentialing (38%), continuum of care (38%), patient assessment (25%), and leadership (25%) (Joint Commission, 2007a).

Based on these findings, the Joint Commission (2007a) conducted an in-depth analysis on three major root causes for health care-associated infections and identified strategies that nurses can adopt to reduce the likelihood of related deaths and serious injuries. Table 1 lists these prevention strategies related to inpatient care.

Challenges for Clinicians in Preventing Health Care-associated Infections

Health care staff providers who provide direct patient care, patients, and their families should all be involved in preventing health care-associate infections. Health care providers must follow hospital policies and clinical practice guidelines to effectively prevent health care-associated infections. On-the-job training is crucial to keep health care providers updated on the most recent guidelines.

Table 1. The major root causes of the reported sentinel events related to health care-associated infections and the corresponding prevention strategies for nurses

Root cause	Prevention strategy

Inadequate orientation and training and unavailability of information (e.g., related to intravascular catheter-related infections)	1. Hospital leaders need to provide up-to-date information about preventing health care-associated infections to health care providers, including physicians and nurses.
	  1.1 Whenever any procedures are revised, health care providers need to be oriented and trained to the revised procedure.
	  1.2 Hospital leaders need to evaluate health care staff members' compliance to the revised procedure.
	2. Nurses can help ensure the other health care providers' compliance with the central line bundle as developed by the Institute for Healthcare Improvement (information available at: http://www.ihi.org/NR/rdonlyres/FEAA3D46-D33E-4244-8ACC-7B01AF0A12EF/0/MIFCLICentralLineBundleCompliance.pdf) and the guidelines for the prevention of intravascular catheter-related infections as initiated by Centers for Disease Control and Prevention (information available at: http://www.cdc.gov/mmwr/PDF/rr/rr5110.pdf).
	  2.1 The five key components in the Institute for Healthcare Improvement's central line bundle were:
	    2.1.1 Hand hygiene
	    2.1.2 Ensuring maximal barrier precautions
	    2.1.3 Using chlorhexidine skin antisepsis
	    2.1.4 Optimal catheter site selection, with subclavian vein as the preferred site for non-tunneled catheters in adults
	    2.1.5 Daily review of line necessity with prompt removal of unnecessary lines

Root cause	Prevention strategy
	2.2 The Institute for Healthcare Improvement also suggested tips for hospitals to aid staff members in complying with the central line bundle: 2.2.1 Placing soap or alcohol-based hand hygiene dispensers in obvious and handy locations and making gloves available only near hand sanitation equipment (e.g., sinks) 2.2.2 Creating a work environment that encourages reminding one another about keeping good hand hygiene 2.2.3 Maintaining a fully stocked cart for central line supplies to facilitate use of maximal barrier precautions 2.2.4 Including chlorhexidine antisepsis kits in carts that store central line supplies 2.2.5 Including daily review of the need for a central line in rounds 2.2.6 Recording the time and date of each central line placement, for record-keeping purposes and to help in decision-making about removal 3. Nursing leaders, managers, and nurses may adopt the *Infusion Nursing Standards of Practice* in practice (information available at: http://www.ins1.org/standards/index.html; this book was published by the Infusion Nurses Society, Norwood, MA, in 2006). 3.1 Nurses may use related references for ongoing infusion site care, maintenance of the infusion lines, and preventing infusion-related complications. 4. When adopting a revised procedure, hospital and nursing leaders must anticipate resistance to change. 4.1 Hospital and nursing leaders should engage health care staff members in planning ways to address the concerns and potential problems with the new procedures.
Inadequate care planning (e.g., to decrease the risk of developing *Clostridium difficile*-associated diarrhea)	1. Nursing leaders, managers, and nurses need to ensure that all health care providers, who may have direct contact with patients, understand the rationale for using prevention strategies to prevent health care-associated infections. 2. Hospital and nursing leaders should ensure that all health care providers perform proper hand hygiene. 3. Nurses should teach patients about proper hand hygiene to protect themselves and what to expect from the health care providers who provide care, treatment, or procedures to them. 3.1 Nurses should encourage patients to ask their health care providers whether they have washed their hands. 4. Hospital leaders and physicians should ensure judicious use of antibiotics. 4.1 For example, the use of antimicrobial medications is the leading risk factor for *C. difficile*-associated diarrhea. 4.2 If antimicrobial medications are ordered inappropriately, supervisory staff, pharmacists, other physicians, or nurses need to address the issue with the prescribing physician. 4.3 Nurses can help colleagues understand the rationale for appropriate and timely use of antimicrobial medications. Nurses can help ensure that they integrate the rationale into their practice. 4.4 Patient education related to medication use can also incorporate the principles of judicious antibiotic use.

Table 1. Continued

Root cause	Prevention strategy
	5. When available, nurses should use disposable equipment or clean equipment carefully before using on different patients.
	5.1 Nurses should avoid use of equipment that may harbor pathogenic organisms between patients.
	6. Nurses and other health care providers should use appropriate contact precautions.
	6.1 Nurses should wear gloves whenever entering a patient room and for delivering all care.
	6.2 Nurses should wear a gown if their working clothes and shoes may become soiled during the processes of delivering care.
	6.3 If a patient has *C. difficile*-associated diarrhea, it is important to place the infected patient in a private room or in a room with another patient who also has *C. difficile*-associated diarrhea to prevent a *C. difficile* outbreak or halt the outbreak.
	7. Nurses should be aware of the risk factors for commonly seen health care-associated infections. Nurses can help identify the pattern of transmission of *C. difficile* infections.
	7.1 If a new strain of *C. difficile* is detected, nurses can participate in monitoring infected patients and contact appropriate infection control staff for changes in the conditions of infected patients.
	7.2 Nurses can also help monitor compliance with strategies to prevent an outbreak or contain the existing outbreak of health care-associated infection.
	8. Nursing leaders, managers, and nurses should ensure that environmental cleaning practices provide proper sanitation and disinfection.
	8.1 When fecal contamination is possible, cleaning and disinfecting frequently touched surfaces and reusable devices are essential.
	8.2 Nurses need to know the types of solutions used for cleaning and disinfecting surfaces and objects on their units and whether the solutions used are effective in eliminating found pathogens on patients.
	8.3 Nurses should regularly disinfect their endoscopes and other devices used for more than one patient, according to the manufacturer's instructions.
	9. Nursing managers and nurses need to be aware of and alert for unintended consequences of contact precautions.
	9.1 For health care providers, the additional time required to use contact precautions can result in not using the precautions properly.
	9.2 Patients for whom contact precautions are implemented may have adverse psychological effects or believe they are being avoided.
	9.3 When a patient is isolated due to infections, nurses must assess the patient's psychological status (e.g., the amount of telephone contact from family or friends) and should not avoid the patient.

Root cause	Prevention strategy
Inadequate assessment on patients who are receiving mechanical ventilation (e.g., related to prevent ventilator-associated pneumonia) *Note:* Some patients who are receiving mechanical ventilation may be in intensive care units. Other patients stay in acute inpatient care units.	1. Nurses can help ensure health care providers' compliance with the guidelines on preventing ventilator-associated pneumonia and the ventilator bundle for reducing the incidence of ventilator-associated pneumonia as developed by the Institute for Healthcare Improvement (information available at: http://www.ihi.org/nr/rdonlyres/d823e3fd-d10b-493e-a6a8-37c767825780/0/vaphowtoguide.doc; published on 2007) and the guidelines for preventing health care-associated pneumonia as initiated by Centers for Disease Control and Prevention (information available at: http://www.cdc.gov/mmwr/preview/mmwrhtml/rr5303a1.htm; published on 2004). 1.1 The four key components in the Institute for Healthcare Improvement's ventilator bundle for reducing the incidence of ventilator-associated pneumonia are: 1.1.1 Elevating the head of the bed to between 30° and 45° 1.1.2 Implementing daily "sedation vacation" and daily assessment of readiness for extubation 1.1.3 Ordering and using prophylaxis for peptic ulcer disease 1.1.4 Using prophylaxis for deep venous thrombosis unless it is contraindicated 1.2 The Institute for Healthcare Improvement also suggests several interventions and strategies to facilitate implementation of the ventilator bundle, including: 1.2.1 Implementing a mechanism to ensure elevation of the head of the bed: 1.2.1.1 Including this intervention on nursing flow sheets 1.2.1.2 Including this intervention as one of the topics at multidisciplinary rounds 1.2.1.3 Nurses should encourage respiratory therapists to notify nursing staff, if the head of the bed is not elevated. 1.2.1.4 Nurses should empower respiratory therapists to place patients in the semirecumbent position with assistance from nursing staff. 1.2.1.5 Physicians should include elevation of the head of the bed in order sets for initiation and weaning of mechanical ventilation.
	1.2.2 If available, the health care team should implement a protocol to lighten sedation daily to assess for neurologic readiness for extubation. 1.2.2.1 It is important to include related precautions on patients in the protocol (e.g., nurses should increase monitoring and vigilance to prevent self-extubation). 1.2.2.2 It is necessary to include a "sedation vacation" strategy in the weaning protocol and in the care plan to wean patients from the ventilator. 1.2.2.3 It is essential for physicians and nurses to avoid patient oversedation. Adopting a sedation scale for assessment of sedation may be necessary.

Table 1. Continued

Root cause	Prevention strategy

	2. Nurses should position patients who are receiving mechanical ventilation in a semirecumbent position. Such positioning may reduce the incidence of gastroesophageal reflux and incidence of ventilator-associated pneumonia.
	3. Nurses should avoid flushing contaminated secretions from the ventilator circuit into the lower airway.
	    3.1 Contaminated secretions can lead to ventilator-associated pneumonia.
	    3.2 Nurses should also avoid flushing medication nebulizers from the ventilator circuit into the lower airway during turning.
	    3.3 Nurses should empty contaminated condensates carefully.
	4. Physicians and nurses should maintain the endotracheal tube cuff pressure at 20 cm H_2O or more to help prevent leakage of secretions around the tube and into the lower airway.
	5. Nurses should observe for signs of hyperglycemia. Hyperglycemia is often associated with increased numbers of complications.
	6. When possible, health care team members should be encouraged to use noninvasive ventilation. Intubation itself does contribute to the risk of infection.

Source: Joint Commission (2007a). Preventing infection-related events. In R. A. Porché, Jr. (Ed.), *Front line of defense: The role of nurses in preventing sentinel events* (2nd ed., pp. 155-166). Oakbrook Terrace, IL: Joint Commission.

In addition, we must understand that hospital staff members (including physicians and nurses) have no financial incentive to modify their practice by, for example, washing their hands between patients and wearing clean gloves. In addition, staff members seldom perceive that good hand hygiene can make any difference on their chance of attracting occupational infectious diseases. Consequently, hospitals must offer sufficient and effective orientation for new staff members and continuous education on hand hygiene to all staff members who provide direct patient care. It is especially important that hospitals have comprehensive supervisory plans in place to periodically monitor staff members' compliance in hand hygiene.

Comprehensive Management and Supervisory Strategies would Make a Difference!

As a matter of fact, having clinical practice guidelines in place will not guarantee good compliance and patient outcome (e.g., low health care-associated infection rates). For each hospital, patient safety and quality care will be guaranteed only if hospitals have detailed managerial strategies to effectively supervise and monitor staff members' practice and performance (e.g., nurses' and physicians' compliance to the hand hygiene guidelines).

It is essential that the possible consequences of poor department, unit, or individual compliance to hand hygiene guidelines should be announced and well communicated before implementing any related supervisory plans. The compliance findings on practicing good hand hygiene should be documented, tracked, and discussed among staff members and their immediate supervisors. Hospital and nursing leaders also need to be informed about the improvement in hand hygiene compliance on a monthly or quarterly basis, including rates of various health care-associated infections. The commitment of hospital executives to promoting good hand hygiene is crucial to prevent health care-associated infections.

Use of Common Sense to Prevent Spreading of Infectious Diseases

In inpatient care units, patients are often frail and susceptible to pathogens of any kind. Consequently, in addition to practicing good hand hygiene, all health care providers must use appropriate contact precautions. For example, health care providers who have direct contact with patients should wear clean gloves whenever entering a patient room and for delivering all care. Health care providers should consider wearing a gown if their working clothes may become soiled during the processes of delivering care. In addition, health care providers should wear masks all the time (e.g., surgical masks), particularly when having close contact with patients, to prevent spreading airborne pathogens and contracting infectious diseases.

In US hospitals, nurses, physicians, and other health care providers are not used to wearing masks, even when they have close contact with patients in ambulatory or inpatient care settings. When we catch the flu, our community members also are not accustomed to wearing masks to prevent spreading germs. We do know that when we sneeze or cough, we should cover our mouth and nose. Likewise, wearing masks should be considered a thoughtful professional practice to prevent spreading airborne germs to others and contracting airborne germs from others (e.g., colleagues, and patients). Obviously, we do not want to have a sick nurse or physician taking care of us during hospitalization.

Hospitals are the place for patients to receive treatments, heal, and regain health and get better, not to become more ill. When we come to hospitals to work as a health care provider, to receive care as a patient, or to visit our hospitalized loved ones as a family visitor, we should wear masks to protect patients and ourselves, especially when we have close contact with patients who can be really frail and susceptible to all kinds of infectious diseases.

To promote good hand hygiene, hospitals should install a voice reminder inside and outside the door of each patient room in all inpatient care units and intensive care units. Voice reminders would replay a recorded message every time a staff member comes in the room, saying, for example, "Wash your hands and wear gloves to protect patients and yourself." Voice reminders would replay another recorded message every time a staff member leaves the room, saying, for instance, "Wash your hands to prevent infections." It is also essential to install voice reminders inside and outside of each outpatient clinic or physician office.

We also believe that health care providers should leave germs at hospitals. As a result, we suggest that all health care providers (including physicians and nurses) who provide direct patient care should only wear their working clothes and shoes at work. Health care providers should wear their nonworking clothes and shoes for coming to work, change to their working outfit at their working unit or department, and change back to their nonworking clothes and shoes before leaving their workplace. This practice is important to prevent health care providers becoming the carriers of infectious diseases within the hospital and between the hospital and the community.

To cultivate this good practice habit and promote a healthy professional lifestyle, hospitals should provide free laundry services for all health care providers' working clothes. Dirty clothes may be collected twice a week from each unit or department, and the clean clothes may be returned in 3 days. In this way, hospital leaders can be sure that their staff members are wearing clean and disinfected working clothes. For disinfection and laundry safety concerns, hospitals may need to limit the styles of working clothes worn, including the types of fabrics and colors. When we discuss patient safety in hospitals, nurses with good hygiene habits and clean working clothes or uniforms are important.

In summary, health care providers must follow and meet the terms indicated in hospital policies and guidelines associated with preventing health care-associated infections. Health care providers also should maintain good hand hygiene and wear a gown and mask to protect their patients and themselves. These professional practices are keys to preventing health care-associated infections and occupational infectious diseases.

Opportunities for Patient and Family Involvement

As for the opportunities for patient and family involvement, the World Health Organization (2007) suggested four strategies for hospitals. We modified these strategies to meet the needs for hospitalized patients who stay in acute inpatient care units. These strategies were:

1. Nursing managers and nurses should produce information for patients and their families that highlights the importance of good hand hygiene.
2. Nurses should raise the awareness of patients and their families of the risks to their health when momentary failures in timely and appropriate hand hygiene occur.
3. Nurses should educate patients and their families on correct hand hygiene technique and indications to ensure that they are aware of the correct moments for keeping good hand hygiene.
4. Hospital and nursing leaders and nursing managers should encourage nurses and the other staff members to clean their hands in the presence of their patient, prior to touching the patient. In addition, patients should be invited and encouraged to ask their health care providers whether they have cleaned their hands prior to treatment.

Table 2 summarizes our suggested prevention strategies for nurses to prevent health care-associated infections in acute inpatient care settings.

Critical Tips for Patients and Families to Prevent Health Care-associated Infections

What we, as patients and families, can do to prevent health care-associated infections is limited, but we may still be able to make a big difference by avoiding contagious disease during our hospital stays. Table 3 outlines tips for patients and families to be involved in the efforts of preventing health care-associated infections. These tips were modified from the Joint Commission's patient safety program, Speak Up™ initiatives (Joint Commission, 2007c).

Table 2. Preventing health care-associated infections:
Critical tips for nurses who work in acute inpatient care units

Dimension	Strategy
Having sufficient orientation and training about prevention of health care-associated infections	1. Nurses' must follow the hospital's clinical practice guidelines and policies associated with prevention of health care-associated infections. 2. Nurses must understand and accept the rationale for using prevention strategies to avoid health care-associated infections. 3. Nurses should be aware the risk factors for commonly seen health care-associated infections. This way, nurses can help prevent an outbreak or contain the existing outbreak of health care-associated infection. 4. Whenever any procedures are revised, nurses should be oriented and trained to the revised procedure. 5. Nursing leaders need to evaluate nurses' compliance to the revised procedures on a regular basis.

Maintaining a safe care environment	1. Nurses must perform proper hand hygiene between patients.
	2. Nurses must use appropriate contact precautions.
	  2.1 Nurses should wear gloves whenever they enter a patient room and for delivering all care.
	  2.2 Nurses should wear a gown if their working clothes may become soiled during the processes of delivering care.
	  2.3 Nurses should wear masks all the time (e.g., surgical masks), particularly when having close contact with patients to prevent spread of airborne pathogens and contract infectious diseases.
	3. When available, nurses should use disposable equipment or cleansed equipment carefully between patients. Nurses should avoid use of equipment that may harbor pathogenic organisms between different patients.
	4. Nurses should help ensure that environmental cleaning practices provide proper sanitation and disinfection.
	  4.1 When fecal contamination is possible, cleaning and disinfecting frequently touched surfaces and reusable devices are essential.
	  4.2 Nurses should regularly disinfect their endoscopes and other devices used for more than one patient.
	5. Nurses should only wear designated working clothes and shoes at work and put on their nonworking clothes and shoes for coming to work and going home.

Table 2. Continued

Dimension	Strategy
	5.1 This practice is important to prevent nurses becoming the carriers of infectious diseases within the hospital and between the hospital and the community.
	5.2 Hospitals should provide free laundry services for nurses' and the other staff members' working clothes. This way, hospital leaders can ensure that their staff members are wearing clean and well-disinfected working clothes.

Ensuring individualized care planning about prevention of health care-associated infections	1. Nurses should teach patients about proper hand hygiene to protect themselves.
	2. Nurses should encourage patients to ask the staff members who have direct contact with them whether they have washed their hands.
	3. Nurses must explain any use of antibiotics and the purposes of antibiotic medications to patients or their families, if any.
	4. Nurses need to be aware and alert for unintended consequences of contact precautions, including:
	    4.1 The additional time required to use contact precautions can result in not using the precautions properly.
	    4.2 Patients for whom contact precautions are implemented may have adverse psychological effects or believe that they are being avoided.
	    4.3 When a patient is isolated due to infections, nurses must assess the patient's psychological status, for example, the amount of telephone contact from family or friends.
	    4.4 When a patient is isolated due to infections, nurses should not avoid the patient.

Table 3. Preventing health care-associated infections: Tips for patients and families

Dimension	Tip
	If I am not well enough to do any of the actions indicated below, I should ask a family or friend to help. These tips can help prevent the spread of colds, the flu, and diseases such as pneumonia, tuberculosis, mumps, rubella (also known as German measles), whooping cough, chickenpox, measles, and strep throat.

Cleaning my hands	1. If I am able to get up, I should wash my hands with soap and water several times a day, especially after hugging or shaking hands with a family or visitor.
	    1.1 I should use soap and water and rub my hands really well for at least 15 seconds.
	2. If I am not mobile or my hands do not look dirty, I can clean my hands with alcohol-based hand sanitizers. I should rub the sanitizer all over my hands, especially under my nails and between my fingers, until my hands are dry.
	    2.1 I should ask my nurse whether I can have a bottle of alcohol-based hand sanitizer at my bedside. If not, I should ask my family to buy one for me.
	3. I should clean my hands before touching or eating food.
	4. I must clean my hands after using the bathroom or bedside commode.
	5. My families must also clean their hands before and after caring for or touching me, using the bathroom, changing my diaper, taking out the trash, etc.

Dimension	Tip

Covering up my mouth and nose	1. I should ask for a mask from my nurse, if available, or purchase my own masks to protect myself from acquiring infectious diseases.
	    1.1 The mask should always cover both my mouth and nose.
	    1.2 I should wear a mask whenever I have interactions with or talk to my health care providers or families during my entire hospital stay.
	    1.3 I should wear a mask on a regular basis to protect myself. I should wear a mask when I am in my own room or in the hallway or another part of the hospital (e.g., hospital restaurants).
	    1.4 When the mask is soiled or wet, I should replace it with a new one.
	2. When I sneeze or cough, I should cover my mouth and nose to prevent spreading pathogens to others (if I am not wearing a mask).
	    2.1 I should keep tissues handy at my bedside and in my pocket. I must be sure to throw away used tissues and clean my hands right away.
	    2.2 If I do not have a tissue, I should cover my mouth and nose with the bend of my elbow or hands. If I use my hands, I must wash them right away.

Helping ensure a safe care environment	6. I should ask health care providers who care for me (e.g., physicians, nurses, and nursing attendants) whether they washed their hands before entering my room and before touching me for performing any treatments or procedures. 7. I should also ask my doctor and nurse to wear gloves and a mask when they have close contact with me. 8. I should ask my doctor and nurse to clean their stethoscopes with alcohol before they use the stethoscope on me. 9. If my family and visitors are sick, I should ask them to stay away from me and go home right away. If my family and visitors who are sick have to stay with me during my hospitalization, I should ask them to wear a mask and maintain good hand hygiene. 10. I must ask my nurse to send housekeeping to clean my room and bathroom as needed. If my bed sheet is soiled, I should ask for a clean one right away. 11. I should not feel embarrassed to use the call light to ask for help with toileting or changing a diaper or sanitary pad. 12. If I get a health care-associated infection, I should ask my doctor and nurse what I can do to get better more quickly.

Source: Joint Commission (2007c). Four things you can do to prevent infection. Available at: http://www.jointcommission.org/NR/rdonlyres/F76BC658-5554-4A82-89ED-67E36F033CF8/0/ Infection_Control_Brochure.pdf (accessed January 11, 2008).

For example, we can ask our health care providers (e.g., physicians, nurses, and nursing attendants) whether they have washed their hands before entering our room and touching us to perform any treatments or procedures. We should also ask our doctors and nurses to clean their stethoscopes with alcohol before they use their stethoscopes on us (Roizen & Oz, 2006).

For patients who have been hesitant to ask their doctors or nurses to wash their hands, stickers saying "Did you wash your hands?" can be made for patients to wear on their hospital gowns (Joint Commission, 2006). However, not all hospitals provide such stickers. If we think we may be hesitant to ask our doctors or nurses to wash their hands and to wear clean gloves and a mask when they have close contact with us, we can simply show them the hand wash reminder located after the Preface of this book that says, "Wash your hands! No infection." We may ask for a sticker of "Did you wash your hands?" if available.

References

Centers for Disease Control and Prevention (2005). Protecting patients (date last modified: November 2, 2005). Available at: http://www.ced.gov/ncidod/dhqp/patient.html (accessed January 10, 2008).

Centers for Disease Control and Prevention (2006). Infectious diseases in healthcare settings (date last modified: May 22, 2006). Available at: http://www.ced.gov/ncidod/dhqp/id.html (accessed January 10, 2008).

Centers for Disease Control and Prevention (2007a). Healthcare-associated infections (HAIs) (date last modified: May 30, 2007). Available at: http://www.ced.gov/ncidod/dhqp/healthDis.html (accessed January 10, 2008).

Centers for Disease Control and Prevention (2007b). Estimates of healthcare-associated infections (date last modified: May 30, 2007). Available at: http://www.ced.gov/ncidod/dhqp/hai.html (accessed January 10, 2008).

Centers for Disease Control and Prevention (2007c). Device & procedure-associated conditions (date last modified: July 18, 2007). Available at: http://www.ced.gov/ncidod/dhqp/dpac.html (accessed January 10, 2008).

Joint Commission (2006). Goal 7: Reduce the risk of health care-associated infections. In A. Grayson. (Ed.), *Meeting the Joint Commission's 2007 National Patient Safety Goals* (pp. 53-66). Oakbrook Terrace, IL: Joint Commission.

Joint Commission (2007a). Preventing infection-related events. In R. A. Porché, Jr. (Ed.), *Front line of defense: The role of nurses in preventing sentinel events* (2nd ed., pp. 155-166). Oakbrook Terrace, IL: Joint Commission.

Joint Commission (2007b). *Patient safety pocket guide* (2nd ed., pp. 15-22). Oakbrook Terrace, IL: Joint Commission.

Joint Commission (2007c). Four things you can do to prevent infection. Available at: http://www.jointcommission.org/NR/rdonlyres/F76BC658-5554-4A82-89ED-67E36F033CF8/0/Infection_Control_Brochure.pdf (accessed January 11, 2008).

Joint Commission (2008). 2008 National Patient Safety Goals: Hospital programs (manual chapter). Available at: http://www.jointcommission.org/NR/rdonlyres/82B717D8-B16A-4442-AD00-CE3188C2F00A/0/08_HAP_NPSGs_Master.pdf (accessed January 9, 2008).

Klevens, R. M., Edwards, J. R., Richards, C. L. Jr., Horan, T. C., Gaynes, R. P., Pollock, D. A., & Cardo, D. M. (2007). Estimating health care-associated infections and deaths in U.S. hospitals, 2002. *Public Health Reports, 122*(2), 160-166.

Lautenbach, E. (2001). Practices to improve handwashing compliance. In K. G. Shojania, B. W. Duncan, K. M. McDonald, & R. M. Wachter (Eds.), *Making health care safer: A critical analysis of patient safety practices* (pp. 119-126). Evidence report/technology assessment: Number 43, AHRQ publication No. 01-E058, July 2001. Rockville, MD: Agency for Healthcare Research and Quality. Available at: http://www.ahrq.gov/clinic/ptsafety/ (accessed January 10, 2008).

Roizen, M. F., & Oz, M.C. (2006). *You the smart patient: An insider's handbook for getting the best treatment* (pp. 193-222). New York, NY: Free Press.

World Health Organization (2007). Improved hand hygiene to prevent health care-associated infections. Patient Safety Solutions, 1 (solution 9) (published on May 2007). Available at: http://www.jcipatientsafety.org/fpdf/presskit/PS-Solution9.pdf (accessed January 11, 2008).

The Impact of Hospital Human Resource Management on Patient Outcomes

Learning from a Legal Case Summary ᴬ

Hospital M provided inpatient and outpatient care in Michigan. Hospital M's registered nurses were represented by a nurse union between February 1998 and February 2001. According to the agreement between the nurse union and Hospital M in December 1998, for 1 year Hospital M was permitted to obligate registered nurses to work overtime when patient safety was involved. Hospital M would pay registered nurses a double-time scheduling premium for forced overtime. During this year, Hospital M required very little forced overtime because registered nurses volunteered for enough extra hours to meet Hospital M's staffing needs.

When the agreement expired in November 1999, the nurse union unsuccessfully tried to negotiate an extension. With the expiration of the double-time scheduling premium for overtime, Hospital M began to rely on forced overtime to meet staff needs in intensive care units and inpatient care units. Some registered nurses attempted to avoid forced overtime. Two registered nurses were allegedly fired for submitting falsified medical documents stating that they could not work overtime.

The nurse union had "No F.O.T." buttons made and Hospital M's registered nurses started to wear them throughout Hospital M. The "No F.O.T." buttons represented a silent protest for "no forced overtime." Shortly after Hospital M leaders learned of these buttons, Hospital M issued a command to ban these buttons. Hospital M thought that the ambiguous message of these buttons would prompt patients to ask questions and might promote discussion of forced overtime between registered nurses and patients.

Hospital M sought review of the National Labor Relations Boards' (abbreviated as Board) decision that Hospital M's prohibition of "No F.O.T." buttons constituted an unfair labor practice in violation of the National Labor Relations Act. The nurse union, responsible for distributing the "No F.O.T." buttons to registered nurses at Hospital M in support of its opposition to forced overtime, sought enforcement of the Board's decision and order.

According to the National Labor Relations Act, employees have a protected right to wear union insignia at work. It is a protected, concerted activity in the situation that employees wear pins or stickers in an effort to encourage their coworkers to support the union's position on a matter. In addition, substantial evidence supported the Board's conclusion that the buttons represented a silent protest of forced overtime and that the nurses' wearing of the buttons was a protected activity. No evidence suggested that by wearing the buttons, these registered nurses engaged in a partial strike, slowdown, or even intermittent work stoppage.

Consequently, the court denied Hospital M's petition for review and granted the Board permission to enforce its order. Hospital M's registered nurses should be allowed to wear the "No F.O.T." buttons.

Source: NexisLexis®Academic: Federal & State Cases (Case number: 01-2263/01-2525; May 15, 2003, decided) (accessed on January 12, 2008).

Learning from a Legal Case Summary

On August 18, 1981, Patient K, a male podiatrist, was admitted to Hospital M for treatment of a duodenal ulcer. Patient K also suffered from pancreatitis, and the symptoms of pancreatitis made it unsafe for him to undergo suggested ulcer surgery. To control the pancreatitis-related symptoms, Dr. T, Patient K's treatment physician, determined that Patient K should receive high caloric IV feeding by a total parenteral nutrition (abbreviated as TPN) line.

An IV feeding by a TPN line starts with insertion of a 4-inch long, large-bore needle into a patient's subclavian vein. The catheter will then pass into the vein, and the catheter will be connected to a drip bottle or pump that supplies the nutrient fluid. The insertion site will be numbed by novocaine (a local anesthetic medication), but the patient will not necessarily be sedated during the insertion process of a TPN line.

On August 28, 1981, Dr. W was assigned to install the TPN line for Patient K. Patient K was nervous and agitated throughout the procedure. Patient K moved his head, cried out, complained of pain, and requested additional injections of novocaine. Dr. W was unable to insert a TPN line on his first attempt. The assisting nurse also witnessed that Patient K was complaining of pain and was moving while Dr. W was attempting to insert the TPN line. This situation showed that Dr. W deviated from the prevailing standard of care in 1981 by attempting to insert a TPN line on a resistant patient, who was not sufficiently sedated. Later in the same day, a TPN line was established.

The next morning after the procedure, Patient K was found semiconscious, with one end of the TPN line disconnected from the nutrient source and open to the air, with the other end of the line remaining in his chest. Patient K exhibited signs of neurologic distress. Later that night, Patient K also suffered seizures. Patient K eventually recovered from his neurologic problems and was discharged on September 9, 1981.

Patient K then filed a medical malpractice action against Dr. W and Hospital M for the permanent injuries he sustained as a result of the negligence in the insertion process of the TPN line and of the negligence in supervision during the procedure. Dr. W was also sued for performing the insertion procedure without obtaining Patient K's informed consent. Patient K claimed that he was no longer able to work as a podiatrist due to his neurologic problems, and as a consequence, he was incapable of supporting his elderly mother and maintaining his own home.

The appellate court affirmed the judgment of the trial court that Patient K should be awarded $460,000 for damages and negligence toward Patient K in the insertion procedure of a TPN line and the negligence in supervision.

Source: NexisLexis®Academic: Federal & State Cases (Case number: 8841, 8851; September 17, 1991, decided) (accessed on January 12, 2008).

Background

Hänecke and associates (1998) found that there would be an exponentially increased accident risk beyond the ninth hour among a German working population. As a matter of fact, many nurses routinely work 12-hour shifts. Any overtime beyond a 12-hour shift is well beyond the threshold identified in Hänecke and associates' study. Errors tend to occur when nurses are tired and sleepy because that fatigue can result in a decline in behavioral performance and physiologic functioning.

Stone and associates (2007) investigated the effects of working conditions on safety outcomes in elderly patients in intensive care units. They concluded that increased overtime was associated with higher rates of catheter-associated urinary tract infections and pressure ulcers. We believe that patients and their families want a nurse who is alert, has not being working for extended hours, and is able to deliver safe care, treatments, and procedures. Consequently, we must demand our hospitals to staff nurses based on the principle of promoting patient safety not just based on the nurse-to-patient ratio.

Reflections on the First Legal Case: Patient Safety and Overtime

In the first legal case, patient safety was practically mentioned as a slogan. The cost to Hospital M on nursing services was indeed the center of this legal case. It was understandable that the nurse union was striving for better benefits and salary scales for their nurse members. In fact, we cannot see even a shadow of patient safety concerns in this case.

Hospital M's assertion was meant to avoid paying a double-time scheduling premium for forced overtime. Banning the "No F.O.T." (no forced overtime) buttons was intended to prevent Hospital M from being pressured to reach such an agreement with the nurse union to pay double-time scheduling premiums for forced overtime.

Hospital M should employ more registered nurses instead of using overtime. It is obvious that using overtime is cheaper for Hospital M and even less expensive if Hospital M does not need to pay for the double-time scheduling premium for forced overtime.

Working in an inpatient care or intensive care unit as a nurse is indeed a physically and psychologically demanding job. Registered nurses are generally tired after finishing their 8-hour or 12-hour shifts. A nurse's productivity during overtime hours can be compromised and patients' safety can also suffer due to a nurse's tiredness.

For example, during overtime hours, nurses may be less diligent in monitoring their patients' conditions and slower or less willing to answer call lights. It is understandable that some nurses may voluntarily work overtime or extra hours for additional income, especially when they are already at work. We questioned: Is it safe to have nurses work overtime after their 8-hour or 12-hour shift?

Hospitalized patients and families know that at least one nurse will be assigned to care for the patient 24 hours a day, 7 days a week, during the entire hospital stay. A patient seldom questions whether a nurse, who is present in the patient room, can practice safely. A safe care environment does include nurses who can practice their tasks and deliver patient care safely.

Hospital and nursing leaders often claim that on the top of the nationwide nursing shortage, the current US hospital environment is extremely cost constrained. They may argue that using overtime is a compromised approach, where patient safety is involved. Should we as patients continue buying such assertions from hospital and nursing leaders? Our answer is no.

Good Human Resource Management Does Make a Difference!

The suitability of health care staff members to do the tasks they are supposed to perform is crucial to safety of patient care. Important staff attributes may include personality, emotional maturity, working attitude, professional training, and competencies. Whether a hospital's human resource management strategies are adequate affects the safety of patients who receive care at the hospital. Human resource management involves the functions of but is not limited to recruitment, providing orientation to new staff and offering on-the-job training, performance appraisal, promotion, retention, and termination of unsuitable staff members.

Nurses' personality, stress, and burnout can be directly or indirectly predictive of patient outcomes. According to our observations, when nurses are at an optimum level of stress, stress can be beneficial to job performance. Stress at an optimum level may lead to arousal and increased attention on the part of staff members. Adequate supervision may result in higher motivation for nurses to improve the quality of their care deliveries.

When a nurse's stress level is above or below the optimum level (e.g., insufficient or overwhelmed), he or she may show increased levels of poor performance, job dissatisfaction, and absenteeism. However, it should be noted that each individual nurse's optimum level of stress can vary due to personality and prior related experiences.

Decaire and associates (2006) examined the relationship between the characteristics of the staff members and the nature of patient-related incidents that occurred in a psychiatric hospital in Canada over a 1-year period. Of the 52 incidents, 42.3% ($n = 22$) were categorized as nonviolent and 57.7% ($n = 30$) as aggressive (verbal and violent). Findings showed that for the linkage between the perceived social climate within the work setting and involved incidents, staff members who perceived having a higher level of clarity in their work environment were present during fewer verbally aggressive incidents. The ones who perceived having more autonomy within their work environment were present during more nonviolent incidents. As for the relationship between staff personality and involved incidents, staff members who perceived themselves as being more open were associated with a greater frequency of nonviolent incidents (Decaire et al., 2006).

The study by Decaire and associates (2006) concluded that staff personality and perceived social climate within the work setting were predictive of staff's job performance. We should interpret Decaire and associates' findings carefully because the characteristics of patients admitted to medical or surgical care units versus the ones admitted into psychiatric hospitals are different. Verbally aggressive and violent incidents mainly occur in behavioral care settings or psychiatric hospitals and rarely happen in medical or surgical care units.

Reporting our Concerns during Hospital Stays

When we are hospitalized in a medical or surgical inpatient care unit, a safe care environment is key to promoting our recovery and healing. Although as patients we may not be able to differentiate whether our nurses perform up to the standard of care, we are absolutely capable of telling (1) whether our nurses respond to our call lights promptly in a timely manner and treat us in respect and (2) whether our patient rooms and bathrooms are kept clean and dry to prevent slipping and falling.

No doubt nurses' attributes (e.g., personality, morale to practice as a nurse, work-associated or life-associated stress level) can have an effect on their performance in practice. If our nurses (including the unlicensed assisting personnel) are rude and thoughtless in their attitude or are performing careless and obviously incorrect tasks on us, we should get angry and complain.

If we are in a Joint Commission-accredited hospital, we may voice our grievance to the Joint Commission's Complaint Line at 1-800-994-6610, 8:30 A.M. to 5:00 P.M. central time, Monday through Friday. We may voice our complaint anonymously if we prefer (Roizen & Oz, 2006).

To solve our immediate safety concerns related to our care, we must ask to talk to the unit nurse manager or the immediate supervisor of the staff nurse who we want to complain about. We may tell the unit clerk or our nurse that we have some concerns about this hospital's care environment and we want to communicate to the unit nurse manager directly as soon as possible. If this method does not work, we should call the hospital's operator and ask for the department that handles patient complaints (e.g., department of risk management). It is important for us to write down the time we make the call and the person we speak to.

However, if we prefer being anonymous, our safety concerns might not be addressed immediately.

Summary

Hospital leaders must first commit to patient safety and quality care before we will be able to receive safe care during our hospitalization. Safe hospital care will not be guaranteed without hospital leaders' commitment to promote a safe care environment. Comprehensive management strategies and evaluation plans must be in place to adequately monitor and supervise staff members' performance on a regular basis. If we unfortunately experience an adverse event or a preventable hospital harm or error (e.g., a fall, development of a pressure ulcer, or medication errors), in most of the situations hospital leaders would be legally responsible and could not exonerate themselves from blame.

References

Decaire, M. W., Bédard, M., Riendeau, J., & Forrest, R. (2006). Incidents in a psychiatric forensic setting: association with patient and staff characteristics. *Canadian Journal of Nursing Research, 38*(3), 68-80.

Hänecke, K., Tiedemann, S., Nachreiner, F., & Grzech-Suklo, H. (1998). Accident risk as a function of hours at work and time of day as determined from accident data and exposure models for the German working population. *Scandinavian Journal of Work and Environmental Health, 24*(3), 43-48.

Roizen, M. F., & Oz, M. C. (2006). *You the smart patient: An insider's handbook for getting the best treatment* (pp. 193-222). New York, NY: Free Press.

Stone, P. W., Mooney-Kane, C., Larson, E. L., Horan, T., Glance, L. G., Zwanziger, J., & Dick, A. W. (2007). Nurse working conditions and patient safety outcomes. *Medical Care, 45*(6), 571-578.

Unsafe Design of Patient Rooms

Making Patient Rooms Safer

To reduce medication errors, health care-associated infections, and patient falls, health care systems in the United States spend an estimated $200 billion each year in the construction and renovation of hospitals (Scott, 2007). What kind of design will make rooms safer for patients? What kind of unsafe design features should patients and families pay attention to?

We believe that the safe design of patient rooms should be as close to a home environment as possible, including beds and mattress, chairs, and toilet and shower areas. When designing the layout of a patient room, hospitals must put themselves in patients' positions and assume that hospitalized patients are frail. Reiling (2007) suggested that facility safety principles for inpatient care areas should be designed around the following latent conditions:

1. Automating where possible (e.g., adopting a computerized physician order entry system)
2. Having immediate accessibility of information, close to the point of service
3. Minimizing staff fatigue
4. Reducing noise
5. Involving patients with care
6. Using scalability, adaptability, and flexibility (e.g., using adaptive systems that would allow function in the future)
7. Standardizing as much as possible (e.g., standardizing location of equipment, supplies, room layout, and care processes)
8. Ensuring patients are visible to staff

Possible features of safe design and considerations for hospital patient rooms, several of which have been adopted in some hospital construction or renovation projects (e.g., Reiling, 2007; Scott, 2007) include:

1. Providing only private patient rooms to prevent health care-associated infections and medication errors due to insufficient patient identification
2. Having a designated family space in each patient room to accommodate overnight stays
3. Standardizing patient rooms when building or renovating them: To promote more effective and efficient care, design features may include having every patient room consistently designed, for example, from the location of the bathrooms, to the location of the power outlets, to bed controls, to the placement of the gloves boxes, to the light switches.
4. Installing lift infrastructures in every patient room to minimize risks and injuries during transfers: The lifting device should have the capacity to transfer a patient from bed to chair, wheelchair or bedside commode, from bed to bathroom, and in the reverse order, and from patient room floor back to bed.
5. For added safety, each patient room should be wired for the use of cameras to assist with monitoring of high-risk patients: Monitor cameras will connect directly to the nurses' station or a centralized location. Monitor cameras will be used only with the consent of the patient.
6. Building in sufficient light sources in patient rooms by using both natural and artificial light: Hospitals may install automatic lights or motion-detecting light switches that go on when a patient attempts to get out of bed or enters the bathroom.
7. Increasing the number of sinks and hand sanitizers in the hallway, installing one additional sink in each patient room (other than the one in the bathroom), and installing hand sanitizers at the bedside
8. Placing the bathroom near the head of the bed with a hand rail from the bed to the bathroom
9. Installing nonslip flooring in patient bathrooms
10. Reducing noise and vibration: Noise can negatively affect the quality of the healing environment for patients, including elevating blood pressure and altering sleep quality. Design features may include, for example, choosing vibration-reducing structural systems, using stronger steel, having sufficient insulation between rooms, having more absorbent ceiling tiles, adopting quiet-engineered mechanical systems, equipment and technology, and eliminating overhead paging.
11. Ensuring air quality: Possible design features include:
    a. Increasing air flow in patient rooms (e.g., the number of times the air is removed and returned from a patient room)
    b. Using ultraviolet filters and ultraviolet lights in inpatient care areas to eliminate airborne pathogens
    c. Using curtains on the windows, instead of blinds, to reduce condensation and the risk of infection
    d. Continuously and carefully monitoring the air quality (e.g., dust and particles in the air) in inpatient care areas whenever any ongoing renovation or construction projects are occurring within the hospital

e. Allowing at least 1 month to let chemical particles from wall painting solvents or adhesives release from the newly renovated or constructed inpatient care areas, especially in patient rooms

f. Monitoring the air humidity, room temperature, any toxic gas, and toxic substance or residuals in inpatient care areas on a regular basis

12. Supplying clean and pathogen-free tap and fountain water for drinking and use in patient room bathrooms and stand-alone sinks

13. Promoting knowledge and the free flow of medical information at bedside: Possible design features should consider allowing for greater participation of patients and their families in the care process and allowing immediate access of information to professionals at the point of service. In addition, patients and their families should be able to access their scheduled medications or other treatments prescribed at bedside.

14. Adding nursing substations between two patient rooms to help nurses spend more time with patients: Each substation should have a locked nurse-server cabinet that holds supplies and patients' bar-coded medications. The supply drawer in each nursing substation should be uniformly stocked throughout the hospital. Substations should also have windows to allow for viewing patients from the charting area.

During acute hospital stays, deconditioning, a complex process of physiologic change, may follow after a period of inactivity, bed rest, or sedentary lifestyle. Deconditioning often has an impact on patients' musculoskeletal system (e.g., diminished muscle mass and decreases in muscle strength by 2-5% per day). The decline in muscle mass and strength has been linked to inpatient falls, functional decline, increased frailty, and immobility (Gillis & MacDonald, 2005). In addition, hospitals must consider the needs of frail patients and the complexity and diversity of patients (e.g., obese, postoperative, blind, and neurologically impaired patients).

To accommodate the needs of patients during hospital stays and promote safer hospital stays, we suggest additional design features toward hospital patient beds, toilets in patient room bathrooms, and grab bars and hand rails.

Patient Bed Design

The Height of Bed by Design

The key to prevent patient falls and fall-related injuries in hospitals is using patient beds that can go as low as possible. Hospital beds should be no higher than home beds. We suggest that the height of the patient beds at the lowest position, including the mattress, should not be higher than 6 to 8 inches from the floor to the top of the mattress.

The patient beds should allow patients to control the overall height of the beds, though we suggest including only the lowering control button for patients to use. The control panel for lowering the overall height of the bed and adjusting the heights of the head and foot portion should be reachable by patients themselves.

Using Voice Reminders to Remind Staff Members to Lower Patient Beds

Nurses and physicians may raise the patient bed when delivering care, treatments, or procedures. After completing the tasks, nurses and physicians must lower the bed to its lowest position. However, most of the nurses and physicians do not have the habit of routinely lowering a patient's bed to its lowest position after completing their tasks. In fact, it is common sense that the height of beds should be maintained in the lowest position to prevent falls and fall-related injuries, especially for patients at high risk for falls.

As a result, we suggest that hospitals should install voice reminders that say "prevent injury, please lower the bed" to remind staff members to lower the overall heights of patient beds. The voice reminder should be installed by the door of the patient room and would be initiated when someone is walking out the patient room.

Bed Width by Design

The current size for hospital patient beds is 34.5 to 36 inches in width. Safe hospital patient beds should be at least 39 to 45 inches in width to be at least comparable to the twin/single size for home beds of 39 inches in width. A wider patient bed can prevent a patient from falling off the bed when turning, especially during sleep.

In other words, when lying on the midline of the bed parallel to the longer side of the bed, having a safe bed width of 45 inches would allow patients to turn freely without fear. Fear of falling may result in decreased self-initiated turning or changing positions, which may further lead to dysfunction and an increased possibility of developing pressure ulcers.

Mattress with Sufficient Air Ventilation by Design

We conducted an investigation on the mattresses designed to go with hospital patient beds, which are available on the US market. We found that except for one specialty mattress (used for patients who have developed serious stage 3 or stage 4 pressure ulcers), almost all the mattresses have a vinyl, waterproof cover to protect the mattress from getting soiled. This airtight mattress cover will provoke excessive perspiration, skin moisture, and increased heat between the skin area and the supporting surface in contact with it.

As one of the standard practices in hospitals, a cotton bed sheet will be applied on top of the vinyl mattress cover. The cotton bed sheet may absorb perspiration but is unable to promote air ventilation between the skin and the mattress. Most of the patient rooms in US hospitals are air-conditioned. However, an air-conditioned environment will not relieve the excessive skin moisture and heat between the skin and the mattress. Only the inpatients who lie on the mattresses know how hot it is and how uncomfortable the current mattress is due to excessive perspiration as provoked by the mattresses.

In addition to patients' clothes or pajamas, the cotton bed sheet can easily and quickly get soiled and wet due to the heat and excessive perspiration. If we are lucky, the cotton bed sheet is changed at least once a day. Without requesting a clean bed sheet, our bed sheet may not be changed at all during our entire hospital stay.

Providing summer sleeping mats to all inpatients is a ready-to-adopt strategy to prevent development of pressure ulcers. The purpose of using summer sleeping mats between the airtight mattress cover and the cotton bed sheet is to relieve the skin moisture and the increased heat between the skin area and the supporting surface in contact with. Summer sleeping mats have been commonly used in many areas in daily life, especially in hot and humid regions (e.g., tropical areas).

The summer sleeping mats can be made of bamboo or any other natural materials. Bamboo sleep mats use 100% natural bamboo as the weaving material. Bamboo is cool, lightweight, and absorbs moisture. The advantage of the bamboo matting is that it is smooth, soft, and cool. With a good bamboo sleeping mat, when patients lie down on the mat, their body temperature will cool down quickly. Also, patients will not feel cold and their hair will not be nipped on it.

Summer sleeping mats should be used for all patients and should be placed between the mattress and the cotton bed sheet to provide a ventilating, cool, and comfortable sleeping surface. Using bamboo sleeping mats can prevent accumulated moisture on skin areas and decrease the heat between the skin and the surface with direct contact. To increase the comfort level, the cotton bed sheet may be used, but it is not always needed depending on patients' preferences. It is also important to ensure that the summer sleeping mats are securely tied to patient beds to avoid mats sliding away from the lying area.

The bamboo sleep mats are washable and air dry quickly. For infection control purposes, even after disinfection, each patient should only use his or her own summer sleeping mat.

Adding High-low Horizontal Grab Bars or Hand Rails to Prevent Falls

Our previous study found that risk factors related to patient room setting and design included the distance and path from the bed to the bathroom, no grab bars in patient rooms to assist moving across the room, insufficient grab bars in the bathroom, and lack of traction on the bathroom grab bars (Tzeng & Yin, 2008). As a result, we suggest that high-low horizontal grab bars or hand rails should be mounted and installed on every part of the patient room walls, every part of the bathroom walls in a patient room, and in the corridors commonly used by patients (e.g., hallways from patient rooms to nurses' stations).

High-low horizontal grab bars or hand rails should be mounted with heights of 26 inches (low) and 36 inches (high) above the floor in all areas commonly used by patients (Figure 1). Such horizontal bars must be easy to grasp and to generate push-up force when needed. Short horizontal bars may be more useful than vertical bars. Some short horizontal bars may be installed as appropriate.

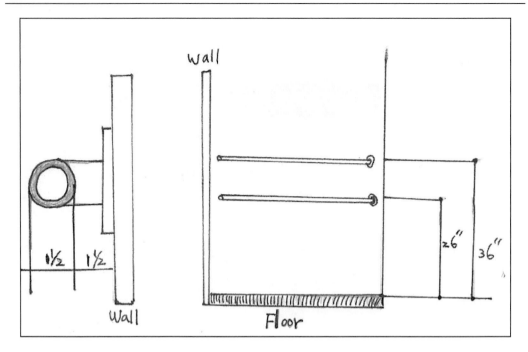

Figure 1. The high-low horizontal grab bars/hand rails. The left illustration shows the suggested specifications for grab bars. The right illustration indicates the suggested positions to mount the high-low horizontal grab bars.

Safer Toileting in Patient Bathrooms

Toileting involves stand-to-sit and sit-to-stand movements. Compared with chairs, a standard toilet in a bathroom usually has no armrest or backrest. A patient may easily lose balance when performing the stand-to-sit movement because of the hollow center and may need to hold on to something to gain upward force and rise from a toilet.

Inpatients do have an urgent need for a special design to meet their special needs and optimize functions during toilet transfers. In addition, the report of *Common ADA Errors and Omissions in New Construction and Alterations* (US Department of Justice, 2002) indicated that people who have mobility disabilities (e.g., walk with a cane, a walker, or crutches or have limited balance) typically find that using a toilet with parallel grab bars mounted on the right and left sides of the toilet is easier and safer than using one that has grab bars installed on one side wall and the back wall. Based on this report and our observations on patients' needs, we suggest that hospitals adopt two toileting safety elements: (1) renovating toilets to a 21.5-inch height from the floor to the top of the seat, and (2) mounting a U-shaped support stand (U-stand) on the bathroom floor around the toilet to be used as hand rails (Figure 2).

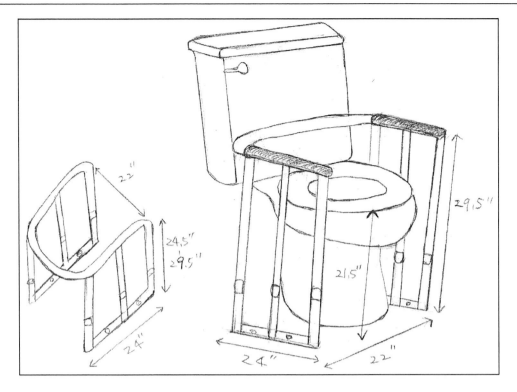

Figure 2. The U-shaped support stand to be used to enhance patient safety when performing the toileting movements.

Toilet Seat Height by Design

The toilet seat height should consider the burden to patients' hip and knee joints. Unfortunately, as we know, no research has investigated the appropriate toilet seat height for healthy or frail patients. Some studies did address the appropriate height of chairs. For example, Demura and Yamada (2007) suggested that the range of a safe chair seat height should be no lower than 80% of the lower leg length. A chair seat height of about 120% of a patient lower leg length was recommended.

After considering the specifications of the toilet-related equipment currently available on the US market, a toilet seat height of 21.5 inches is recommended. Hospitals may install new toilets with a high profile of 21.5 inches. Another option is to mount a standard toilet on the top of a product, such as a "toilevator," to raise the toilet base. As an alternative, hospitals may include raised toilet seats as standard toilet equipment in patient rooms.

Installing a U-shaped Support Stand around the Toilet

This U-stand was designed to be used as a hand rail and to resolve risk factors when a patient is performing the toileting movement (Figure 2). It is intended to provide parallel armrests and a backrest to support users (a three-sided support) and to be used to help generate needed push-up force when the patient is performing the sit-to-stand movement from the toilet seat.

Such a design would fit most toilets, with or without water tanks. A U-stand should be mounted to the floor of the bathroom to increase sturdiness. A fixed floor-mounted U-shaped stand is preferred because it would be steadier and could offer better support than a removable one. In addition, the frame of this U-stand should be made of 1-inch steel tubing to bear the weight of a patient up to 400 pounds and have an adjustable armrest height (24.5-29.5 inches). This U-stand may be used on a standard toilet with a toilet seat height of 16.5 to 21.5 inches.

The height of the U-stand should be adjusted to fit the users. If the armrests are too high, the user may not be able to use the U-stand to produce an upward force to lift his or her body from the toilet seat. The armrest height should be adjusted to be about 8 inches above the toilet seat; if the seat height is 17 inches, the U-stand should be adjusted to 25 inches. Foam padding should extend to the entire length of the armrest for added comfort and protection. The suggested width between the armrests is 22 inches, including the width of the armrests.

As an alternative to install a U-stand, hospitals may place a bedside commode on the top of the toilet. The purpose, the same as installing a U-shaped support stand around the toilet, is to ease the physical exertion when trying to get up from the toilet seat. If a bedside commode is used, the sturdiness and the amount of weight-bearing of the commode must be evaluated carefully before use to avoid potential risks of slipping and falling.

Reporting our Concerns about Unsafe Patient Rooms

When we are hospitalized in a medical or surgical unit, an intensive care unit, or a psychiatric hospital, a safe care environment is key to promoting our recovery and healing. If we are in a Joint Commission-accredited hospital, we may voice our grievance to the Joint Commission's Complaint Line at 1-800-994-6610 on weekdays, 8:30 A.M. to 5:00 P.M. central time; we can call anonymously, if we prefer (Roizen & Oz, 2006).

To solve our immediate safety concerns related to our care environment (e.g., wet floor, poor lighting, broken equipment, a unsteady IV stand with wheels, malfunctioning bed, and unsteady bedside chair), we must talk to our nurse or request the opportunity to discuss our concerns with the unit nurse manager. Our nurse may replace the malfunctioning equipment or furniture by other items that are in good condition.

Unfortunately, poor equipment and little furniture maintenance are commonly seen in hospitals. For instance, a broken bed may not be replaced by a good one immediately because no back-up systems are in place and scheduled inspection and preventive maintenance are lacking. This is definitely a problem in hospital management. For our safety, we must complain and speak up.

We may tell the unit clerk or our nurse that we have some concerns about this hospital's care environment and we want to communicate this to the unit nurse manager directly as soon as possible. If this method does not work, we should call the hospital's operator and ask for the department that handles patient complaints (e.g., department of risk management). It is important for us to write down the time we place the call and the person we speak to.

After all, a safe care environment with a safe patient room design is a must to ensure our physical safety during hospital stays. If we complain for a condition of unsafe care environment, we may not benefit from the improvement right away. However, without our input and urge for changes in the US hospital environment, our families and friends or even ourselves may suffer in a future use of hospital inpatient services. Long before we start to judge whether we are receiving good quality of care during our hospitalization, we should first ask for a safe patient room. Indeed, maintaining a safe care environment is one of the primary responsibilities of nursing leaders and nurses.

Referentes

Demura, S., & Yamada, T. (2007). Height of chair seat and movement characteristics in sit-to-stand by young and elderly adults. *Perceptual and Motor Skills, 104*(1), 21-31.

Gillis, A., & MacDonald, B. (2005). Deconditioning in the hospitalized elderly. *Canadian Nurse, 101*(6), 16-20.

Reiling, J. G. (2007). Creating a culture of patient safety through innovative hospital design. In Agency for Healthcare Research and Quality (publisher), *Advances in patient safety: From research to implementation* (Vol. 2, *Concept and methodology*, pp. 425-438). Available at: http://www.ahrq.gov/downloads/pub/advances/vol2/Reiling.pdf (accessed January 16, 2008).

Roizen, M. F., & Oz, M. C. (2006). *You the smart patient: An insider's handbook for getting the best treatment* (pp. 193-222). New York, NY: Free Press.

Scott, D. E. (2007). Designing safer patient rooms. *American Nurse*, 2007(November/December), 7.

Tzeng, H. M., & Yin, C. Y. (2008). The extrinsic risk factors for inpatient falls in hospital patient rooms. *Journal of Nursing Care Quality, 23*(3) (in press).

US Department of Justice (2002). Common ADA errors and omissions in new construction and alterations. Washington, D.C.: US. Department of Justice, Civil Rights Division, Disability Rights Section. (Accessed November 6, 2007, at http://www.usdoj.gov/crt/ada/errors.pdf.)

Section III: Knowing Why

Say NO to Poor Care Safety I: Poor Communication among Health Care Providers

Promoting Effective Communications among Health Care Providers

As indicated in the National Patient Goals for 2008, Goal 2-Requirement 2E, and the *2008 Comprehensive Accreditation Manual for Hospitals: The Official Handbook* (Joint Commission, 2007), the Joint Commission requires hospitals to implement a standardized approach to hand-off communications among health care providers, and this approach should include an opportunity for health care providers to ask and respond to questions. Hand-off refers to passing necessary patient information from one health care provider to another. This requirement applies to general hospitals, psychiatric hospitals, and the units that provide behavioral health care.

The several types of patient hand-off include but are not limited to:

1. A nurse transfers responsibility of a patient to the other nurse during the change of nursing shift or from one unit to the other unit.
2. A physician transfers the complete responsibility of a patient to the other physician.
3. A physician transfers on-call responsibility to the other physician.
4. A staff member (e.g., a physician, nurse, or nursing attendants) temporarily transfers responsibility to the other staff to be able to leave the unit for a short time.
5. An anesthesiologist reports to a postanesthesia recovery room nurse.
6. The responsible nurse or physician transfers a patient from the emergency room to an inpatient care unit, a different hospital, a nursing home, or home health care agency.

7. The critical laboratory or radiology results are sent to a physician's office.
8. In a behavioral health care unit or facility, hand-offs may occur at change of shift, from clinical staff to program staff, or from teacher to child care worker.

The purpose of this requirement is to ensure that accurate information about a patient's current condition, care plan, treatment, and any recent or anticipated changes is communicated during a hand-off (Joint Commission, 2007). To effectively complete a hand-off, nurses must allocate specific time to perform the hand-off communications and allow time to ask and respond questions (Joint Commission, 2006).

The Expectations from the Joint Commission

The Joint Commission (2007) listed five implementation expectations to achieve Goal 2, Requirement 2E:

1. A hospital's process for effective hand-off communications must involve interactive communications that allow for the opportunity for questioning between the giver and receiver of patient information.
2. A hand-off communication should include the up-to-date patient care plan, treatment, condition, and any recent or anticipated changes.
3. A hand-off communication must involve a process for verification of the received information as appropriate (e.g., repeat-back or read-back).
4. A hand-off communication should provide an opportunity for the receiver of the hand-off information to review the patient's relevant historical data (e.g., previous care plans and treatment).
5. Interruptions during the hand-off process should be limited to avoid ineffective communication or incomplete exchange of information.

These five expectations also apply to psychiatric hospitals and the psychiatric units in general hospitals that provide inpatient care services 24 hours day, 7 days a week.

Possible Solutions to Improve Hand-off Communication

Verbal reports that occur at shift changes are often hurried. The off-duty staffs (e.g., nurses or physicians) are frequently eager to leave. As a result, the Joint Commission suggested that each hospital should standardize its approach on how the information is exchanged during hand-off communications to ensure that information about a patient's condition and care plan are not lost or forgotten.

As a matter of fact, communication failures have been identified as one of the root causes for 65% of all sentinel events reported to the Joint Commission. As one of the hospital accreditation requirements, hospitals are currently under pressure to make communications among health care providers complete, accurate, timely, and clear (Joint Commission, 2006).

One of the main concerns to effective communication is the difference in communication styles used between nurses and physicians. Nurses often take more of a narrative and descriptive approach to explaining a medical situation (e.g., changes in a patient's condition). However, when answering a call from a nurse, a physician typically wants to hear only the main headings of a situation from the nurse, as a professional habit or simply to shorten the communication time.

To bridge this gap in the communication styles between nurses and physicians, the Joint Commission (2006) suggested that when a nurse is calling a physician for a situation, this nurse should convey the patient's needs by using medical diagnoses and offer options as appropriate. The Joint Commission further recommended using the situational briefing model of communication as developed at Kaiser Permanente of Colorado (also called the SBAR technique).

The situation-background-assessment-recommendation (SBAR) technique provides clinical nurses a framework for communicating with physicians about a patient's condition (Institute for Healthcare Improvement, 2007). For example, when a nurse is contacting a physician, the SBAR process can be followed to enhance communication:

1. Situation: What is the situation I am calling about?
    1.1. I must identify myself, my unit, the patient I am calling about, and the room number.
    1.2. I should briefly describe the problem, when it occurred or started, and how severe it is as I have observed.
2. Background: What background information is important to the situation of the patient I am calling for? Any of the following information may be included but is not limited to:
    2.1. The admitting diagnosis and date of admission
    2.2. List of current medications and treatments, allergies, and critical laboratory results
    2.3. Most recent vital signs
    2.4. Code status
3. Assessment: What is my assessment of the situation?
4. Recommendation: What do I recommend or what do I want the physician to decide?

Summary: Communication Is Crucial in the Effort of Promoting Patient Safety

The SBAR technique can be a format used to frame any conversation, especially critical ones that require a physician's immediate attention and action (Institute for Healthcare Improvement, 2007). Nurses may also use the SBAR technique to communicate with not only physicians and the other health care providers, but also patients and their families in the process of providing patient education.

The SBAR technique is an easy-to-remember, concrete mechanism to convey information. Patients and families may also want to adopt this model in the process of understanding their own or their hospitalized loved one's physical and psychological status.

References

Institute for Healthcare Improvement (2007). SBAR technique for communication: A situation briefing model. Available at: http://www.ihi.org/IHI/Topics/PatientSafety /SafetyGeneral/Tools/SBARTechniqueforCommunicationASituationalBriefingModel.ht m (accessed December 12, 2007).

Joint Commission (2006). Goal 2: Improve the effectiveness of communication among caregivers. In A. Grayson. (Ed.), *Meeting the Joint Commission's 2007 National Patient Safety Goals* (pp. 17-36). Oakbrook Terrace, IL: Joint Commission.

Joint Commission (2007). *2008 Comprehensive accreditation manual for hospitals: The official handbook*. Oakbrook Terrace, IL: Joint Commission Resources.

Say NO to Poor Care Safety II: Incorrect Patient Identification in the Process of Providing Care

Background

The Joint Commission (2006) used a story published in the *Chicago Sun-Times* on May 11, 2005 (Fischer, 2005) to illustrate the importance of using at least two patient identifiers to avoid wrong-patient errors.

> A female patient had a mastectomy in February 2005 after a biopsy, which indicated that she had breast cancer. Several weeks later, this patient learned shocking news that her surgeon had removed her healthy breast because the laboratory had substituted another woman's biopsy results for hers.

When we are hospitalized, we are supposed to receive the care, treatment, or procedures that our primary responsible physician has ordered for us for the medical, surgical, or emotional problems that resulted in this particular hospitalization. In some ways, it is hard for patients and families to imagine that we may suffer preventable hospital harms and errors as a consequence of incorrect patient identification.

Ensuring correct patient identification in the process of inpatient care provision is indeed the obligation of the health care provider who implements the order. However, wrong-patient errors occur in inpatient care settings. The Joint Commission (2007) claimed that wrong-patient errors occur in practically all aspects of diagnosis and treatment. Such errors are not a hospital legend!

Preventing Wrong-Patient Errors

As indicated in the National Patient Goals for 2008, Goal 1 Requirement 1A, and the *2008 Comprehensive Accreditation Manual for Hospitals: The Official Handbook* (Joint Commission, 2007), the Joint Commission demanded that hospitals use at least two patient identifiers when providing care, treatments, or services. It is crucial to reliably identify the patient as the one for whom the care or treatment is intended and to match the care or treatment to the correct patient.

Two pieces of patient-specific information can be, for example, the patient's name and date of birth. The Joint Commission accepts the use of the information indicated on a patient's undamaged, identification wristband, being worn by the patient (Joint Commission, 2006).

The Joint Commission (2007) also listed five implementation expectations to achieve Goal 1 Requirement 1A:

1. Hospitals must use two patient identifiers when administering medication or blood products.
2. Hospitals should use two patient identifiers when collecting blood samples or other specimens for clinical or diagnostic tests (e.g., biopsy). It is essential for hospitals to establish the workflow to maintain each individual patient sample's identity through the pre-analytical, analytical, and post-analytical processes (e.g., ensuring the correct label on the specimen tube or vial).
3. Hospitals are required to use two patient identifiers when providing treatment or procedures other than the ones indicated in expectations 1 and 2.
4. It is crucial that a patient's room number or physical location not be used as an identifier.
5. The container used for blood and other specimens should be labeled in the presence of the patient.

Patient Verification Immediately before the Start of any Invasive Procedure

The Joint Commission (2006) also urged hospitals to conduct a final verbal verification process to confirm the correct patient, procedure, site, and availability of appropriate documents, immediately prior to the start of any invasive procedure. This process should be an active communication technique and must involve the entire surgical team.

A final verbal verification process should be conducted prior to the following procedures involving (Joint Commission, 2006):

1. Puncture or incision of the skin (e.g., an operation, a bone marrow collection, or a fine-needle aspiration)
2. Insertion of an instrument or a foreign material into the body

3. Percutaneous aspirations
4. Biopsies
5. Cardiac and vascular catheterization

In this final verbal verification process, it is essential to ensure four correct identifications and one agreement (Joint Commission, 2006):

1. Correct patient identity
2. Correct procedure and site
3. Correct patient position
4. Ensuring the availability of the correct implant, special equipment, or requirement to be used for the procedure
5. Agreement reached between the patient or family and the primary responsible doctor (e.g., the surgeon) on the procedure to be done

A patient's identity should be re-established if the in-charge health care provider (e.g., a surgeon, nurse, or laboratory technician) leaves the patient's room or location prior to initiating the procedure. For instance, it is essential for the surgeon to mark the procedure site, unless the surgeon is in continuous attendance from the time of the decision to do the procedure and the patient consents to the initiation of the procedure. However, this situation may not always occur. Consequently, re-establishing patient identity is necessary if the in-charge health care provider leaves the patient's room or location prior to initiating the procedure.

Minor procedures may not need an extensive final verification process. Minor procedures include peripheral IV line placement or insertion of a nasogastric (NG) tube or Foley catheter (Joint Commission, 2006). Still, at least two patient identifiers should be verified before starting a procedure.

The Joint Commission (2006) further emphasized that anyone (including physicians, nurses, or laboratory personnel) who collects samples should use at least two identifiers to ensure correct patient identification. It is important to label the specimen container in the presence of the patient.

In other words, no prior labeling of collection container should be permitted in the laboratory and in inpatient care units. If possible, hospitals should enforce using the same two identifiers across inpatient care units and departments.

A hospital's laboratory should also establish written guidelines for rejecting the specimens that are received in the laboratory without complete identification. When this situation occurs, a cautionary statement on the laboratory report should be documented that the specimen was received without complete identification (Joint Commission, 2006).

Summary: Save ourselves by Identifying ourselves to our Health Care Providers

From a patient or a family's perspective, ensuring correct patient identification in the process of receiving inpatient care is taken for granted. Wrong-patient errors should never occur to us. Such errors should not ever happen at all!

What can patients do to prevent wrong-patient errors? Prior to receiving any medication, treatment, or procedures, we may verify ourselves to the nurse, physician, or laboratory personnel by telling our health care provider: (1) who we are (first and last names) and (2) our primary medical problem for this hospitalization. This action, as an active involvement in our care, can be the key to saving ourselves from wrong-patient errors.

Another thing we can pay attention to is the blue wristband. At the time we are admitted to the hospital, we are given a blue wristband, which is more or less like our name tag. However, errors have often been detected on patients' blue wristbands (e.g., a wrong name or a wrong hospital registration number). As a must-do safety tip, we should always make sure that the information printed on our blue wristband is correct, readable, and intact throughout the entire hospital stay. If our blue wristband falls off or becomes unreadable, we should tell our nurse right away. Our nurse should make a new one for us immediately.

Sometimes, hospital staff or nurses in our inpatient care unit may put more wristbands with different colors on us to signify that we are, for example, at high risk for falling. Regardless of how many wristbands we have, we must ask for the purpose of each wristband and the significance of the color we are wearing.

References

Fischer, B. (2005). U of C hospitals sued for error that resulted in removal of breast. *Chicago Sun-Times,* May 11, 2005.

Joint Commission (2006). Goal 1: Improve the accuracy of patient identification. In A. Grayson. (Ed.), *Meeting the Joint Commission's 2007 National Patient Safety Goals* (pp. 9-16). Oakbrook Terrace, IL: Joint Commission.

Joint Commission (2007). *2008 Comprehensive accreditation manual for hospitals: The official handbook.* Oakbrook Terrace, IL: Joint Commission Resources.

Learning the Facts from Research I: The Family Involvement Culture in the US Hospital Environment

Background

Family involvement in inpatient care is increasingly emphasized to provide safe and error-free care (Remen, 2006). As indicated in the National Patient Safety Goals for 2008, Goal 3, the Joint Commission (2007) emphasized the need to define and communicate ways for patients and their families to report concerns about safety and encourage them to do so. As the first step, hospitals and clinicians should encourage family members to visit their loved ones frequently. However, the roles of family members and the economic burdens on families have not been well addressed in the US communities or studied by researchers (Tzeng, 2004).

Family visitors can provide psychological support and physical care to patients but cannot replace nurses in preventing incidents and injuries (e.g., inpatient falls, suicides, and pressure ulcers). There is no doubt that family visitors can increase the safety of the inpatient care provision by, for example, providing one-on-one constant observation to the high-risk patients for fall or suicide. Family visitors may also assist nurses in cleaning and repositioning the patient to prevent pressure sores.

Due to the enormous gap in medical knowledge of patient care between patients and clinicians (e.g., physicians, nurses, or pharmacists), clinicians, especially nurses, are fully obligated to inpatients' safety, with or without the presence of families. Depending on the capabilities and responsibilities of patients' families, family visitors can contribute to positive patient outcomes. For example, a family companion who is a professional nurse or physician can most likely prevent a fall and enhance patient safety during a hospital stay (Tzeng, 2004; Tzeng & Yin, 2007).

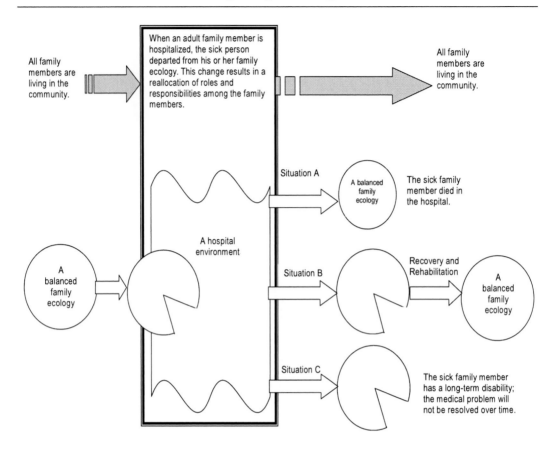

Figure 1.The dynamic balance model of family ecology: In the scenario where an adult loved one is hospitalized.

1. A circle indicates that a balance is reached in family ecology (e.g., successful reallocation of family matter-related obligations among family members). A circle with an indentation means that at least one family member cannot perform his or her roles within the family (e.g., economic responsibility) and may expect another family member to care for him or her (e.g., during rehabilitation or recovery). If a family member dies, the diameter of the circle decreases to indicate the shrinkage in the total number of members included in the family ecology. If a new family member is added (e.g., an infant, an adult through marriage), the diameter of the circle would increase. If the newly added member requires care by another member (e.g., an infant), this circle is indented.

2. Three situations, as examples, are graphed into this figure to illustrate the dynamic balance in family ecology. Situation A: If the hospitalized family member died before being discharged, the circle diameter would decrease as the total number of family members decreases. Situation B: If the loved one lives after a hospital discharge and returns to the community, the family ecology would not be able to immediately reach a balance because this sick family member may still need someone to care for him or her during rehabilitation or recovery. A balance may not be reached until this sick family member recovers to the extent that he or she can perform previously assumed roles and obligations before the most recent hospital admission. Situation C: If the sick loved one lives after a hospital discharge and returns to the community with a permanent disability (e.g., quadriplegia after a car accident), the family ecology would not be able to reach a balance because this sick family member still needs care.

Family Ecology: What's Happening when a Loved One is Hospitalized?

The concept of family ecology was developed based on previous studies related to family involvement (Tzeng, 2004; Tzeng & Yin, 2007; Tzeng et al., 2007) and research in social ecology (McLeroy et al., 1988). Family ecology deals with the spatial and temporal interactions within a family, which may include as few as two members or be as extensive as a clan. Because members of the same family ecology are interdependent, an invisible ecology chain links all the members together as a joint operation coexistent entity.

Family members often have to juggle their time and energy among their various obligations, roles, and relationships with, for example, their economic and social organizations. Over someone's life span, seeking ways to find a balance in a family ecology is required. In fact, we are constantly balancing our life among various tasks needing to be completed.

Figure 1 uses the scenario of an adult loved one being hospitalized to illustrate the dynamic balance in family ecology among the rest of the family members. A family's ecology is assumed to change over time because of birth, aging, disease, and death. Its dynamic balance may be reached when the ecologic chain is modified.

When an adult from the same family ecology is hospitalized, the balance of this family ecology is inevitably disturbed. Some or all of the rest of the family members have to find time to visit this person (the patient). The patient's previously assumed responsibilities must be reallocated to the other family members. The rest of the family members may need to share financial, housekeeping, and caring responsibilities to keep the routine family activities running.

If the hospitalization demands out-of-pocket medical-related expenses (e.g., a surcharge for staying in a private room, copayment for medications), the financial burden to the other family members would increase. Added economic responsibility to a working person may result in, for example, more overtime hours for extra income. The other family members must strive to regain the balance of their disturbed family ecology.

An Empirical Study of the Family Involvement Culture in the United States

Do US hospitals have a culture of family involvement? We could not find an answer for this question. As a result, we conducted a study to investigate the extent to which family members visit their loved ones during hospital stays in a US hospital environment. This descriptive study was conducted in two acute medical units (A unit and B unit) and one pediatric medical and rehabilitation unit (C unit) of a Michigan medical center in early 2007. The head counts of family visitors at bedside on two weekdays and two weekend days at three time points a day were recorded. Each patient room was visited only once at each data collection time point. The institutional review board of the University of Michigan reviewed and approved this study.

Table 1. Descriptive information on family involvement-related variables

Variable/Frequency	Unit A: Adult medical care unit	Unit B: Adult medical care unit	Unit C: Pediatric care unit
No. of occupied beds	358 (93.2%)	362 (94.3%)	430 (81.4%)
Patient gender: Male	218 (60.9%)	158 (43.6%)	246 (57.5%)
Having a sitter at bedside	7 (2.1%)	9 (2.6%)	0 (0%)
Having at least one family visitor (all data)	79 (23.2%)	82 (24.0%)	254 (67.2%)
Data collected on*			
Weekdays	33 (19.4%)	35 (20.0%)	144 (73.1%)
Weekend days	47 (27.5%)	47 (28.1%)	112 (61.2%)
Data collected at:			
Morning (9:00 A.M. to 10:30 A.M.)	17 (14.2%)	21 (17.8%)	96 (71.6%)
Afternoon (2:00 P.M. to 3:30 P.M.)	36 (33.3%)	28 (26.2%)	80 (65.0%)
Evening (7:00 P.M. to 8:30 P.M.)	26 (23.2)	33 (28.2%)	78 (64.5%)

* Data were collected on two weekdays and two weekend days.

Main Study Findings

A total of 1296 observations were recorded and 1150 (88.7%) were occupied beds. Among the occupied beds, 622 patients (53.9%) were male and 531 (46.1%) were female. Only 16 patients (1.5%) had a hospital-paid sitter at the bedside. A total of 418 patients (39.3%) had family visitors. Among these 418 observations, 294 (70.5%) had only one family visitor, 86 (20.6%) had two, 24 (5.8%) had three, 7 (1.7%) had four, 2 (0.5%) had five, 3 (0.7%) had six, and 7 (0.2%) had seven. Table 1 illustrates additional descriptive information to compare the differences across three study units.

We found that among adult patients, 23.2% to 24% had at least one family visitor. More family visitors came during weekend days and in the afternoon or evening. Among pediatric patients, 67.2% had at least one family visitor and more family visitors came to be with sick children during the weekdays.

These finding suggested that the study hospital had a popular culture of family involvement for hospitalized sick children. However, only about 24% of the adult patients had at least one family visitor. In other words, adult patients were expected to have at least one family member visit every other day. Because this study did not survey the relationships between the patients and the visitors, family visitors could be relatives, neighbors, friends, or colleagues.

Lessons Learned from this Study

When a Child is Hospitalized

As a study limitation, this study did not collect family composition information in detail (e.g., socioeconomic status, ethnic background, religious and cultural values, and total number of household members). We inferred that when the sick family member was a child, most families would spare at least one adult family member to accompany the patient for the entire hospital stay.

A common belief is that having at least one familiar face accompany the sick child may promote the healing process and may decrease stress levels caused by staying in an unfamiliar surrounding and receiving medical treatments and procedures. To spend time at bedside, these family members most likely have to be either working a flexible schedule, taking personal or vacation leave from work, or be unemployed (e.g., retirees or homemakers). When a child is hospitalized, the economic burden and time commitment on the adult family members are significant.

When an Adult Family Member is Hospitalized

Compared with pediatric patients, study findings showed that family visitors were almost two thirds less common for adult patients. Regardless of health status before hospital admission, these patients were frail and may have had life-threatening medical problems. Family members may perceive their adult loved one as being less vulnerable than a sick child. Consequently, compared with pediatric inpatients, having family visitors for adult inpatients was less popular.

In addition, when an adult loved one is hospitalized, the rest of the family members have to seek a balance by redistributing various family-related responsibilities (Figure 1). Regardless of ethnic and cultural background, the phenomenon of involving family members in their loved one's inpatient care is a complicated ecologic concept that involves each individual's personal life and the relationship with economic and social entities.

The Expected Roles of Family Visitors in Inpatient Care

Hospital care is assumed to fulfill each inpatient's physiologic needs (Maslow's level 1—human needs). If this assumption is true, more research is needed to investigate whether family involvement can promote Maslow's level 2 human needs—safety. Having family visitors during a hospital stay undoubtedly can fulfill Maslow's level 3 human needs—love and socialization.

However, Kalisch's study (2006) concluded that some patients' physiologic needs in acute care settings have been missed by nurses and nursing attendants. In addition, previous studies (Tzeng & Yin, 2007; Tzeng et al., 2007) suggested that most of the family visitors assumed their responsibility to fulfill their loved one's physiologic needs during hospital stays. As a matter of fact, researchers have limited understanding about the expected roles of family visitors in participating in inpatient care from their own points of view.

Private Rooms versus Semiprivate Rooms: The Patients Staying in the Semiprivate Rooms Had More Visitors!

Among the adult patients who stayed in private rooms, 14.2% ($n = 97$) had at least one family visitor and 37.2% ($n = 254$) had no family visitors; for those who stayed in semiprivate rooms, 9.5% ($n = 65$) had at least one family visitor, and 39.1% ($n = 267$) had no family visitors. Study findings suggested that staying in a private room did not correlate with having more frequent family visits than staying in a semiprivate room.

According to our observations, the competition in the extensiveness of family involvement among the patients who stayed in semiprivate rooms may result in a certain social pressure on their family members. For example, family members may feel obligated to visit the hospitalized loved one more often than before. In addition, a patient may have certain expectations from the family members (e.g., staying longer at bedside with the patient). An adult or a pediatric patient may indicate that the other patients in the same room had more family visitors than he or she had. This patient may ask family members to visit and may expect a comparable number of visitors as the other patients in the same room.

Most patients have to pay an extra charge for a private room. This may indicate that these patients are financially secure enough to pay for privacy. If a patient in a private room is wealthier than one in a semiprivate room, the wealthy patient would likely have more family visits. However, the competition for love and socialization between patients in the same semiprivate room may be the main contributor to a higher family visit frequency; this would not apply to patients staying in private rooms.

If this assumption is true, staying in a private room should not mean increased family involvement. A semiprivate room has limited designated space for family visitors, however. Still, we may see more frequent family visitors in semiprivate rooms than in private rooms.

Regulations Related to the Design of Patient Rooms: Private Rooms are Preferred!

As indicated in the *2006 Guidelines for Design and Construction of Health Care Facilities* (Facility Guidelines Institute, 2006), single-bed rooms are the minimum standard for medical/surgical and postpartum nursing units in general hospitals. The executive summary of *The Use of Single Patient Rooms versus Multiple Occupancy Rooms in Acute Care Environments* (American Institute of Architects, 2003) addressed the rationale of having single-bed rooms as the minimum standard. This report claimed that private or single-occupancy rooms, which have been the trend in hospital design, may improve patient care and satisfaction and reduce the risk of contracting health care-associated infections (American Institute of Architects, 2003).

After considering other organizational and patient outcomes (e.g., operational costs per patient day and inpatient fall rates), it is still unknown whether patients and insurance companies are willing to pay an extra charge for private rooms. Especially, the US health care environment is currently under enormous pressure to improve the safety and quality of patient care and restrain the increasing health care-related expenses at the same time.

A safe patient room design should consider a hospital's capital cost, operating costs and corresponding income, patients' and insurance companies' willingness to pay an extra charge, and patients' privacy preferences. Here we ask: Is having all private rooms in hospitals the answer to promote a culture of family involvement? The answer to this question may vary depending on patients' socioeconomic status and family ecology.

Innovative Patient Room Design Ideas to Promote Family Involvement

Space in a private or semiprivate room is precious. When promoting a culture of family involvement in acute care settings (e.g., adding seating furniture for family members), hospitals need space-saving ideas to efficiently use the available space in each patient room, especially for semiprivate rooms.

We suggested that each inpatient care unit should have enough sofa beds or recliners for family visitors. Ideally, each private room should have a recliner as standard furniture, and each semiprivate room should have two recliners; these recliners should not be removed from patient rooms. In Asian countries (e.g., Taiwan, China, Japan, etc.), one recliner always goes with a patient bed in acute, medical, or surgical inpatient units. These recliners can be used as bedside chairs and may convert to a flat bench for sleeping.

When purchasing sofa beds or recliners for family visitors, hospital and nurse leaders should consider how to store these sofa beds or recliners. If these sofa beds or recliners will not be kept in patient rooms, it would be helpful to incorporate such furniture into the interior design of the family rooms or the public areas within an inpatient care unit for better maintenance and equipment management (e.g., lightweight sofa beds with wheels).

As for the room design, a love seat designed to be used as a twin bed may be mounted to the patient room wall (similar to a folding shower chair). When someone needs to use the seat, it can be pulled down. After use, the seat can be easily folded back. Such innovative design ideas may be economical and save the precious space in both semiprivate and private rooms.

References

American Institute of Architects (2003). Executive summary: The use of single patient rooms versus multiple occupancy rooms in acute care environments. Available at: http://www.aia.org/SiteObjects/files/05_Pilot_Study_on_Assessment.pdf (accessed October 3, 2007)

Facility Guidelines Institute (2006). *Guidelines for design and construction of health care facilities*. Washington, DC: The American Institute of Architects.

Joint Commission (2007). *2008 Comprehensive accreditation manual for hospitals: The official handbook*. Oakbrook Terrace, IL: Joint Commission Resources.

Kalisch, B. J. (2006). Missed nursing care: a qualitative study. *Journal of Nursing Care Quality, 21*(4), 306-313.

McLeroy, K. R., Bibeau, D., Steckler, A., & Glanz, K. (1988). An ecological perspective on health promotion programs. *Health Education Quarterly, 15*(4), 351-377.

Remen, R. N. (2006). Including your patients in a culture of safety. In M. McGreevey (Ed.), *Patients as partners: How to involve patients and families in their own care* (pp. 7-31). Oakbrook Terrace, IL: Joint Commission.

Tzeng, H. M. (2004). Roles of nurse aides and family members in acute patient care in Taiwan. *Journal of Nursing Care Quality, 19*(2), 169–175.

Tzeng, H. M., & Yin, C. Y. (2007). Involving family visitors, sitters, or volunteers in preventing inpatient falls. *Journal of Nursing Administration, 37*(7-8), 329-334.

Tzeng, H. M., Yin, C. Y., Tsai, S. L., Lin, S., & Yin, T. J. C. (2007). Patient falls and open visiting hours: A case study in a Taiwanese medical center. *Journal of Nursing Care Quality, 22*(2), 145-151.

Learning the Facts from Research II: Historical Human Resource Issues Related to Hospital Nursing

Background

In the 1990s, the importance of human resource systems and related strategies surfaced. Regardless of the types of business and service industries, current human resource systems primarily emphasize individual human resource functions, including recruitment, selection, training, compensation, and performance appraisals. These functions have been aligned with each other and linked to the overall strategies of the organization (Khatri et al., 2006).

Previous studies in health care institutions have added to our understanding of the links between nursing staffing levels and mix and outcome indicators (e.g., fall rates, length of stay, mortality; Aiken, Clarke, & Sloane, 2002; Needleman et al., 2002). Buchan (2004) claimed that research on magnet hospitals has been ongoing for over 20 years. Findings have highlighted positive links between good human resource practices (e.g., being successful in recruiting, retaining, and motivating nursing staff), staffing characteristics, and outcomes of care. However, these studies did not directly address specific human resource management interventions (Buchan, 2004).

Magnet Recognition and Good Human Resource Practice

The American Nurses Credentialing Center (2007a-d) first started the magnet research study in 1983 and formally established the Magnet Recognition Program in 1997. Magnet recognition was meant to acknowledge hospitals with good human resource practice. This program focused on advancement toward three goals:

1. Promoting quality in a setting that supported professional practice
2. Identifying excellence in the delivery of nursing services to patients

3. Disseminating best practices in nursing services

The requirements for designation as a magnet hospital included 14 forces of magnetism, as follows (American Nurses Credentialing Center, 2007a):

1. Quality of nursing leadership
2. Organizational structure
3. Management style
4. Personnel policies and programs
5. Professional models of care
6. Quality of care
7. Quality improvement
8. Consultation and resources
9. Autonomy
10. Community and the health care organization
11. Nurses as teachers
12. Image of nursing
13. Interdisciplinary relationships
14. Professional development

Dimensions of Human Resource Management

On the basis of Donabedian's (1966) structure, process, and outcome model, we further categorized the 14 forces of magnetism, as identified by American Nurses Credentialing Center (2007a), into three orientations:

1. The structural orientation: Forces of organizational structure, management style, consultation and resources, and community and the health care organization
2. The process orientation related to employers and employees: Forces of quality of nursing leadership, professional models of care, quality improvement, autonomy, nurses as teachers, interdisciplinary relationships, and professional development
3. The outcome orientation: Forces of quality of care and image of nursing

For health care sectors, Buchan (2004) suggested three groups of human resource management-related indicators:

1. Activity-related indicators (e.g., occupied beds)
2. Staffing-related indicators (e.g., job satisfaction, absence, overtime, retention, accidents or injuries, assaults on staff, vacancy rates, and use of temporary staff)
3. Care-related indicators (e.g., patient length of stay, readmission rates, mortality rates, urinary tract infections, pneumonia, pressure ulcers, cross-infections, and patient satisfaction)

We assumed that human resource issues at the hospital and executive levels (e.g., organizational structure, strategic management, and culture) would have an influence on human resource allocations, management practices, and effectiveness. Strategic management in human resource practices may lead to different nursing care-related outcomes. As a result, defining the crucial components of human resource management in nursing is needed. It is also important to acknowledge imperative human resource management components by analyzing the human resource management-related issues that have been addressed in published research and non-research reports.

Identifying the Historical Human Resource Issues Related to Hospital Nursing in the Past 30 Years (1977–2006)

We conducted a descriptive study to identify the historical human resource issues related to hospital nursing in the past 30 years. Development of the historical trends in human resource issues of hospital nursing would allow us to capture the picture of discoveries, generalized knowledge, and gaps in knowledge. The journal articles published in the three oldest nursing journals were the sources of data: *American Journal of Nursing, Nursing Outlook*, and *Nursing Research*. Content analyses were conducted. A typology of human resource issues in hospital nursing was developed.

Primary Findings

A total of 10,691 records were reviewed, resulting in 1799 valid records (16.8%) that addressed human resource issues related to hospital nursing. In the years 1981, 1992, 1994, from 1998 to 2001, and from 2003 to 2006, more than 60 human resource management-related articles were published per year.

In the developed typology of human resource management in hospital nursing, we identified a total of 30 human resource issues and grouped these issues into eight themes (Table 1). The eight themes were:

1. Recruitment and retention
2. Personnel
3. Staffing and scheduling
4. Work content and flow
5. Professional development
6. Work environment
7. Occupational hazards and staff safety
8. Productivity, care quality, and patient safety

**Table 1. Descriptive information on the eight human resource themes
and corresponding issues**

Themes and corresponding issues	Total records from the three journals	*American Journal of Nursing*	*Nursing Outlook*	*Nursing Research*
1. Recruitment and retention	**150**	**86**	**50**	**14**
1.1. Nursing shortage	47	23	24	7
1.2. General recruitment and selection	66	43	16	0
1.3. International recruitment and selection	13	9	4	7
1.4. Staff retention	24	11	6	0
2. Personnel	**115**	**74**	**26**	**15**
2.1. Staff orientation	4	2	2	0
2.2. Performance appraisal	24	6	7	11
2.3. Salary, benefits, and non-monetary rewards	32	19	9	4
2.4. Promotion and clinical ladders	5	3	2	0
2.5. Disciplinary action and termination	9	9	0	0
2.6. Licensures and credentials	30	24	6	0
2.7. Nurses' rights (e.g., Family and Medical Leave Act, Americans with Disabilities Act, protected against discharge without cause, right to work/HIV-positive nurses, and right to be unionized and right to strike)	11	11	0	0
3. Staffing and scheduling	**118**	**94**	**14**	**10**
3.1. Staffing	84	64	13	7
3.2. Scheduling	34	30	1	3
4. Work content and flow	**301**	**220**	**32**	**49**
4.1. Work analysis and content	201	157	7	37
4.2. Interaction and partnership with physicians and other health care providers	16	11	4	1
4.3. Workflow	84	52	21	11
5. Professional development	**249**	**139**	**70**	**40**
5.1. General nursing competencies	102	54	26	22
5.2. Career development and growth	101	60	25	16
5.3. Evidence-based practice	46	25	19	2
6. Work environment	**243**	**112**	**83**	**48**
6.1. Employers' leadership and managerial skills	67	31	24	12
6.2. Working atmosphere and hospital facility	106	50	34	22
6.3. Gender issues (e.g., men in nursing)	18	8	8	2
6.4. Diversity in nursing (e.g., a culture-sensitive environment for nurses and patients)	52	23	17	12
7. Occupational hazards and staff safety	**254**	**210**	**20**	**24**
7.1. Occupational hazards and diseases	109	95	11	3
7.2. Workplace safety	82	76	3	3
7.3. Nurses' mental health	54	33	5	16
7.4. Nurses' physical health	9	6	1	2
8. Productivity, care quality, and patient safety	**369**	**281**	**41**	**47**
8.1. Monitoring nursing care quality	100	72	3	25
8.2. Medical errors, accidents, and incidents	123	106	10	7
8.3. Professional ethics, dilemmas, and obligations	146	103	28	15
No. of valid records	**1799**	**1216**	**336**	**247**

Productivity, work content and flow, and occupational hazards were the three most often reported themes. The total number of human resource-related records for each of these eight themes is shown in Table 1. The historical trends of these eight emerged themes by year are presented in Table 2.

Table 2. Descriptive information on the eight identified human resource themes by year

Year	Frequency by Theme							
	1	2	3	4	5	6	7	8
	Recruitment and retention	Personnel	Staffing and scheduling	Work content and flow	Professional development	Work environment	Occupational hazards and staff safety	Productivity, care quality, and patient safety
1977	0	4	0	7	8	3	4	8
1978	4	6	1	9	15	10	1	7
1979	3	4	3	14	15	10	5	3
1980	4	5	3	6	6	13	7	12
1981	7	6	4	8	7	11	6	17
1982	2	4	3	6	7	7	9	15
1983	8	4	4	5	2	6	8	9
1984	4	6	3	7	4	9	1	10
1985	5	4	0	10	5	5	7	8
1986	5	3	2	9	8	6	7	9
1987	2	1	1	11	8	6	5	11
1988	10	3	4	8	4	4	10	9
1989	8	7	2	6	3	13	5	14
1990	4	3	0	14	7	8	11	6
1991	4	1	2	11	3	6	4	4
1992	2	3	5	11	6	13	15	7
1993	3	1	2	12	4	10	9	12
1994	2	3	2	17	7	9	8	19
1995	5	2	0	9	6	4	4	13
1996	4	2	3	9	4	9	4	14
1997	4	2	4	9	5	11	5	15
1998	2	1	2	9	16	14	7	14
1999	5	8	5	7	8	9	9	17
2000	8	4	7	19	7	6	16	18
2001	3	5	9	6	14	4	11	15
2002	12	2	2	5	10	6	10	11
2003	10	5	9	21	9	4	12	18
2004	6	2	18	12	11	5	11	18
2005	6	2	10	11	17	8	28	21
2006	8	12	8	13	23	14	15	15
Total	150	115	118	301	249	243	254	369

For each human resource theme, frequencies greater than 10 are shown in boldface.

Lessons Learned from this Study

In this study, the typology of human resource management in hospital nursing summarized the human resource management issues, based on the nursing literature published in the past 30 years. The importance of addressing human resource issues in hospital nursing emerged since 1998, which somehow corresponds to the Magnet Recognition Program established by the American Nurses Credentialing Center in 1997.

These identified themes also correspond to Donabedian's (1966) structure, process, and outcome model. The eight themes identified in our study were matched with the three structure, process, and outcome orientations in Donabedian's (1966) model as follows (Table 1):

1. Involving both structure and process orientations: Theme 1 (recruitment and retention), Theme 2 (personnel), and Theme 6 (work environment)
2. Having a process orientation: Theme 3 (staffing and scheduling), Theme 4 (work content and flow), and Theme 5 (professional development)
3. Engaging both process and outcome orientations: Theme 7 (occupational hazards and staff safety) and Theme 8 (productivity, care quality, and patient safety)

Productivity and Patient Safety

In 1996, the Institute of Medicine launched a health care quality initiative focused on assessing and improving the nation's quality of care. From 1996 to 1998, the first phase focused on understanding the scope of issues as one of overuse, misuse, and underuse of health care services. From 1999 to 2001, the second phase of this initiative targeted the demands on the health care system and called for related policy environment transformations to close the gap between what is known to be good-quality care and what actually existed in practice. The current phase, begun in 2002, focuses on reforming three different overlapping levels of the system: the environmental level, the level of the health care organization, and the interface between clinicians and patients (Institute of Medicine, 2006).

As indicated in Tables 1 and 2, Theme 8 (productivity and patient safety) was the most reported human resource theme with the highest number of records. From 1993 to 2006, 216 (n = 369; 58.5%) Theme 8 (productivity, care quality, and patient safety) articles were published. During the same period, 87 (n = 123; 70.7%) code 8.2 (medical errors, accidents, and incidents) records were obtained. In addition, as early as 1993, there was a dramatic increase in reporting issues related to monitoring nursing care quality (code 8.1). We believe that in the past 10 years, the Institute of Medicine has played an important role in leading the directions of health care service research, especially in the areas of nurses' productivity and care quality and the linkage between nursing care and patient safety.

Individual Human Resource Functions

Khatri and colleagues (2006) claimed that in the 1990s, strategic human resource management issues in the hospital surfaced. The current human resource systems in hospital nursing emphasize primarily individual human resource functions that have been linked to delivering high-quality patient care. However, according to the information presented in Table 2, Theme 1 (recruitment and retention), Theme 2 (personnel), and Theme 5 (professional development) did not show any obvious historical trends.

Safe Practice and Nurses' Occupational Diseases

Another individual human resource function concerning staff safety and safe practice should be highlighted. The issue of occupational hazards and diseases (code 7.1) has been discussed sporadically over time. Since 1999, the issue of work safety (code 7.2) emerged as an important one. In comparison, nurses' mental health (code 7.3) was discussed more frequently in the 1980s.

Staffing, Scheduling, Work Content, and Flow

Theme 4 (work content and flow) showed an emphasis over the past 30 years. In comparison with the other human resource issues, the issue of work analysis and content (code 4.1) was the most reported human resource issue. This finding suggested that nurses' functions have been gradually expanded and nurses' roles in hospital care teams have been clarified gradually over the past 30 years. These phenomena indicated that the nursing profession has been growing within.

It should also be noted that since 2000, staffing (code 3.1) has emerged as an important human resource issue. The global shortage of nurses and the increased emphasis on patient safety may have contributed to this trend, such as linking skill mix or nurse-to-patient ratios to patient safety and clinical outcomes.

Summary: Expecting a Better Hospital Human Resource Allocation and Management

Despite the fact that the nursing profession is growing, human resource issues have not changed in a dramatically significant way in the past 30 years. Certainly, each hospital's structural-level human resource policies or strategic management (e.g., executives' decisions and preferences) would have an impact on human resource practices and effectiveness. The effectiveness of human resource practices (e.g., staff nurses' qualifications and training and nurse-to-patient ratios) may consequently lead to different care-related outcomes Often, as a feedback loop, these outcomes may further influence the structural-level decisions related to human resource allocation for the purposes of improving patient safety during hospital stays.

In other words, human resource management in hospital nursing should no longer emphasize only the individual human resource functions. Taking both the macro and micro approaches to address human resource management issues is a must to ensure safe patient care deliveries. Safe hospital stays demand not only having high-quality nursing staff who are compliant with professional practice standards, as a micro approach, but also each hospital's operational system that supports safe practice, as a macro approach.

References

Aiken, L., Clarke, S., & Sloane, D. (2002). Hospital staffing, organization, and quality of care: Cross national findings. *International Journal for Quality in Health Care, 14*(1), 5-13.

American Nurses Credentialing Center (2007a). Forces of magnetism. Available at: http://www.nursecredentialing.org/magnet/forces.html (accessed May 26, 2007).

American Nurses Credentialing Center (2007b). Goals of the magnet program. Available at: http://www.nursecredentialing.org/magnet/goals.html (accessed May 26, 2007).

American Nurses Credentialing Center (2007c). History of the magnet program. Available at: http://www.nursecredentialing.org/magnet/history.html (accessed May 26, 2007).

American Nurses Credentialing Center (2007d). What is the Magnet Recognition Program? Available at: http://www.nursecredentialing.org/magnet/index.html (accessed May 26, 2007).

Buchan, J. (2004). What difference does ("good") HRM make? *Human Resources for Health, 2*(1), 6 [Electronic version].

Donabedian, A. (1966). Evaluating the quality of medical care. Milbank Memorial Fund *Quarterly, 44*(2), 166-206.

Institute of Medicine (2006). Crossing the quality chasm: The IOM health care quality initiative. Available at: http://www.iom.edu/CMS/8089.aspx?printfriendly=true&redirect=0 (accessed May 26, 2007).

Khatri, N., Wells, J., McKune, J., & Brewer, M. (2006). Strategic human resource management issues in hospitals: A study of a university and a community hospital. *Hospital Topics, 84*(4), 9-20.

Needleman, J., Buerhaus, P., Mattke, S., Stewart, M., & Zelevinsky, K. (2002). Nurse-staffing levels and the quality of care in hospitals. *New England Journal of Medicine, 346*(22), 1715-1722.

Learning the Fact from Research III: The Linkage between Nurse Staffing and Inpatient Fall Rates

Background

When patients are hospitalized for acute health conditions, they need professional care to heal and recover. Not meant to offend, nursing attendants, hospital-hired sitters, or family visitors with their wits and efforts combined are certainly not equivalent to a professionally trained nurse (Tzeng & Yin, 2007a).

Hospital and nursing leaders often have a financial pressure to decrease the amount of nursing personnel cost per patient day. In the current US hospital environment, engaging unlicensed assistive personnel in inpatient care is a commonly adopted solution to be used to ease some of workload of the licensed nurses. Of course, it is much cheaper to hire a full-time nursing attendant than a full-time registered nurse.

In fact, hospital and nursing leaders often assume that more nursing staff and higher total number of nursing hours per patient day would lead to safer inpatient care because more nursing staff may refer to more nursing hours available to address patients' needs at the bedside. As defined by the American Nurses Association (2007) in the report of the National Database of Nursing Quality Indicators (NDNQI), the total nursing hours per patient day include both licensed and unlicensed nursing hours. Unlicensed assistive personnel refer to hospital-hired nursing attendants or nurse aides.

In most of the Asian countries (e.g., Taiwan, China, Japan, Korea, etc.), a registered nurse has to care for 8 to 10 patients per day shift in an acute inpatient care unit in a medical center. In contrast, in the United States, a registered nurse often only cares for 4 to 6 patients per day shift in an acute inpatient care unit in a medical center. Would a patient staying in a US hospital receive more bedside nursing hours than one who stays in a hospital in Asian countries? Unfortunately, no empirical study has ever addressed this issue.

Being naive or not, we asked another question: When the total nursing hours per patient per day increases, would the total number of nursing hours spent at the bedside increase as well? We believe that in acute inpatient care units, the number of bedside nursing hours per patient- day, not the total nursing hours per patient-day, is the key variable to be linked to patient fall rates and pressure ulcer rates. However, no study has ever investigated the linkage between the number of bedside nursing hours per patient-day and patient outcomes (e.g., patient fall rates and pressure ulcer rates). As a matter of fact, no research has yet addressed the concept of bedside nursing hours.

Would More Total Nursing Hours per Patient-day Contribute to Safer Hospital Stays?

If the roles and functions of professional nurses can be replaced, we would have no need for patients to be hospitalized at 24-hour inpatient units. Licensed nurses (including registered nurses and licensed practical nurses) are obligated to monitor patients' conditions periodically and report changes to responsible physicians. In some way, professional nursing training ensures that a patient's condition would be appropriately monitored. Nursing attendants, hospital-hired sitters, or family visitors may have certain medical knowledge. However, such knowledge may not be sufficient to conduct medically appropriately monitoring.

We questioned: When the total nursing hours per patient-day are increased by including unlicensed assistive personnel to share nurses' workload in acute inpatient care settings, would the bedside nursing hours per patient-day provided by licensed nursing personnel increase? Would the increase in the total nursing hours lead to fewer patient falls? The answers to both questions are arguably negative. Nevertheless, no empirical studies have addressed either question.

In addition, human nature related to the dynamic of responsibility sharing among licensed nurses and unlicensed assistive personnel needs to be considered. For example, it is often unclear whether nurses or nursing attendants have to answer call lights.

Can we Replace or Supplement Professional Nurses' Roles by addIng Unlicensed Assistive Caregivers?

Without safety, there is no quality. Hospital delivery systems such as staffing patterns must be designed to improve patient safety (e.g., prevent falls; Tzeng & Yin, 2007b). Increasing total nursing hours per patient-day is commonly seen as a way to improve patient safety in acute care settings.

We claim that using unlicensed assistive caregivers (unlicensed assistive personnel, hospital-hired sitters, or family visitors) for inpatient care is not an effective way to ensure patient safety by preventing falls, for example (Tzeng & Yin, 2007a; Tzeng et al., 2007). If these caregivers could effectively prevent falls, fall prevention tasks should not be categorized as professional nursing tasks and consequently should be delegated to unlicensed assistive caregivers.

According to our observation, in Asian countries, the family involvement culture in acute care settings is popular (e.g., China, Taiwan, Thailand, Japan, Korea, and the Philippines). If family members are not available to accompany their hospitalized loved ones, often they may hire an aide for the entire hospital stay (Tzeng & Yin, 2007a). The aides hired by families may have some basic health care training before being eligible to be hired. They are often delegated to perform some nursing tasks (e.g., bathing, cleaning, repositioning, feeding, and assisting in ambulation, transferring patients, and ambulation).

It should also be noted that acute hospitals in Asian countries rarely use nursing attendants or sitters to assist professional nurses. In addition, nursing attendants are not considered to be part of the nursing workforce.

One of our previous studies (Tzeng, et al., 2007) investigated the links between patient falls and open visiting hours in an acute hospital in Taiwan. Results were abstracted from fall incident reports and survey data completed by the nurses who reported the fall incidents. We found that when patient falls occurred, 38 (27.0%) of accompanying members were sleeping in patient rooms, 22 (15.6%) were not in the patient care unit at that moment (though nurses were told that they would accompany patients), 5 (3.5%) were using patient room bathrooms, 26 (18.4%) were near the patient but not watching the patient, and 50 (35.6%) were watching the patient but unable to get to the patient in time or were improperly supporting the patients when the patient was falling or losing balance.

A total of 103 (73.0%) accompanying family members had received health education related to prevention of patient falls, but these patients still fell. In addition, 11 (7.8%) family members had taken formal courses on patient fall prevention (e.g., training for becoming a certified nursing aide), but these 11 patients still fell (Tzeng, et al., 2007).

Another study (Tzeng & Yin, 2008b) investigated the impact of family and personal caregivers on inpatient fall-related injuries in a Taiwanese medical center. This study used the same data sources as the previous study (Tzeng, et al., 2007). Study findings showed that if no family members were present when a patient fell, the fall-related injury was less serious. In other words, having a family member present when a fall occurred did not lessen the severity of fall-related injuries.

One possible explanation for the lower severity of injury in those without family companions may be that the patient is more careful about ambulation and transfers because no one is in the room to help with these. Moreover, the companions may not have provided safe assistance because they were not trained in these techniques. Without appropriate assistance, the patient may be placed in more danger of severe injury (Tzeng & Yin, 2008b).

As a matter of fact, families are not prepared and not able to share nurses' responsibilities in inpatient care. Families were there primarily to offer psychological support. In addition, as we have observed, nurses tend to depend on family members to help assist in a patient's physical care (e.g., toileting and repositioning), and even count on family members to provide constant observation on patients at high risk for falling. Regardless of whether an inpatient has a family member present, frequent bedside nursing visits are important to prevent falls.

An Empirical Investigation into the Relationship between Fall Rates and Nursing Hours

To further understand the linkage between nurse staffing and patient outcomes, we conducted a descriptive study to illustrate the relationship between fall rates (fall rate and fall injury rate per 1000 patient-days) and nurse staffing (total nursing hours, registered nurse [RN] hours, and unlicensed assistive personnel hours per patient-day) at two acute, medical inpatient care units of a medical center in Michigan. These two units were comparable (32 beds) in size and patient characteristics; Unit A used only RNs and nursing attendants, and Unit B used RNs, licensed practical nurses, and nursing attendants.

A preexisting dataset, the NDNQI report (American Nurses Association, 2007; the second quarter of 2005 to the first quarter of 2007), was the data source for the analyses. This project was approved by the Institutional Review Board of the University of Michigan to protect human subjects.

Primary Findings

When all available data points ($n = 16$) were used, the results showed that the total nursing hours per patient-day (Spearman's rho $= .59$, $p = .02$) and the unlicensed assistive personnel hours per patient-day (Spearman's rho $= .56$, $p = .03$) were statistically and significantly correlated with the number of injury falls per 1000 patient-days. In other words, when the total nursing hours and the unlicensed assistive personnel hours per patient-day were increased, the fall injury rates also increased.

Using only the data of Unit A, no associations between staffing patterns and fall rates were found. For Unit B, the unlicensed assistive personnel hours per patient-day were statistically and significantly correlated with the number of total falls per 1000 patient-days (Pearson r $= .82$, $p = .01$; Spearman's rho $= .79$, $p = .02$; $n = 8$). This finding implies that in Unit B, when the unlicensed assistive personnel hours per patient-day were increased, the total fall rates would also increase.

Lessons Learned from this Descriptive Study

Regardless of limited data points, this study's significant findings suggested that when the total nursing hours and the unlicensed assistive personnel hours per patient-day are increased, the fall rates and the fall injury rates also increased. It indicated that more personnel resources may not lead to fewer falls or fall injuries in acute care settings. Consequently, having more nursing hours per patient-day is arguably not an appropriate quality indicator to be linked to patient outcomes or safer hospital stays.

Total Nursing Hours versus Bedside Nursing Hours

The total nursing hours per patient-day generally involve three major activity categories: (1) bedside hours (working directly with patients); (2) patient care-related administrative hours (time spent preparing patient treatments and procedures and documenting charts); and (3) assorted administrative hours (time spent on activities that are not related to patients). We propose that the bedside nursing hours per patient-day, instead of the total nursing hours, are keys to promote safer hospital stays. However, no studies have ever measured or documented the bedside hours per patient-day that nursing staff actually work directly with their patients.

Ethical Concerns Related to Nursing Practice

Given the nursing shortage, possible strategies to retain qualified nurses include ensuring safe working environments to minimize occupational hazards, providing flexible work arrangements to accommodate family considerations, and reducing incentives that encourage early retirement. Being a staff nurse in an acute inpatient care setting is physically demanding (Chen et al., 2006; Tzeng & Yin, 2007a). From the viewpoint of the acute hospital, reducing the workload of nurses in clinical care by adding unlicensed assistive personnel seems to be a rational way to retain nurses.

However, it is argued that using nursing attendants to share nurses' workloads and requesting hospital-hired sitters and family visitors to constantly observe patients at high risk for falls and those at high risk for suicide attempts is self-destructive for the nursing profession. Using unlicensed assistive caregivers to substitute for or supplement licensed nursing personnel is to deny the necessity and irreplaceable roles of nurses in acute inpatient care (Tzeng, 2006).

It may be inappropriate to assume that having reasonable (or as high as possible) total nursing hours per patient-day will ensure patient safety, reduce patient deaths, help recruit new nurses, and prevent nurses already on the job from suffering "burnout" and exiting the profession (Tzeng & Yin, 2008a). When the nursing community and nursing executives accept that unlicensed assistive caregivers can share professional nursing functions, the nursing profession is committing suicide by killing the image of nurses as perceived by the public. If professional nursing functions are replaceable by unlicensed assistive caregivers, nursing ought not to be called a profession and there is no need to have professional nursing schools, professional training, and licensures.

The current cost-containment hospital environments are inevitably business oriented and market driven. Some hospital and nursing leaders may claim that using unlicensed assistive personnel is a short-term strategy that is meant to accommodate the ongoing worldwide nursing workforce shortage by decreasing nurses' workloads and increasing total nursing hours per patient day for better patient care. If this statement is acceptable, the nursing profession has lost its way.

If this trend of using unlicensed assistive caregivers to supplement total nursing hours continues, nursing professionals will lose their identity and be less respected by the public. It is the same as declaring that the roles of professional nurses are not important in the process of delivering acute inpatient care (Tzeng, 2006; Tzeng & Yin, 2007c).

Summary

If our car has a flat tire and we do not know how to replace it with the spare tire, we have to ask a friend or call the gasoline station to send someone to change the tire. If we cannot start the engine, we are in big trouble, and we need to have a tow truck tow our car to the garage for professional services. Similarly, if we have a fever, runny nose, and minor congestion, we or our families can take care of the problem at home.

However, if we have major abdominal surgery, we would prefer to stay in a high-quality hospital until we are well enough to be discharged. This is the time we need professional nursing care. Nurses are respected because of their professional training and irreplaceable roles in inpatient care, both of which are desperately needed when we are ill.

If all nurses stay at the nurses' station, it is not right because nursing care is based on observation not on reviewing charts. The number of bedside nursing hours should be the most critical factor for quality nursing care (e.g., fall rates) in inpatient care settings. Using unlicensed assistive caregivers should not replace bedside licensed-nursing hours per patient-day that are most needed for hospitalized patients. Nursing is an irreplaceable profession in acute inpatient care settings. A business-driven nursing care model that includes unlicensed assistive caregivers on the care team will eventually reverse the development of the nursing profession.

References

American Nurses Association (2007). The national database. Available at: http://www. nursingworld.org/MainMenuCategories/ThePracticeofProfessionalNursing/ PatientSafetyQuality/NDNQI/NDNQI_1.aspx (accessed September 9, 2007).

Chen, L., Evans, D., Evans, T., Sadana, R., Stilwell, B., Travis, P., Van Lerberghe, W., & Zurn, P. (2006). *Working together for health: The world health report 2006*. Geneva, Switzerland: The World Health Organization.

Tzeng, H. M. (2006). Testing a conceptual model of the image of nursing in Taiwan. *International Journal of Nursing Studies, 43*(6), 755-765.

Tzeng, H. M., & Yin, C. Y. (2007a). Using family visitors, sitters, or volunteers to prevent inpatient falls. *Journal of Nursing Administration, 37*(7-8), 329-334.

Tzeng, H. M., & Yin, C. Y. (2007b). No safety, no quality: Synthesis of research on hospital and patient safety (1996–2007). *Journal of Nursing Care Quality, 22*(4), 299–306.

Tzeng, H. M., & Yin, C. Y. (2007c). Seeing the nursing profession from a different perspective: Nurstry? Why not! *Nursing Forum, 42*(4), 185-188.

Tzeng, H. M., & Yin, C. Y. (2008a). What's our philosophy? *Journal of Professional Nursing, 24*(1), 5-6.

Tzeng, H. M., & Yin, C.Y. (2008b). Inpatient falls: The impact of family and personal caregivers. *Applied Nursing Research* (in press).

Tzeng, H. M., Yin, C. Y., Tsai, S. L., Lin, S., & Yin, T. J. (2007). Patient falls and open visiting hours: A case study in a Taiwanese medical center. *Journal of Nursing Care Quality, 22*(2), 145-151.

Epilogue

Adverse events in health care facilities are a leading cause of death and injury in the United States. The National Quality Forum (2006) is devoted to improving the quality of American health care by setting national priorities and goals for performance improvement and promoting the attainment of national goals through education and outreach programs. The National Quality Forum, a nonprofit organization, is a voluntary consensus standard-setting organization.

On October 16, 2006, the National Quality Forum endorsed a list of 28 serious reportable events in health care that are largely preventable and of concern to both the public and health care professionals and providers. These events have been clearly identifiable and measurable and, therefore, the risk of occurrence is significantly influenced by the policies and procedures of the health care facilities (e.g., hospitals). Based on the National Quality Forum (2006), these 28 serious reportable events (also called never events) were:

1. Abduction of a patient of any age
2. Any occurrence of care ordered by or provided by someone pretending to be a physician, nurse, pharmacist, or other licensed health care provider
3. Any related incident that a line designated for oxygen or other types of gas to be delivered to a patient contained the wrong gas or was contaminated by toxic substances
4. Artificial insemination with the wrong donor sperm or donor egg
5. Death or serious disability, such as kernicterus (a form of brain damage caused by excessive jaundice), associated with failure to identify and treat hyperbilirubinemia in neonates
6. Death or significant injury of a patient or staff member resulting from a physical assault, such as battery, that occurred within a health care facility
7. Infant discharged to the wrong person
8. Intraoperative or immediate postoperative death in a normal healthy patient
9. Maternal death or serious disability related to labor or delivery in a low-risk pregnancy when being cared for in a health care facility

10. Patient death or serious disability associated with a medication error, including errors involving the wrong medication, wrong dose, wrong patient, wrong time, wrong rate, wrong preparation, or wrong route of administration

11. Patient death or serious disability associated with the use of restraints or bed rails when being cared for in a health care facility

12. Patient death or serious disability associated with the use or function of a device in patient care when the device was used or functioned other than as intended

13. Patient death or serious disability due to spinal manipulative therapy

14. Patient death or serious disability linked to an electric shock or elective cardioversion when being cared for in a health care facility

15. Patient death or serious disability linked to hypoglycemia, the onset of which occurred when being cared for in a health care facility

16. Patient death or serious disability linked to patient elopement or disappearance

17. Patient death or serious disability linked to the use of contaminated medications, devices, or biologics provided by the health care facility

18. Patient death or serious disability related to a burn incurred from any source when being cared for in a health care facility

19. Patient death or serious disability related to a fall, while being cared for in a health care facility

20. Patient death or serious disability related to a hemolytic reaction due to the administration of ABO-incompatible blood or blood products

21. Patient death or serious disability related to intravascular air embolism that occurred when being cared for in a health care facility

22. Patient suicide or attempted suicide resulting in serious disability when being cared for in a health care facility

23. Pressure ulcers, stage 3 (the skin breakdown showing a crater in which damage is evident to the tissue below the skin) or stage 4 (the pressure ulcer becoming so deep that there is damage to the muscle and bone, and sometimes tendons and joints), acquired after being admitted to a health care facility

24. Sexual assault on a patient within a health care facility

25. Surgery performed on a wrong body part

26. Surgery performed on a wrong patient

27. Unintended retention of a foreign object within a patient's body after surgery or other procedure

28. Wrong surgery or procedure performed on a patient

Any of these 28 adverse events are preventable and should not occur to us during our hospital stay. The United States and health insurers (e.g., Medicare, Aetna, and WellPoint) are trying to end reimbursements to hospitals for treatment that results from serious medical errors. In other words, health insurers are taking actions to improve patient safety and reduce health care costs by trying to ban paying for or letting their patients be billed for hospital errors (Fuhrmans, 2008).

For example, in August 2007, the federal Medicare program (Centers for Medicare & Medicaid Services, 2008) announced that starting October 1, 2008, Medicare will no longer pay the extra cost of certain hospital errors and preventable injuries to patients, including the conditions of:

1. Object left in during surgery
2. Air embolism
3. Blood incompatibility
4. Catheter-associated urinary tract infections
5. Pressure sores
6. Vascular catheter-associated infections
7. Surgical site infections-mediastinitis after coronary artery bypass graft surgery
8. Falls and trauma fractures, dislocations, intracranial injuries, crushing injuries, and burns

Based on the same report (Centers for Medicare & Medicaid Services, 2008), conditions being considered for the year of 2009 by Medicare include:

1. Ventilator-associated pneumonia
2. *Staphylococcus aureus* septicemia (also called hospital-acquired blood infections)
3. Deep vein thrombosis and pulmonary embolism

Private health insurers are looking first at banning reimbursements for only the gravest mistakes, that is, the 28 never events compiled by the National Quality Forum. It is believed that this movement will trigger hospital safety improvement and savings for patients. Hopefully, these efforts will stop these preventable adverse events from occurring in the first place (Fuhrmans, 2008).

Currently, hospitals have a financial incentive to invest in reducing preventable hospital harms and errors by promoting a safer care environment. For instance, health care staff members must be trained to follow hospital policies and clinical practice guidelines to effectively prevent health care-associated infections. To promote a safer care environment, hospitals must offer sufficient and effective orientation for new staff members and on-the-job training on hand hygiene to all staff members who provide direct patient care.

However, having clinical practice guidelines in place will not guarantee good compliance and patient outcome (e.g., low health care-associated infection rates). It is especially important that hospitals have comprehensive supervisory plans in place to periodically monitor staff members' compliance in hand hygiene. Patient safety and quality care will be guaranteed only if hospitals have detailed managerial strategies to effectively supervise and monitor staff members' practices and performances.

Hospitals in the United States have advanced medical technologies to cure or extend our lives, and many have good policies in place already. Our doctors and nurses are well trained and equipped with the competencies required to deliver safe care. However, the key to preventing hospital harms and errors is having comprehensive supervisory strategies to monitor staff members' performances and the associated patient outcomes. Only outstanding management and supervisory plans can motivate staff members to deliver safe care. In other words, a safe care environment should include not only a well-designed, risk-free hospital setting, but also hospital leaders' commitment to patient safety, adequate and appropriate human resource allocation with a patient safety-first mission in mind, and a set of comprehensive supervisory strategies to monitor staff members' performance.

No hospital safety, no care quality! Patient safety should be more than a slogan in hospital care. Hospitals should have zero tolerance for preventable patient harms, errors, and complications. We are hospitalized to cure, to heal, to regain our health, or simply to extend our lives. No matter what, we must say no to any preventable hospital harms and errors.

References

Centers for Medicare & Medicaid Services (2008). Hospital-acquired condition. Available at: http://www.cms.hhs.gov/HospitalAcqCond/06_Hospital-Acquired%20Conditions.asp (accessed January 15, 2008).

Fuhrmans, V. (2008). Insurers stop paying for care linked to errors (published on January 15, 2008 in *The Wall Street Journal*). Available at: http://online.wsj.com/article/SB12 0035439914089727.html?mod=googlenews_wsj (accessed January 15, 2008).

National Quality Forum (2006). National Quality Forum updates endorsement of serious reportable events in health care (published on October 16, 2006). Available at: http://s.wsj.net/public/resources/documents/WSJ_PRSeriousReportableEvents10-15-06.pdf (accessed January 15, 2008).

Glossary of Terms
Commonly Used in Hospital Care

Accreditation: A process whereby an institution or a program is recognized by an external body as meeting certain predetermined standards. This external organization is often created for the purpose of ensuring the quality of the accredited institution or program. Accreditation may be either permanent or given for a specified period of time.

Acute care: Medical treatment delivered by acute care facilities to individuals whose illness or health programs are of a short-term nature or an acute episodic nature of a chronic disease.

Acute disease: A disease that is characterized by a single episode of a relatively short duration from which the patient returns to his or her normal previous level of activity.

Advanced practice nurses: Professionals who are qualified by education at an accredited school of nursing, have a master's degree or higher, and are licensed by state law to practice nursing (e.g., nurse anesthetists, nurse clinical specialists, nurse practitioners, and nurse midwives).

Adverse event: An injury or death that results from a medical intervention.

Agency for Healthcare Research and Quality (abbreviated as AHRQ): AHRQ is a public health service agency within the US Department of Health and Human Services that reports to the Secretary. AHRQ was created in December in 1989 as the Agency for Health Care Policy and Research, and reauthorized in December 1999 as the Agency for Healthcare Research and Quality. AHRQ's mission is to support research designed to improve the outcomes and quality of health care, reduce health care costs, address patient safety issues and medical errors, and broaden access to effective services. Available at: http://www.ahrq.gov/.

Allied health personnel: Specially trained and licensed health care workers other than physicians, dentists, optometrists, chiropractors, podiatrists, and nurses. However, this term has no constant or agreed-on detailed meaning.

Ambulatory care: Health services that provide outpatient-based health care services. A patient must travel to a location to receive services that do not require an overnight stay. Such a patient is called an outpatient.

Ancillary services: Supplemental health services that include laboratory, radiology, physical therapy, and inhalation therapy. These services are provided in conjunction with ambulatory or inpatient care.

Centers for Disease Control and Prevention (abbreviated as CDC): This government agency is in charge of protecting the nation's public health by providing direction in the prevention and control of communicable (e.g., acquired immunodeficiency syndrome) and other diseases (e.g., injury, environment and occupational hazards, behavioral risks, and chronic diseases), and responding to public health emergencies. Available at: http://www.cdc.gov/.

Centers for Medicare & Medicaid Services (abbreviated as CMS): This government agency, under the Department of Health and Human Services, directs the Medicare and Medicaid programs, and conducts research to support those programs. Available at: http://www.cms.hhs.gov/.

Certified nurse aide (abbreviated as CNA): Assisting nursing personnel who have completed required state training and competency testing in the skills required to work as a nurse aide or nursing attendant.

Chronic care: Health care and treatment rendered to individuals whose health problems are of a long-term and continuing nature. Chronic care facilities include rehabilitation facilities, nursing homes, and psychiatric hospitals.

Chronic disease: A disease that has one of more of the follow characteristics: being permanent; leaving residual disability; being caused by nonreversible pathologic alternation; requiring special training of the patient for rehabilitation; or being expected to require a long period of medical attention, supervision, observation, or care.

Clinical laboratory personnel: Health care professionals, technicians, and assistants employed in a health care facility where specimens are collected, grown, tested, or evaluated and the results are recorded.

Critical care: A subspecialty of medicine related to the diagnosis, treatment, and medical support of patients with multiple organ dysfunctions during a medical emergency or crisis.

Cultural competence: A health care provider's or institution's understanding of and sensitivity to the cultural background and primary language of patients in any component of service delivery, involving direct patient care, patient education materials, health care facility settings, and public health campaigns.

Direct patient care: Activities rendered by a health care professional involving direct patient interaction in the process of delivering treatments or procedures, administering medications, or implementing care plans.

Family practice: A medical specialty that provides continuing comprehensive primary health care for the entire family.

Health care providers (also called health care personnel): Individuals working in the provision of health services as individual practitioners or employees of health care institutions or programs. They may or may not be professionally trained and may or may not be subject to public regulation.

Health education: Any combination of learning opportunities designed to facilitate voluntary adaptations of behavior contributing to health.

Health status: The state of health of a specified individual or population. It may be measured by obtaining people's subjective assessment of their health, by using the incidence or prevalence of major diseases, or by one or more indicators of mortality and morbidity in the population (e.g., longevity or maternal and infant mortality).

Healthcare Cost and Utilization Project Quality Indicators (abbreviated as HCUP QIs): HCUP QIs, developed by the Agency for Healthcare Research and Quality, comprise a set of 33 clinical performance measures that inform: (1) hospitals' self-assessments of inpatient quality of care and (2) state and community assessments of access to primary care. HCUP QIs cover three dimensions of care: (1) potentially avoidable hospital admissions; (2) potentially inappropriate use of hospital procedures; and (3) potentially avoidable adverse hospital outcomes. Available at: http://www.ahrq.gov/data/hcup/.

Hospital: An institution whose primary function is to provide inpatient diagnostic services and surgical and nonsurgical therapeutic services for a variety of medical conditions. Most hospitals provide emergency care and some outpatient services.

Human factors research: The study subjects of the interrelationships between humans, the tools they use, and the environment in which they live and work.

Inpatient: An individual who has been admitted at least overnight to a hospital for the purpose of receiving diagnostic treatment or other health services. The hospital is responsible for the individual's room and board.

Institute for Healthcare Improvement (abbreviated as IHI): IHI is a not-for-profit organization that was created in 1991 to help lead the improvement efforts of health care systems for the purpose of increasing their quality and value. Measures of improvement include: better clinical outcomes, improved health status, lower cost, broadened access, greater ease of use, and higher satisfaction for individuals and their communities. Available at: http://www.ihi.org/ihi.

Institute of Medicine (abbreviated as IOM): A private, non-for-profit institution that provides objective, timely, and authoritative information and advice relating to health and science policy to the government, corporate sector, professions, and public as a component of the National Academy of Sciences under a congressional charter. Available at: http://www.iom.edu/.

Institute of Medicine care needs: Institute of Medicine identified four care needs: (1) *end of life care*: care concerned with those not expected to survive more than 6 months; (2) *getting better*: care associated with acute illness or injury; (3) *living with illness*: care for chronic or recurrent illness; and (4) *staying healthy*: care concerned with healthy populations or the general health needs of non-healthy populations (e.g., early detection by screening and treatment of presymptomatic diseases, risk factor assessment, disease prevention, and health promotion).

Institute of Medicine domains: Institute of Medicine identified three domains: (1) *effectiveness*: as associated with providing care processes and achieving outcomes as supported by scientific evidence; (2) *patient centeredness*: as related to meeting patients' needs and preferences and providing health education and support; (3) *safety*: concerning actual or potential bodily harm; and (4) *timeliness*: about obtaining needed care while minimizing delays.

Joint Commission: A national private, nonprofit organization whose purpose is to foster the attainment of uniformly high standards of institutional medical care. This organization establishes guidelines for the operation of hospitals as well as the other health care facilities and conducts survey and accreditation programs for these health care institutions. Available at http://www.jointcommission.org/.

Malpractice: Professional misconduct or failure to apply ordinary skills or standards in the performance of a professional act. To prove malpractice requires that a patient demonstrate some injury and that the injury was caused by negligence.

Mandatory reporting: A system under which health care professionals are required by law to inform health authorities when a specified event occurs (e.g., the diagnosis of a certain disease, and a medical error; see also *Sentinel event*).

Medical error: An error or omission occurring to a patient in the process of delivery of medical care. Such errors can occur in diagnosis, treatment, or preventive monitoring or in the failure of the operational system or a piece of medical equipment. Medical errors may result in adverse events such as injury or death.

Medicare: A US health insurance program for people aged 65 and over, for individuals eligible for Social Security disability payments for 2 years or longer, and for persons who need kidney transplantation or dialysis. This program consists of two parts: hospital insurance (Part A) and supplementary medical insurance (Part B). Available at http://www.cms.hhs.gov/.

Morbidity: The extent of illness, injury, or disability in a defined population that is usually expressed in general or specific rates of incidence or prevalence.

Mortality: Term for death, used to describe the relationship of deaths to the population in which they occur. The mortality rate expresses the number of deaths in a unit of population within a given time. It may be expressed as a crude death rate or as a death rate specific for diseases, age, sex, or other attributes.

National Guidelines Clearinghouse (NGC)™: The NGC™ is a publicly available electronic repository for clinical practice guidelines and related materials. Available at www.guideline.gov.

Near miss: A medical error or omission that does not result in harm.

Nurse: Professionals qualified by education at an accredited school of nursing and licensed by state law to practice nursing. They are trained to care for the sick, aged, or injured, or for those requiring medical attention in recovering or maintaining their physical or mental health.

Nurse practitioner: A registered nurse qualified and specially trained to provide primary care, including primary health care in homes and in ambulatory, long-term, and other health care institutions. This individual generally functions under the supervision of a physician but not necessarily in the physician's presence.

Nursing: The professional practice that provides care and services essential to the promotion, maintenance, and restoration of health by attending to a patient's needs.

Patients: Individuals involved in the health care system for the purpose of receiving preventive, diagnostic, or therapeutic procedures.

Pharmacists: Professionals qualified by education and training to engage in the practice of pharmacy.

Physicians: Professionals licensed to practice medicine (including physician specialists).

Occupational health services: Services concerned with the physical, mental, and social well-being of individuals in relation to their working environment and with the adjustment of these individuals to their work. Such services apply to the safety of the workplace and these individuals' health and job satisfaction.

Outcome: This term refers to the findings of a given diagnostic procedure and may also refer to cure of the patient, restoration of function, or extension of life. When used for populations or the health care systems, it may refer to the changes in birth or death rates.

Patient safety: Measures and procedures to make sure patients are free from accidental injury during the process of receiving health care services. Ensuring patient safety may involve the establishment of operational systems and processes that minimize the likelihood of errors and maximize the likelihood of capturing errors when they occur.

Performance measures: Methods or instruments used to estimate the extent to which the actions of health care providers conform to practice guidelines, medical review criteria, or standards of quality.

Quality improvement: The aggregate of all the activities that created a desired change in quality. Quality improvement in the health care facilities requires a feedback loop that involves the identification of the patient care patterns, the analysis of those patterns to identify opportunities for improvement, and then the development of the actions to improve the care quality for future patients.

Quality of care: The level to which delivered health services meet the established professional standards and the judgments of value to the consumer by maximizing the probability of beneficial health outcomes and minimizing errors and harms.

Report card: A report designed to inform patients and health care purchasers (e.g., private insurance companies and government insurance programs) about the quality of health services (e.g., the performance of the practitioners and health care institutions).

Root cause analysis: A process used to identify the basic or causal factors that underlie variations in performance (e.g., the occurrence or possible occurrence of a medical error).

Safety net: The network of health care providers and institutions that provide low-cost or free medical care to medically needy, low-income, or uninsured populations for hospital and ambulatory care.

Sentinel event: An unexpected occurrence or variation involving deaths or serious physical or psychological injuries that require immediate attention. A serious injury may involve loss of a limb or function.

Tertiary care: Services provided by highly specialized physicians and health care professionals and frequently require highly sophisticated equipment and support facilities.

References

AcademyHealth (2007). Glossary of terms commonly used in health care. Available at: http://www.academyhealth.org/publications/glossary.htm (accessed November 6, 2007).

National Guideline Clearinghouse (2007). Glossary. Available at: http://www. guideline.gov/resources/glossary.aspx (accessed November 6, 2007).

Index

A

abduction, viii, 50, 303

abortion, 234

academics, 176

access, 39, 41, 44, 59, 119, 138, 141, 143, 145, 153, 154, 171, 183, 187, 193, 209, 261, 307, 309

accessibility, 28, 259

accidents, 288, 290, 292

accountability, 22, 160, 179

accreditation, 32, 34, 47, 49, 60, 63, 65, 66, 92, 97, 122, 125, 133, 145, 175, 192, 273, 274, 278, 286, 310

accuracy, 32, 36, 58, 149, 154, 170, 171, 185, 224, 278

achievement, 75

acidic, 103

acidosis, 103

acquired immunodeficiency syndrome (AIDS), 7, 179, 180, 231, 232, 233, 308

activity level, 104, 110, 111

acute lung injury, 180, 189

acute renal failure, 188

acute respiratory distress syndrome, 69

ADA, 264, 267

adaptability, 259

adaptation, 194

adhesives, 261

adjustment, 54, 311

administration, 9, 23, 30, 32, 34, 54, 56, 61, 120, 149, 150, 151, 152, 153, 154, 155, 158, 159, 160, 161, 162, 165, 166, 167, 170, 171, 172, 179, 180, 181, 185, 186, 219, 221, 304

administrators, 52, 81, 108

adolescence, 236

adolescent female, 236

adolescent patients, 125

adolescents, 137

adults, 102, 233, 236, 240, 267

adverse event, vii, 16, 26, 34, 37, 38, 40, 42, 43, 48, 57, 58, 64, 65, 166, 177, 188, 206, 207, 208, 209, 210, 216, 217, 220, 221, 227, 258, 304, 305, 310

Africa, 112

afternoon, 135, 165, 282

age, xi, 26, 51, 56, 73, 84, 86, 123, 140, 152, 198, 200, 303, 310

agent, 106

aggression, 120

aggressive behavior, 123

aging, 71, 281

air embolism, 304

air quality, 260

airborne, 234, 245, 247, 260

airflow, 48

airways, 219

alarms, 12, 48, 52, 83, 85, 87, 127, 130

alcohol, 138, 223, 226, 227, 235, 238, 239, 241, 248, 249

alertness, 197, 200

allergic reaction, 153, 188

allergy, 174, 220

alternative(s), 84, 118, 121, 127, 129, 130, 131, 133, 142, 265, 266

Alzheimer's disease, 7

ambulation, 72, 77, 297

American Association of Suicidology, 136, 138, 145

American Nurses Association, 21, 23, 27, 28, 295, 298, 300

American Nurses Credentialing Center, 287, 288, 292, 294

Americans with Disabilities Act, 290

amniotic fluid, 103

amputation, 7
anemia, 99
anesthesia-related, viii, 57
anesthesiologist, 219, 271
aneurysm, 24
antibiotic(s), 217, 219, 221, 224, 227, 229, 233, 234, 236, 237, 241, 248
antibody, 231, 232, 233
anticoagulation, 33, 158
anti-inflammatory agents, 74
antimicrobial(s), 229, 237, 238, 241
anxiety, 128, 138, 211, 213
appendectomy, 24, 117
appendix, 25
arousal, 256
arrest, 129, 220
arrhythmia, 205
arterioles, 103
artery, 24, 193, 218
arthritis, 73, 191, 234, 236
aseptic, 230
Asia, 236
Asian countries, 285, 295, 297
asphyxia, 118
aspiration, 126, 276
aspirin, 173
assault, 138, 303, 304
assessment, ix, 9, 48, 51, 54, 55, 74, 81, 82, 84, 86, 87, 90, 100, 104, 105, 106, 107, 108, 110, 115, 121, 124, 126, 127, 128, 130, 135, 137, 138, 139, 140, 141, 143, 144, 154, 163, 166, 181, 183, 184, 187, 198, 200, 206, 207, 208, 209, 210, 215, 216, 220, 222, 223, 224, 225, 240, 243, 250, 273, 309
assessment techniques, 82
assessment tools, 82
assignment, 182, 186
assistive personnel, 295, 296, 298, 299
asymptomatic, 188, 236
atmosphere, 290
atrial fibrillation, 99
attacks, 73, 235
attention, x, 9, 10, 11, 15, 34, 35, 42, 82, 106, 142, 152, 170, 180, 188, 198, 200, 201, 208, 212, 215, 222, 256, 259, 273, 278, 308, 310, 311
attitudes, 48
authority, 16, 192, 198
autonomy, 93, 257, 288
autopsy, 99
availability, 51, 154, 183, 195, 198, 200, 207, 209, 220, 223, 276, 277

awareness, 27, 82, 83, 87, 122, 246
axial skeleton, 103

B

back pain, 39, 179, 188
background information, 273
bacteremia, 237
bacteria, 99, 234, 235, 237
bacterial, 180, 189, 236
bacterium, 229, 234
barriers, 104, 105, 106, 184, 239
baths, 101, 217
battery, 231, 303
bedsore, 99
behavior, 76, 124, 127, 130, 135, 138, 139, 141, 144, 308
behavioral change, 129, 132
behavioral disorders, 33, 136, 144
benefits, 19, 161, 255, 290
benign, 189
beverages, 235
Bible, 20
bilirubin, 50
biomedical, 51
biopsy, 135, 212, 218, 275, 276
bipolar disorder, 138
birth, 7, 24, 167, 178, 234, 276, 281, 311
bladder, 73, 128
blame, 53, 86, 163, 209, 258
bleeding, 69
blind, 7, 168, 169, 261
blood, 35, 42, 50, 99, 101, 103, 128, 177, 178, 179, 180, 181, 182, 183, 184, 185, 186, 187, 188, 189, 212, 217, 221, 232, 233, 234, 235, 260, 276, 304, 305
blood flow, 103
blood group, 50
blood pressure, 260
blood safety, 180
blood transfusion(s), 42, 177, 178, 179, 180, 181, 182, 184, 185, 186, 187, 188, 189
bloodstream, 99, 233, 238
body aches, 235, 236
body fluid, 114
body temperature, 114, 263
body weight, 103, 107
bone, 102, 103, 104, 276, 304
bone marrow, 276
bowel, 73, 128

braille, 168, 169

brain damage, 303

breakdown, 76, 99, 101, 102, 104, 111, 112, 132, 304

breakfast, 69

breast, 179, 275, 278

breast cancer, 275

bronchoscopy, 237

bronchus, 218

bulbs, 79, 89

Burkholderia, 234

burn, 128, 304

burnout, 48, 256, 299

buttons, 239, 253, 254, 255

bypass graft, 24

C

C. difficile, 229, 234, 241, 242

California, 18, 19, 226

campaigns, 43, 308

Canada, 257

cancer care, 148

cancer treatment, 137

capital cost, 285

capsule, 102, 167

cardiac arrest, 148, 218

cardiac catheterization, 24, 196

cardiac surgery, 195, 219

cardiopulmonary, 123, 180, 215

cardiovascular disease, 147

care model, 300

caregivers, 32, 58, 86, 87, 213, 274, 296, 297, 299, 300, 301

carotid artery, 193

carotid endarterectomy, 193

carpal tunnel, 192

case study, 98, 286, 301

categorization, 75

cathartics, 74

catheter, 36, 149, 196, 215, 218, 226, 227, 238, 240, 254, 255, 305

catheter tube, 70

catheterization, 277

catheters, 36, 129, 132, 229, 240

CDC, 33, 308

cell, 103, 189

cell death, 103

cell transplantation, 189

certainty, 230

certificate, 49, 99

cervical, 191, 229

cervical laminectomy, 191

cesarean section, 195

channels, 221, 225

chemical, 261

chemotherapy, 38, 57, 161

Chicago, 278

Chicago Sun-Times, 275

childbirth, 26

childhood, 236

children, 92, 233, 236, 282

China, 236, 285, 295, 297

Chinese, 114, 169

chloride, 35, 156

cholecystectomy, 24

Christmas, 93

chronic diseases, 308

chronic illness, 18, 56, 73

ciprofloxacin, 229

circulation, 123

classification, 75, 76, 77, 78, 79, 80

cleaning, 223, 242, 247, 279, 297

clinical judgment, 21

clinicians, 1, 2, 32, 37, 42, 44, 45, 92, 155, 174, 199, 202, 208, 279, 292

Clostridium difficile-associated diseases, 229

coccyx, 99

Code of Ethics, 21, 22, 23

codes, 39, 41, 44, 161

coding, 81, 161, 163, 170, 185

coercion, 124

cognition, 128

cognitive, 47, 53, 71, 82, 84, 86, 95, 128, 129, 132, 198, 200

cognitive impairment, 82, 84, 86, 198, 200

colds, 248

colitis, 234

collaboration, 34, 60, 65, 199

collagen, 103

colonoscopy, 215, 216

colorectal, 219

coma, 69

commercial, 17

commode, 71, 72, 77, 79, 88, 89, 248, 260, 266

communication, x, 20, 31, 32, 35, 36, 44, 48, 52, 54, 55, 58, 60, 65, 75, 76, 81, 82, 84, 85, 95, 138, 141, 143, 145, 149, 151, 153, 159, 164, 171, 180, 181, 183, 187, 194, 196, 197, 198, 200, 201, 203,

207, 209, 210, 211, 213, 215, 220, 221, 222, 223, 224, 225, 239, 272, 273, 274, 276
community, vii, 10, 20, 22, 23, 27, 55, 138, 141, 143, 145, 199, 232, 245, 246, 248, 280, 288, 294, 299, 309
compassion, 9, 22
compensation, 287
competence, 22, 127, 139, 151, 154, 184, 198, 200, 208, 210, 222, 223, 224, 308
competency, 51, 130, 142, 181, 240, 308
competition, 284
complexity, 48, 106, 158, 261
compliance, ix, 34, 48, 49, 53, 54, 105, 129, 136, 151, 165, 166, 197, 207, 220, 221, 223, 239, 240, 242, 243, 244, 247, 250, 305
complication(s), viii, x, 9, 25, 26, 31, 34, 43, 50, 57, 58, 64, 156, 178, 180, 188, 189, 217, 218, 219, 220, 221, 223, 224, 225, 226, 227, 229, 231, 236, 239, 241, 244, 306
components, 185, 194, 219, 222, 240, 243, 289
composition, 283
Comprehensive Accreditation Manual for Hospitals, 60, 92, 126, 271, 276
concentrates, 34, 152
concentration, 156
conceptual model, 300
concrete, 9, 56, 274
condensation, 260
confidentiality, 38, 44, 58, 124
conflict, 231
confusion, 65, 83, 118, 120, 127, 129, 130, 150, 156, 157
congestive heart failure, 19, 43, 189
conjunctivitis, 236
consciousness, 148, 197, 200
consensus, 26, 34, 37, 41, 43, 45, 57, 194, 232, 303
consent, 12, 63, 191, 192, 196, 202, 231, 260
construction, 259, 260, 267, 286
consultants, x
consulting, 17, 225
consumption, 235
contamination, 180, 184, 187, 189, 235, 238, 242, 247
content analysis, 37, 85
continuity, 31, 36, 211
contraceptives, 158
control, 38, 41, 43, 57, 58, 61, 64, 65, 75, 76, 79, 83, 89, 93, 94, 95, 110, 114, 124, 125, 149, 160, 161, 219, 221, 237, 242, 254, 261, 263, 308
coronary angioplasty, 24

coronary artery bypass graft, 305
coronavirus, 236
corporate sector, 31, 309
corrosion, 114
costs, 14, 17, 19, 179, 180, 285
cotton, 109, 110, 112, 114, 262, 263
cough, 235, 236, 237, 245, 249
coughing, 235
counseling, 20, 53
coverage, 71, 223
covering, 193
creativity, 53
credentials, 290
credit, 163
Creutzfeldt-Jakob disease, 234
critical analysis, 250
critical value, 207, 211
crying, 148
cues, 107
cultural values, 283
culture, ix, x, 8, 38, 48, 53, 54, 55, 58, 65, 97, 197, 199, 216, 267, 281, 282, 285, 286, 289, 290, 297
curing, ix
curriculum, 176
cystic fibrosis, 234

D

danger, 231, 297
data collection, 61, 281
database, 37, 39, 126, 137, 300
deaf, 7
death(s), viii, x, 17, 33, 38, 50, 57, 58, 64, 99, 118, 120, 126, 128, 129, 130, 131, 133, 135, 136, 137, 138, 149, 162, 180, 205, 207, 218, 221, 233, 235, 240, 250, 281, 299, 303, 304, 307, 310, 311
death rate, 310, 311
death sentence, 137
decisions, 14, 15, 16, 63, 120, 293
deconditioning, vii, 10, 101, 261
decubitus ulcer, 101, 115
deep venous thrombosis, 220, 243
defense(s), 50, 55, 66, 85, 97, 129, 133, 138, 141, 145, 150, 155, 175, 184, 189, 199, 204, 209, 213, 223, 227, 238, 244, 250
deficiency, 188
deficits, 56, 73
deformation, 108
dehydration, 103, 107, 128
delay in treatment, viii, 50, 58

delirium, 82, 117
delivery, 10, 24, 25, 42, 45, 49, 50, 61, 109, 111, 160, 162, 178, 217, 287, 296, 303, 308, 310
demand, 2, 166, 167, 194, 199, 222, 255, 294
dementia, 83, 87, 198
demographic characteristics, 152
dentists, 307
Department of Health and Human Services, 308
Department of Justice, 264, 267
depressants, 82
depression, 138
deprivation, 44, 84
derivatives, 183
dermatitis, 107, 230, 231
dermatologist, 230
dermis, 102
desire, 14, 82, 95, 212
destruction, 102, 188
detection, 30, 44, 205, 309
detergents, 239
diabetes, 73, 101, 147, 221
dialysis, 310
diarrhea, 71, 229, 234, 235, 236, 241, 242
diet, 31, 173
dignity, 22, 84, 120, 122, 139
directives, 63
disability, 139, 140, 144, 280, 303, 304, 308, 310
discharges, 55, 101
discipline, 21, 27, 124
discomfort, 109, 127, 128, 130, 212, 216, 226, 236
disfigurement, 70
disinfection, 21, 114, 235, 242, 246, 247, 263
disorder, 234
dissatisfaction, 9
distress, 123, 189, 193, 254
distribution, 55, 149
diversity, 261
dizziness, 111
doctors, 9, 11, 12, 14, 33, 39, 44, 57, 64, 192, 203, 226, 249, 305
domestic violence, 138
donors, 11
doors, 133, 142, 239
dosage, 165, 167
dosing, 158, 160
drainage, 104, 106, 112, 216, 226, 227
dressing, 216, 223, 225, 226, 227
drug reactions, 90
drug resistance, 234, 237
drug treatment, 65

drug use, 138
drugs, 13, 36, 87, 140, 201, 209, 210, 232
drying, 106, 110, 112
duodenal ulcer, 254
duplication, 157
duration, 307
duties, ix, 20, 21, 22, 23, 55

E

early retirement, 299
ears, 169
eating, 248
Ebola, 234, 237
ecology, 280, 281, 285
economic status, 22
edema, 189
education, 20, 23, 53, 54, 60, 61, 62, 80, 83, 95, 105, 124, 127, 131, 143, 149, 158, 161, 165, 166, 167, 168, 173, 175, 217, 219, 241, 244, 274, 286, 303, 307, 308, 310
educational programs, 108
egg, 303
elastin, 103
elbows, 103, 106
elderly, xi, 17, 24, 72, 85, 89, 101, 117, 128, 147, 191, 192, 255, 267
electric shock, 304
electrocautery, 218
electroconvulsive, 120
electrolyte(s), 35, 36, 128, 149
electrolyte imbalance, 128
embolism, 305
emotion, 75, 98
emotional disorder, 138
emotional distress, 231, 232, 233
employees, 54, 179, 180, 254, 288, 308
employment, 22
endocarditis, 234
endoscopic, 218
endotracheal intubation, 236
energy, 88, 165, 281
environment, vii, x, 1, 7, 8, 14, 22, 27, 29, 39, 44, 51, 53, 54, 56, 59, 63, 64, 80, 81, 84, 87, 89, 92, 93, 94, 96, 122, 127, 128, 130, 131, 133, 137, 139, 142, 144, 155, 159, 160, 184, 185, 187, 201, 209, 210, 225, 227, 247, 249, 256, 257, 258, 259, 260, 262, 266, 267, 281, 285, 289, 290, 291, 292, 295, 305, 306, 308, 309, 311
environmental conditions, 155

environmental factors, 104
epidermis, 102, 103
equipment, viii, 10, 12, 21, 35, 39, 44, 56, 59, 61, 64,
    72, 73, 74, 75, 77, 78, 79, 80, 83, 85, 88, 89, 90,
    92, 96, 104, 109, 110, 112, 128, 129, 131, 132,
    133, 142, 150, 155, 164, 182, 184, 187, 194, 196,
    197, 198, 201, 205, 206, 209, 210, 223, 225, 237,
    241, 242, 247, 259, 260, 265, 266, 277, 285, 310,
    311
ergonomics, 47, 48, 66, 133, 145
esophageal, 24
ethics, 21, 23, 28, 62, 63, 163, 290
ethnic background, 283
ethnicity, 123
etiology, 108
evening, 118, 135, 168, 222, 282
evidence, 9, 24, 36, 42, 43, 48, 54, 65, 93, 221, 230,
    233, 254, 309
execution, 60
exercise, 148, 203
exertion, 75, 266
expertise, 166
exposure, 39, 59, 101, 103, 106, 179, 231, 232, 233,
    234, 235, 258
eyes, 169

F

fabric, 114
failure, 47, 55, 75, 76, 80, 98, 153, 164, 197, 205,
    216, 230, 303, 310
fainting, 99
fall, viii, 2, 71, 74, 76, 80, 81, 82, 86, 90, 92, 295,
    298
family, viii, ix, x, 2, 8, 12, 16, 22, 31, 39, 50, 51, 52,
    54, 58, 59, 60, 61, 62, 63, 77, 80, 82, 83, 85, 86,
    87, 92, 95, 98, 107, 108, 110, 111, 112, 114, 120,
    124, 125, 127, 129, 130, 131, 132, 133, 138, 140,
    141, 142, 143, 144, 145, 153, 157, 158, 164, 171,
    173, 174, 188, 192, 197, 198, 200, 201, 202, 203,
    211, 212, 213, 226, 230, 232, 242, 245, 246, 248,
    249, 260, 277, 279, 280, 281, 282, 283, 284, 285,
    286, 295, 296, 297, 299, 300, 301, 308
Family and Medical Leave Act, 290
family members, 51, 52, 54, 62, 63, 83, 92, 95, 107,
    108, 114, 124, 129, 131, 132, 133, 138, 142, 143,
    144, 145, 158, 164, 232, 279, 280, 281, 283, 284,
    285, 286, 297
family violence, 39, 59
far right, 91, 113

farsightedness, 96
fascia, 102
fatal arrhythmia, 205
fatigue, 44, 48, 155, 222, 255, 259
fear, 51, 94, 109, 110, 232, 233, 262
fecal, 103, 105, 235, 236, 242, 247
feedback, 293, 311
feelings, 82, 93, 111, 139, 141, 226
feet, 91, 94, 113, 114
fever, 188, 189, 216, 235, 236, 237, 300
fifth disease, 236
films, 104, 111, 112
filters, 260
financial resources, 137
fire, viii, 59
firearms, 138
first aid, 123
flexibility, 55, 259
float, 104
floating, 147
flooring, 260
fluid, 13, 103, 107, 128, 218, 254
fluoroscopy, 50
focusing, 53, 180
folding, 285
food, 83, 95, 108, 130, 132, 158, 235, 248
Food and Drug Administration, 237
footwear, 56, 73, 74, 76, 85, 96
foreign object, 50, 304
forgetting, 75
four-point restraints, 118
fractures, 73, 93, 305
freedom, 119, 140
friction, 103, 104, 105, 107, 108, 111, 112
frustration, 84
furniture, 96, 127, 266, 285
fusion, 191, 225

G

gait, 56, 73, 75, 84, 86
gasoline, 300
gastric, 69
gastroenteritis, 236
gastroesophageal reflux, 244
gastrointestinal bleeding, 99
gel, 226, 227, 239
gender, 123, 152, 282
general surgery, 217
Geneva, 300

geriatric, 152, 170

German measles, 248

gestures, 140

glass(es), 96, 142

glaucoma, 73

gloves, 216, 229, 230, 238, 241, 242, 244, 245, 247, 249, 260

glucose, 128, 217, 219, 221

glycoprotein, 234

goals, 32, 33, 34, 35, 41, 42, 49, 53, 219, 287, 294, 303

government, 31, 308, 309, 311

grading, 75

gravity, 103

gross domestic product, 71

group work, 32, 85

groups, 12, 25, 288

growth, 22, 290

guardian, vii, 16, 33

guessing, 75

guidance, 125, 127, 130

guidelines, 9, 33, 35, 38, 41, 42, 43, 44, 47, 58, 62, 65, 104, 117, 120, 140, 158, 181, 204, 206, 221, 222, 224, 238, 239, 240, 243, 244, 246, 247, 277, 305, 310, 311

guilt, 136

H

hallucinations, 117

hands, 1, 2, 11, 34, 216, 223, 224, 226, 227, 229, 230, 231, 235, 238, 239, 241, 244, 245, 246, 248, 249

handwriting, 13, 153

harm, 30, 33, 34, 35, 36, 42, 43, 44, 56, 58, 74, 80, 83, 97, 114, 124, 137, 149, 158, 231, 258, 309, 310

Harvard, 17, 227

Hawaii, 112

hazardous materials, 63

hazards, 37, 39, 40, 41, 44, 59, 60, 76, 84, 88, 89, 97, 139, 142, 144, 180, 289, 290, 291, 292, 293, 299, 308

head, 69, 78, 81, 84, 104, 106, 107, 129, 132, 148, 220, 230, 232, 243, 254, 260, 261, 281

head injury(ies), 129, 132

headache, 235, 236

healing, x, 7, 8, 14, 15, 30, 39, 92, 257, 260, 266, 283

health care costs, 96, 218, 304, 307

health care professionals, 11, 108, 303, 310, 311

health care sector, 288

health care system, 29, 31, 42, 65, 163, 259, 292, 309, 310, 311

health education, 10, 297, 309

health expenditure, 71

health information, 44, 48, 63

health insurance, 71, 310

health problems, 20, 22, 44, 99, 308

health services, 29, 120, 308, 309, 311

health status, 51, 52, 57, 69, 108, 283, 309

heart, 7, 24, 25, 118, 189

heart attack, 7, 118

heart failure, 24

heat, 101, 109, 110, 112, 114, 262, 263

height, 46, 72, 74, 78, 90, 91, 94, 98, 261, 262, 264, 265, 266

helmets, 120

hematocrit, 183

hematoma, 25, 26

hematuria, 99

hemoglobin, 177, 179, 183

hemorrhage, 24, 25, 26, 103, 178

hepatitis, 36, 179, 180, 232, 234, 235

hepatitis B, 235

herbs, 13, 173, 174

higher quality, 14

hip, 25, 70, 83, 225, 227, 265

hip replacement, 225

Hispanic, 192

HIV, 7, 36, 179, 230, 231, 232, 233, 234, 235, 290

HIV test, 230, 231, 232

HIV/AIDS, 179, 235

homicide, viii, 50, 58

hopelessness, 137, 138, 139

hospice, 30

hospital-hired sitters, 295, 296, 299

hospitalization, 1, 9, 10, 14, 15, 20, 24, 25, 26, 31, 34, 39, 65, 71, 73, 93, 96, 109, 139, 171, 173, 175, 180, 206, 216, 229, 245, 249, 258, 267, 275, 278, 281

host, 189

human dignity, 22

human errors, 48

human nature, 199, 296

Human Resource Management, 253, 256, 288

human resources, 63

human subjects, 298

humidity, 48, 92, 261

humiliation, 70

husband, 77, 232
hydration, 99, 107, 123
hydrocortisone, 148
hygiene, 33, 35, 36, 123, 223, 224, 225, 238, 239,
    240, 241, 244, 245, 246, 247, 248, 249, 251, 305
hyperalimentation, 221
hyperbilirubinemia, 50, 303
hyperglycemia, 244
hypoglycemia, 304
hypotension, 73, 147, 189
hypotensive, 177
hypoxia, 156
hysterectomy, 178

I

iatrogenic, 26
identification, x, 11, 32, 36, 38, 53, 58, 61, 104, 105,
    128, 129, 147, 161, 170, 177, 180, 181, 182, 183,
    184, 185, 186, 187, 197, 198, 199, 200, 203, 224,
    238, 260, 275, 276, 277, 278, 311
identity, 55, 196, 198, 201, 276, 277, 300
illumination, 56, 73, 74
images, 91, 113, 194
imaging, 209, 211, 212, 218, 223
immobility, vii, 10, 101, 105, 109, 261
immobilization, 120
immune system, 188, 230, 234, 236
immunity, 235
impairments, 73
implants, 194, 196, 198
implementation, 46, 80, 93, 100, 105, 141, 143, 153,
    163, 171, 194, 199, 204, 209, 243, 267, 272, 276
incentives, 299
incest, 138
incidence, 26, 96, 100, 101, 105, 216, 235, 243, 244,
    309, 310
incidents, 258
inclusion, 37
income, 71, 256, 281, 285, 311
incompatibility, 180, 188, 305
independence, 111
indication, 9, 160, 191
indicators, 23, 24, 25, 26, 27, 28, 287, 288, 309
indirect measure, 24
induction, 218, 237
industry, 31
infant mortality, 309
infants, 36, 196, 198, 200, 232
infection-related, viii, 58

infection(s), x, 1, 2, 8, 9, 11, 15, 17, 25, 26, 27, 30,
    33, 35, 36, 38, 39, 42, 43, 51, 58, 59, 61, 64, 65,
    102, 110, 114, 188, 216, 217, 218, 219, 221, 224,
    225, 226, 227, 229, 230, 233, 234, 235, 236, 237,
    238, 239, 240, 241, 242, 244, 245, 246, 247, 248,
    249, 250, 251, 259, 260, 263, 284, 288, 305
infectious disease(s), 10, 39, 44, 234, 237, 238, 244,
    245, 246, 247, 248, 249
inflation, 71
information exchange, 213
information systems, 206
information technology, 61
informed consent, 16, 191, 194, 197, 198, 200, 201,
    202, 203, 255
infrastructure, 36, 37, 38, 40, 41, 42, 43, 44, 57, 58
initiation, 121, 124, 125, 141, 158, 243, 277
injections, 254
injury(ies), viii, x, 1, 2, 9, 25, 27, 38, 39, 42, 44, 57,
    58, 59, 64, 69, 70, 71, 80, 86, 90, 93, 94, 96, 97,
    104, 105, 107, 111, 112, 120, 126, 129, 130, 131,
    133, 140, 162, 193, 205, 207, 218, 221, 240, 255,
    260, 261, 262, 297, 279, 288, 297, 298, 303, 305,
    307, 308, 309, 310, 311
innovation, 30, 98, 115
inpatient falls, vii, x, 10, 56, 66, 72, 73, 75, 77, 78,
    80, 85, 88, 90, 92, 93, 98, 120, 129, 261, 267,
    279, 286, 300
inpatients, vii, ix, x, 1, 20, 39, 72, 93, 109, 112, 126,
    136, 166, 167, 220, 262, 263, 279, 283
insertion, 195, 196, 218, 229, 230, 254, 255, 277
instability, 84, 86
Institute for Healthcare Improvement, 29, 30, 31, 42,
    43, 45, 64, 71, 97, 100, 101, 102, 105, 107, 114,
    115, 216, 218, 219, 227, 240, 241, 243, 273, 274,
    309
institutions, vii, viii, ix, 32, 49, 60, 65, 101, 102,
    287, 308, 310, 311
instruments, 234, 235, 311
insulation, 260
insulin, 43, 156
insurance, 71, 96, 285, 310, 311
integrity, 22, 23, 27, 61, 101, 103, 104, 106, 108,
    111, 112
intensity, 74
intensive care unit, 52, 69, 70, 99, 117, 148, 163,
    164, 217, 220, 229, 233, 234, 236, 243, 245, 253,
    255, 256, 266
interaction(s), 9, 47, 48, 72, 121, 139, 140, 153, 157,
    158, 160, 163, 173, 249, 281, 290, 308
interdependence, 194, 199

interface, 32, 42, 160, 170, 292
internist, 191, 225
interpretation, 212
interrelationships, 309
intervention, 34, 84, 85, 86, 87, 88, 89, 90, 93, 101,
    104, 124, 140, 243, 307
intervention strategies, 85, 93
interview, 78, 85, 93, 158
intestinal perforation, 229
intimidation, 124
investment, 20
iron, 189
irrigation, 218
ischemia, 103
IV, 13, 74, 75, 79, 88, 89, 120, 129, 131, 132, 148,
    155, 156, 161, 167, 172, 174, 189, 203, 211, 217,
    226, 227, 229, 230, 236, 238, 254, 266, 277

J

Japan, 285, 295, 297
jaundice, 303
job dissatisfaction, 256
job performance, 256, 257
job satisfaction, 288, 311
job training, 240
jobs, 52
joints, 265, 304
judgment, 19, 22, 83, 118, 148, 149, 185, 225, 231,
    255
justification, 120, 121

K

Kaiser Family Foundation, 71, 96
Kentucky, 100, 216
kidney(s), 178, 189, 310
killing, 299
knee replacement, 191
knees, 89, 191
knots, 128, 130
Korea, 295, 297

L

labeling, 48, 149, 155, 171, 182, 277
labor, 253, 303
laceration, 25, 26, 218
language, 15, 41, 95, 131, 143, 308

laptop, 161, 185
laundry, 110, 246, 248
laws, 62
lead, 9, 29, 30, 34, 36, 48, 51, 54, 82, 90, 94, 103,
    120, 122, 127, 128, 130, 149, 156, 189, 199, 206,
    208, 230, 244, 256, 262, 289, 293, 295, 296, 298,
    309
leadership, 53, 62, 181, 240, 288, 290
leadership style, 53
leakage, 244
learning, 10, 54, 62, 231, 308
learning styles, 54
lesions, 111, 230
leukemia, 148
licensed, 32, 60, 162, 163, 295, 296, 298, 299, 300,
    303, 307, 310, 311
life span, 281
lifestyle, 50, 216, 246
life-threatening, vii, 10, 71, 188, 189, 205, 283
likelihood, 29, 33, 140, 153, 158, 171, 185, 206, 207,
    208, 209, 221, 240, 311
limitation, 75, 283
linkage, x, 257, 292, 296, 298
links, 164, 281, 287, 297
liquids, 178
literacy, 169
literature, 292
liver, 189, 218, 235
liver cancer, 235
liver cirrhosis, 235
liver failure, 235
local anesthetic, 254
location, 55, 139, 154, 171, 196, 205, 206, 259, 260,
    276, 277, 307
locus, 75
longevity, 309
love, 144, 283, 284, 285
low risk, 232
loyalty, 22
lubricants, 104, 111, 112
lumbar laminectomy, 191
lung, 135, 233, 234, 238
lung cancer, 135
lung disease, 234
lying, 93, 101, 109, 111, 112, 135, 189, 262, 263
lymph, 236
lymphadenopathy, 236

M

magnet, 287, 288, 294

Magnet Recognition Program, 287, 292, 294

magnetism, 288, 294

maintenance, 61, 63

malaise, 236

malnourishment, 102

malnutrition, 103, 128

malpractice, 118, 148, 179, 193, 310

management, 48, 61, 62, 65, 107, 115, 206, 208, 210, 238, 256, 258, 266, 285, 288, 289, 292, 294, 306

management practices, 289

manpower, 75, 77, 79, 80

manufacturer, 162

market, 36, 94, 109, 114, 262, 265, 299

marriage, 280

mastectomy, 225, 275

meals, 107, 111

measles, 248

measurement, 28, 49, 72, 156

measures, 9, 21, 23, 24, 25, 26, 27, 38, 53, 58, 63, 76, 78, 81, 83, 95, 309, 311

mechanical ventilation, 219, 236, 243, 244

mechanical ventilator, 117

media, 36, 38, 58

median, 71

mediastinitis, 305

mediation, 123

Medicaid, 10, 17, 305, 306, 308

medical care, vii, ix, 14, 25, 26, 37, 39, 40, 59, 60, 117, 167, 282, 294, 310, 311

Medical Examiners, 230, 232

medical malpractice, x, 193, 230, 255

medical technicians, x, 9

Medicare, 10, 19, 28, 71, 125, 304, 305, 306, 308, 310

medication, x, 1, 3, 8, 9, 10, 13, 14, 17, 19, 30, 33, 34, 35, 36, 38, 39, 41, 48, 51, 54, 56, 58, 61, 73, 82, 83, 90, 95, 139, 147, 148, 149, 150, 151, 152, 153, 154, 155, 156, 157, 158, 159, 160, 161, 162, 163, 164, 165, 166, 167, 168, 170, 171, 172, 173, 174, 175, 176, 181, 185, 189, 202, 217, 219, 220, 232, 241, 244, 254, 258, 259, 260, 276, 278, 304

medication error, viii, 50, 57, 58

medicine, 7, 8, 11, 19, 28, 33, 154, 158, 171, 179, 180, 182, 185, 225, 308, 311

memory, 65, 73, 192, 222, 224

men, 20, 128, 290

meningitis, 237

mental cognition, 128

mental health, 141, 290, 293, 310

mental impairment, 129, 132

messages, 164

methicillin-resistant, 43, 216, 221, 224

methicillin-resistant Staphylococcus aureus (MRSA), 221, 224, 235

microorganisms, 238

milligrams, 165

Minnesota, 179, 230, 231, 232

miscommunication, 36, 224

mobility, 73, 104, 105, 106, 107, 110, 111, 120, 229, 264

models, 31, 239, 258, 288

moisture, 78, 101, 103, 104, 105, 106, 107, 109, 110, 112, 114, 262, 263

money, 14, 202

mood, 138, 144

mood change, 138

mood disorder, 138

morale, 257

morbidity, 237, 309

morning, 135, 165, 168, 178, 179, 192, 201, 232, 254

morphine, 156

mortality, 24, 25, 39, 59, 189, 218, 237, 287, 288, 309, 310

mortality rate, 24, 189, 288, 310

motion, 104, 110, 123, 260

motivation, 75, 98, 256

movement, 36, 103, 119, 264, 265, 267, 305

multidrug-resistant tuberculosis, 237

mumps, 236, 248

muscle mass, vii, 10, 261

muscle strength, vii, 10, 111, 129, 261

musculoskeletal, vii, 10, 48, 56, 73, 261

musculoskeletal system, vii, 10, 56, 73, 261

myocardial infarction, 19, 24, 28, 42, 215

myopathy, 73

N

narcotic, 160

narcotics, 43, 156

National Database of Nursing Quality Indicators (NDNQI), 295, 298, 300

National Labor Relations Act, 253, 254

National Patient Safety Goals, 32, 33, 46, 49, 57, 58, 59, 62, 66, 74, 80, 92, 97, 102, 115, 136, 145, 157, 175, 204, 238, 250, 274, 278, 279

National Quality Forum, 303, 305, 306

nearsightedness, 96

neck, 118, 135, 218

necrosis, 102, 103

necrotic, 230

needle(s), 36, 182, 229, 230, 232, 233, 234, 235, 254, 276

negative consequences, 51

neglect, 165

negligence, 17, 19, 99, 118, 148, 149, 164, 174, 179, 210, 217, 227, 255, 310

neonate, 25

neonates, 25, 303

nervous system, 82

network, 311

neurosurgery, 148

neurovascular, 229

New England, 17, 227, 294

New York, 75, 98, 175, 180, 189, 217, 227, 250, 258, 267

noise, 48, 84, 89, 259, 260

not-for-profit, 19

nurses' station, 89, 118, 127, 130, 133, 142, 154, 156, 205, 260, 300

nursing care, vii, 9, 10, 17, 27, 55, 95, 132, 163, 208, 286, 289, 290, 292, 300

nursing home, 271, 308

nutrition, 99, 104, 106, 107, 108, 123

nutritionists, 9, 108

O

obesity, 196

obligate, 253

obligation, 22, 44, 275

observations, 132, 141, 256, 264, 282, 284

omission, 157, 310

on-the-job training, 54, 80, 185, 256, 305

operating room, 104, 177, 178, 191, 192, 194, 195, 196, 197, 198, 199, 200, 202, 203, 215, 217, 218, 219, 220, 221, 222, 224

operating system, 223

operator, 257, 266

organ, 11, 195, 308

organization(s), vii, 29, 32, 42, 47, 48, 50, 55, 60, 66, 90, 97, 145, 204, 287, 288, 292, 294, 303, 307, 309, 310

orientation, ix, 54, 62, 84, 86, 127, 138, 139, 151, 170, 184, 185, 197, 198, 200, 208, 223, 224, 240, 244, 247, 256, 288, 290, 292, 305

orthopedic surgeon, 70, 217

osteoporosis, 128, 130

otitis media, 237

outpatients, vii, 10, 126, 167, 220

outreach programs, 303

overload, 189, 218

oversight, 180

overtime, 253, 254, 255, 256, 281, 288

oxygen, 88, 101, 218, 303

P

packaging, 36, 149

pain, 9, 15, 38, 41, 57, 70, 83, 95, 99, 102, 111, 127, 128, 130, 138, 161, 193, 202, 212, 215, 221, 226, 254

pain management, 128, 130, 161, 221

palliative care, 30

pancreas, 189

pancreatitis, 254

Parkinson's disease, 73

parotitis, 236

particles, 260, 261

partnership, 290

pathogenic, 242, 247

pathogens, 7, 180, 229, 234, 235, 242, 245, 247, 249, 260

patient care, 9, 14, 21, 22, 30, 31, 35, 36, 39, 48, 52, 53, 54, 56, 57, 60, 62, 63, 72, 79, 110, 123, 124, 127, 130, 131, 142, 156, 164, 206, 221, 222, 224, 240, 244, 245, 256, 272, 279, 284, 285, 286, 293, 294, 297, 299, 304, 305, 308, 311

patient-controlled analgesia (PCA), 155, 156, 161

patient handling, 39, 48

patient rights, 140

patient-centered, 30, 31, 52, 71, 72

pediatric, 25, 26, 82, 92, 120, 125, 152, 170, 232, 281, 282, 283, 284

pediatric care, 282

pediatric patients, 26, 125, 152, 170, 282, 283

penicillin, 236

peptic ulcer disease, 220, 243

perception(s), 9, 17, 104, 105, 128, 129, 132, 136

perforation, 218

performance, 47, 48, 49, 60, 62, 63, 65, 108, 120, 121, 122, 123, 124, 125, 154, 163, 164, 193, 221,

222, 224, 244, 255, 256, 257, 258, 287, 303, 306, 309, 310, 311

performance appraisal, 256, 287

perfusion, 103

perinatal, viii, 58

peritonitis, 218, 234

permit, 35, 209

personal, 16, 22, 70, 76, 78, 85, 92, 139, 142, 154, 164, 231, 283, 297, 301

personal life, 283

personal responsibility, 154

personality, 256, 257

pharmaceutical, 166, 167

pharmacists, ix, x, 9, 26, 38, 58, 64, 65, 80, 108, 150, 155, 159, 160, 162, 163, 166, 167, 171, 181, 241, 279

pharmacology, 7, 162, 163, 166, 171

philanthropy, 29

Philippines, 297

phlebotomy, 179, 184

phobia, 232

phosphate, 35, 156

physical abuse, 123, 124

physical activity, 119

physical environment, vii, 10, 47, 48, 56, 63, 72, 73, 76, 87

physical health, 290

physical restraints, x, 64, 117, 119, 130

physical therapist, x, 83, 110, 111

physical therapy, 308

physicians, 20, 26, 111, 150, 152, 167, 206, 243, 244, 311

physiology, 84

pills, 138, 148

planning, ix, 60, 63, 81, 83, 84, 90, 136, 141, 220, 241, 248

plasma, 183

plastic surgeon, 179

platelet count, 183

platelets, 183

pneumonia, 19, 42, 219, 233, 234, 236, 237, 238, 243, 244, 248, 288, 305

pneumothorax, 25, 26, 215, 222

podiatrists, 307

poor, x, 56, 57, 73, 93, 155, 162, 169, 244, 256, 266

poor performance, 162, 256

population, 20, 26, 33, 58, 71, 80, 84, 101, 120, 136, 145, 309, 310

positive behaviors, 199

postanesthesia, 177, 216, 217, 218, 220, 223, 271

postoperative, viii, x, 50, 57, 58, 64, 177, 201, 216, 217, 218, 219, 220, 221, 222, 223, 224, 225, 226, 227, 261, 303

potassium, 35, 156

power, 16, 71, 260

practical nurses, 162, 296

prediction, 105

pregnancy, 26, 303

premiums, 255

pressure, x, 1, 3, 14, 21, 30, 43, 64, 78, 83, 87, 94, 100, 101, 102, 103, 104, 105, 106, 107, 108, 109, 110, 111, 112, 114, 115, 197, 244, 255, 258, 262, 263, 273, 279, 284, 285, 288, 295, 296, 304

pressure sore, 107, 114, 279

pressure ulcers, 101, 102, 104, 105, 106, 109

prevention, 20, 39, 42, 43, 44, 53, 59, 61, 62, 63, 69, 71, 80, 81, 83, 84, 86, 92, 93, 95, 100, 104, 105, 106, 107, 108, 110, 112, 115, 121, 127, 137, 138, 139, 142, 145, 151, 154, 162, 175, 181, 182, 194, 197, 199, 207, 210, 217, 221, 237, 240, 241, 246, 247, 248, 296, 297, 308, 309

price index, 98

privacy, 63, 139, 284, 285

probability, 311

productivity, 164, 256, 292

profession, 8, 20, 21, 22, 23, 28, 293, 299, 300

professional development, 288, 292, 293

professional growth, 22

professions, 31, 309

profit, 29, 31, 309

program, 10, 14, 19, 33, 46, 59, 62, 66, 69, 79, 80, 84, 85, 86, 96, 100, 105, 108, 132, 161, 163, 167, 236, 237, 247, 272, 287, 294, 305, 307, 310

programming, 156, 161

promote, x, 1, 8, 15, 20, 29, 32, 33, 44, 53, 54, 56, 64, 71, 112, 159, 166, 174, 207, 211, 239, 245, 246, 253, 258, 260, 261, 262, 283, 285, 299, 305

prophylactic, 217, 221

prophylaxis, 219, 220, 243

protein, 234

protocol(s), 38, 39, 41, 42, 43, 54, 58, 59, 65, 80, 107, 121, 122, 140, 189, 194, 204, 217, 219, 243

protozoa, 235

psychiatric hospitals, 33, 122, 126, 127, 129, 136, 142, 257, 271, 272, 308

psychiatric patients, 140

psychological problems, 7

psychologist, 141

psychosocial, 137

psychotropic medications, 129

public health, 307, 308
puerperium, 26
pulmonary edema, 189
pulmonary embolism, 25, 305
pulse, 117
pumps, 159, 161, 170, 172, 184, 187
punishment, 53
pyoderma gangrenosum, 230

Q

qualifications, 60, 92, 122, 293
quality control, 154
quality improvement, 29, 30, 55, 63, 71, 288
quality of life, 203
query, 46
questioning, 159, 162, 163, 272

R

radiotherapy, 38, 50, 57
range, 64, 101, 104, 110, 123, 233, 265
rape, viii, 50, 58
rash(es), 103, 106, 236
reality, 19, 65, 162
recall, 93, 191, 215
recognition, 33, 58, 183, 237, 287
reconcile, 33, 57, 152, 157, 158, 173
reconciliation, 30, 36, 155, 156, 158, 159, 170, 219
recovery, 8, 14, 39, 58, 199, 215, 216, 217, 218, 222, 229, 257, 266, 271, 280
recruiting, 287
red blood cells, 180, 188, 189
Red Cross, 179
redistribution, 107
reduction, 33, 53, 62, 80, 86, 90, 133, 139, 179
refining, 30
regional, 28
registered nurses, 162, 253, 296
regulation, 46, 98, 120, 308
rehabilitation, 20, 99, 126, 280, 281, 308
relationship(s), 22, 53, 213, 257, 281, 282, 283, 288, 298, 310
relatives, 70, 282
relevance, 34, 123
reliability, 48
religion, 15
repair, 7, 24, 85, 89, 92
repair system, 7

research design, 307
resection, 24
residential, 72
residuals, 261
resistance, 241
resolution, 53
resource allocation, x, 14, 289, 293, 306
resource management, x, 27, 37, 39, 40, 44, 48, 59, 60, 64, 256, 287, 288, 289, 292, 293, 294
resource policies, 293
resources, 14, 184, 185, 288, 298, 306, 312
respiratory, x, 25, 99, 126, 189, 218, 220, 236, 243
respiratory arrest, 126, 218
respiratory failure, 25, 99, 218
respiratory therapist, x, 243
response time, 95
restaurants, 249
retention, viii, 30, 50, 57, 62, 64, 256, 288, 289, 290, 291, 292, 293, 304
retirees, 283
returns, 280, 307
rewards, 290
risk assessment, 71, 74, 80, 104, 105, 106, 108, 136, 140, 145
risk factors, 54, 56, 57, 65, 66, 72, 73, 74, 75, 76, 77, 78, 80, 84, 85, 93, 98, 103, 105, 106, 108, 136, 137, 138, 139, 154, 155, 156, 242, 247, 263, 265, 267
risk management, 48, 62, 64, 257, 267
risk profile, 36
risk-taking, 138
RNA, 236
Robert Wood Johnson Foundation, 29
robotics, 161
rods, 139, 142, 144
rolling, 84
room design, 48, 78, 80, 267, 285
room temperature, 109, 261
rubber, 78, 88
rubella, 248

S

sacrum, 103, 106
saliva, 236
sample, 37, 40, 181, 186
sanitation, 241, 242, 247
SARS-CoV, 236
satisfaction, 8, 9, 14, 17, 19, 27, 96, 284, 288, 309
Save-Our-Skin, 100

savings, 305

scalability, 259

scheduling, 39, 59, 253, 255, 256, 289, 290, 291, 292

schizophrenia, 138

school, 179, 299, 307, 310

science, 8, 20, 21, 31, 43, 309

scores, 74

searching, 7, 160

security, ix, 15, 52, 63, 120, 138, 150, 153, 160, 171, 239

sedative(s), 43, 76

sedentary lifestyle, vii, 10, 261

seizures, 73, 254

selecting, 61

self-assessment, 75, 309

self-destructive behavior, 138

self-healing, 7, 8

self-interest, 231

sensation, 103

sensitivity, 63, 308

sepsis, 25, 99, 229

series, 17, 42, 60, 219, 230

severity, 80, 180, 297

sex, 310

sexual abuse, 138

sexual contact, 50

shaping, 23

sharing, 79, 90, 232, 235, 296

shear, 103, 104, 105, 107, 111, 112

short supply, 118

shortage, 256, 290, 293, 299

shortness of breath, 189

showers, 217

side effects, 13, 42, 56, 61, 83, 153, 171, 174, 202, 232

signaling, 52

signals, 87

sign(s), 12, 15, 16, 19, 81, 86, 123, 132, 137, 139, 140, 143, 144, 145, 156, 183, 187, 191, 201, 202, 216, 222, 233, 244, 254, 273

sites, 12, 197, 201, 230, 233

situation-background-assessment-recommendation (SBAR), 273, 274

skills, 21, 51, 53, 54, 75, 92, 96, 104, 109, 110, 123, 139, 148, 184, 208, 210, 222, 290, 308, 310

skin, 27, 99, 100, 101, 102, 103, 104, 105, 106, 107, 108, 109, 110, 111, 112, 114, 115, 132, 195, 216, 217, 221, 223, 230, 234, 235, 238, 240, 262, 263, 276, 304

sleep apnea, 220

slowdown, 254

smiles, 9

smoke, 128

social context, 21

social organization, 281

social policy, 23

Social Security, 310

socialization, 283, 284

society, 21, 71

socioeconomic status, 283, 285

sodium, 35, 156

soil, 234

solvents, 261

sounds, 12, 79

species, 8

specificity, 21

speed, 160, 197

sperm, 303

spinal fusion, 24

spine, 194, 195

sputum, 212, 237

stability, 75, 76, 77, 78, 79, 80, 88, 129

stabilization, 126

staff development, 62

staffing, 20, 55, 63, 75, 77, 80, 84, 95, 122, 127, 131, 140, 143, 155, 164, 184, 208, 210, 223, 225, 253, 287, 292, 293, 294, 296, 298

stages, 102, 115, 160, 162

standards, vii, 9, 10, 13, 19, 23, 32, 48, 49, 97, 120, 122, 125, 126, 170, 224, 225, 226, 241, 294, 307, 310, 311

Staphylococcus aureus, 43, 216, 221, 224, 230, 235, 237, 305

statistics, viii, xi, 45, 59, 66, 138, 145, 180

steel, 260, 266

stenosis, 193

sterile, 33, 158, 230

stethoscope, 227, 249

stimulus, 164

stock, 154, 156, 160

storage, 61, 63, 78, 89, 150, 151, 153, 154, 170, 171, 178, 184, 187

strain, 70, 242

strategic management, 289, 293

strategies, vii, 10, 51, 61, 72, 80, 81, 83, 84, 86, 90, 95, 100, 105, 106, 107, 121, 127, 138, 139, 151, 154, 162, 181, 182, 194, 197, 207, 210, 221, 225, 240, 241, 242, 243, 244, 246, 247, 256, 258, 287, 299, 305

strength, vii, 10, 73, 83, 96, 129, 261

stress, 39, 44, 48, 59, 86, 215, 222, 256, 257, 283

stress test, 215, 216

stretching, 103

stroke, 229

students, 61

subcutaneous tissue, 102

substance abuse, 82

suffering, 36, 70, 99, 118, 193, 231, 299

suicidal ideation, 140, 141, 142, 143, 145

suicidal risk, 137

suicide, viii, x, 33, 50, 58, 64, 135, 136, 137, 138, 139, 140, 141, 142, 143, 144, 145, 217, 279, 299, 304

suicide attempts, 299

suicide rate, 136

summer, 110, 112, 114, 263

supervision, 20, 84, 127, 141, 142, 144, 255, 256, 308, 310

supervisor(s), 84, 85, 95, 127, 131, 140, 143, 155, 182, 183, 187, 197, 208, 210, 245, 257

supply, 101, 110, 164, 261

Supreme Court, 231, 233

surgeons, 192, 194, 199, 203

surgeries, vii, 10, 12, 36, 71, 191, 193, 203, 218, 220, 225

surgery, viii, x, 1, 3, 7, 11, 25, 35, 38, 48, 50, 51, 54, 57, 58, 64, 69, 71, 90, 120, 135, 177, 178, 179, 191, 192, 193, 194, 195, 196, 197, 198, 199, 200, 201, 202, 203, 204, 216, 217, 218, 219, 220, 221, 222, 224, 225, 226, 227, 229, 230, 231, 232, 254, 300, 304, 305

surgical site infections, 42, 216, 219, 233

surgical unit, 117, 135, 216, 266

surveillance, 61

survival, 19, 208

sweat, 109

Switzerland, 300

symbols, 32, 152, 169, 170

symptom(s), ix, 73, 127, 130, 137, 156, 174, 183, 187, 226, 235, 236, 254

syndrome, 189, 236

syringe, 148

systems, viii, 7, 8, 17, 27, 30, 32, 38, 39, 41, 42, 44, 45, 52, 54, 58, 59, 60, 61, 65, 92, 94, 152, 159, 160, 161, 164, 166, 167, 170, 184, 185, 187, 196, 209, 259, 260, 266, 287, 293, 296, 311

T

Taiwan, 169, 285, 286, 295, 297, 300

tanks, 266

teachers, 288

teaching, 19

team members, 151, 198, 199, 201, 202, 203, 215, 244

technician, 118, 141, 178, 183, 186, 277

technological change, 28

technology, 7, 8, 19, 20, 21, 24, 47, 159, 161, 163, 170, 185, 209, 210, 250, 260

telemetry, 118, 205

telephone, 32, 35, 167, 210, 223, 242, 248

temperature, 48, 84, 88, 89, 92, 102, 109, 177, 230

temporal, 281

tendon(s), 102, 304

terminal illness, 138

Texas, 70

Thailand, 297

theft, 153, 171

theory, 75, 76, 98, 232

therapeutic(s), 82, 119, 129, 131, 150, 151, 152, 154, 163, 170, 217, 309, 310

therapists, x, 108

therapy, 33, 74, 75, 108, 111, 120, 127, 130, 150, 151, 152, 158, 166, 170, 174, 183, 189, 203, 230, 238, 304, 308

threatening behavior, 123

threats, 8, 53

threshold, 255

thromboembolism, 219

thrombosis, 25, 30, 305

time commitment, 283

time frame, 159, 170, 205, 208, 210, 217, 222, 223

time periods, 218

time pressure, 197, 222

timing, 217, 221

tissue, 101, 102, 108, 230, 235, 238, 249, 304

toddlers, 198, 200

toilet, 56, 72, 77, 78, 79, 89, 94, 96, 132, 144, 259, 264, 265, 266

total joint replacements, 216, 217

total parenteral nutrition, 38, 57, 254

toxic shock syndrome, 234

toxic substances, 303

toxicity, 156, 180

toxin, 103

trachea, 218

training, ix, 10, 12, 21, 39, 48, 54, 59, 61, 62, 64, 84, 86, 100, 123, 127, 138, 139, 140, 151, 152, 153, 161, 162, 163, 165, 167, 170, 183, 184, 186, 187, 197, 198, 200, 208, 209, 210, 219, 222, 223, 224,

240, 247, 256, 287, 293, 296, 297, 299, 300, 308, 310

transcription, 150, 152, 153, 160, 162, 170

transcripts, 93

transformation(s), 30, 31, 292

Transforming Care at the Bedside, 29, 30, 31

transfusion, x, 36, 38, 50, 58, 177, 178, 179, 180, 181, 182, 183, 184, 185, 186, 187, 188, 189

transfusion error, viii, 50, 58

transfusion reactions, 178, 183, 187, 188, 189

transition(s), 30, 36, 52, 140, 142, 144, 149, 159, 197, 199, 201

transmission, 61, 208, 231, 232, 234, 235, 236, 237, 238, 242

transplantation, 238, 310

trauma, 25, 305

treatment delays, x, 187, 206, 207, 208, 209, 210, 212, 213

trees, 114

trend, 19, 42, 141, 284, 293, 300

trial, 99, 178, 179, 255

trochanter, 104

trust, ix, 8, 33

tuberculosis, 39, 44, 237, 248

turnover, 55

typology, 37, 75, 77, 80, 289, 292

U

ulcer(s), x, 1, 3, 21, 25, 30, 43, 64, 94, 100, 101, 102, 103, 104, 105, 106, 107, 108, 109, 110, 111, 112, 114, 115, 230, 254, 255, 258, 262, 263, 279, 288, 296, 304

ultrasound, 193

ultraviolet light, 260

uniform, 140, 221, 224

uninsured, 311

United States, 8, 19, 32, 34, 35, 72, 102, 114, 136, 149, 159, 233, 235, 237, 259, 281, 295, 303, 304, 305

unlicensed, 257, 295, 296, 298, 299, 300

urinary tract infection, 229, 233, 238, 255, 288, 305

urine, 70, 89, 103, 128, 188, 212

urticaria, 177

US Department of Health and Human Services, 307

users, 101, 265, 266

uterus, 178

V

vaccination, 236

vaccine(s), 36, 235

validation, 54, 161

values, 22, 23, 31, 32, 83, 183, 187, 211

vancomycin, 237

variable(s), 282, 296

variation, 28, 121, 208, 311

vein, 25, 30, 229, 240, 254, 305

venereal disease, 179

ventilation, 84, 88, 101, 109, 112, 219, 244, 262

ventilator, viii, 57, 219, 238, 305

ventricular fibrillation, 118

ventricular tachycardia, 205

vibration, 48, 260

victims, 128

village, 21

vincristine, 148, 155

violence, 39, 59

viral, 180, 234, 236

viral hemorrhagic fever, 234

viral infection, 180

virus(es), 36, 179, 233, 234, 235, 236, 237

vision, 56, 57, 62, 73, 165

vitamins, 13, 173, 174

voice, 52, 245, 257, 262, 266

W

waking, 96

walking, 82, 90, 111, 262

Wall Street Journal, 306

Washington, 267, 286

weakness, 69

weapons, 140

wear, 83, 202, 230, 235, 239, 242, 245, 246, 247, 249, 253, 254

weight loss, 107

well-being, 47, 120, 311

wheelchair, 74, 77, 88, 101, 127, 130, 260

whey, 112

whooping cough, 248

Wikipedia, 188, 189

windows, 133, 260, 261

women, 20, 101, 234

work environment, 30, 39, 41, 44, 46, 59, 163, 164, 241, 257, 292

work stoppage, 254

workers, 48, 234, 307
workflow, 276
working conditions, 48, 255, 258
working hours, 31
working population, 255, 258
workload, 48, 76, 164, 295, 296, 299
workplace, 245, 311
World Health Organization (WHO), 33, 34, 35, 36,
    46, 175, 238, 246, 251, 300
worry, 1, 11, 211
wound dehiscence, 25, 26
wound infection, 217
writing, 138, 168, 169, 181
wrong body part, 50, 193, 304
wrong patient, 50, 161, 181, 186, 193, 304
wrong-site, viii, 50, 57, 58, 64, 193, 194, 199
wrong-site surgery, 191, 193, 194, 197, 199, 200,
    202, 203

X

x-ray, 212, 215